# WOMEN AND HEALTH

*Cultural and Social Perspectives*

# Any Friend
## of the
# MOVEMENT

## Networking for Birth Control
## 1920–1940

Jimmy Elaine Wilkinson Meyer

THE OHIO STATE UNIVERSITY PRESS

Columbus

to my newest loves,
Judah Ahmet Duran and Malcolm Nazim Duran,
I dedicate this work, with fervent hope for a peaceful world,
one that treasures difference.

Library of Congress Cataloging-in-Publication Data

Meyer, Jimmy Elaine Wilkinson.
    Any friend of the movement : networking for birth control, 1920–1940 / Jimmy
Elaine Wilkinson Meyer.
        p.  cm.  — (Women and health : cultural and social perspectives)
Includes bibliographical references and index.
    ISBN 0-8142-0954-8 (hardcover: alk. paper) — ISBN 0-8142-9034-5 (CD-ROM)
    1. Birth control—United States—History—20th century. 2. Maternal Health
Association of Cleveland, Ohio. 3. Birth control clinics—United States. I. Title. II.
Women & health (Columbus, Ohio)

    HQ766.5.U5 M484 2004
    363.9'6'09730904—dc22
                        2003019937

Jacket design by Janna Thompson Chordas.
Text design by Jennifer Forsythe.
Type set in Adobe Caslon.


The paper used in this publication meets the minimum requirements of the American
National Standard for Information Sciences—Permanence of Paper for Printed Library
Materials. ANSI Z39.48-1992.

9  8  7  6  5  4  3  2  1

# Contents

# List of Figures

# Foreword

We are very pleased to be publishing Jimmy Elaine Wilkinson Meyer's *Any Friend of the Movement: Networking for Birth Control 1920–1940*. Focused on the founding and operations of the Maternal Health Association of Cleveland, a birth control clinic, this book tells an important story about one local institution. In so doing, it illuminates the complex history of maternalist reform and women's health needs. Through this insightful case study we learn the motivations and strategies of key women in bringing birth control to their community. As Meyer notes in her introduction, this work "highlights the critical role of gender in voluntary activity, policy making, and state building." *Any Friend of the Movement* is significant in its careful delineation of the financial and organizational trials of the clinic, but it is much more than an institutional history. The narrative is particularly powerful because it contains the voices not only of the organizers of the Maternal Health Association, but also of the clinic's clients. Meyer uncovered a cache of letters from clients that provide an extraordinary window into the private needs that stimulated and supported the unfolding of the birth control movement. The correspondence between organizers and clients highlights the crucial role that each played in this critical public movement in the first half of the twentieth century.

— RIMA D. APPLE AND JANET GOLDEN, SERIES EDITORS

# *Preface*

In the 1920s my grandmother Helen bore two children within twenty months of her wedding day. Upon discovering that she was pregnant for the second time, Helen realized that her naive notions of birth control held serious flaws. A few years later her third and last child died shortly after birth.

In the 1950s, although equipped with more information and options, my mother, Elaine, endured six pregnancies, at least three of those unplanned. Mom bore five living children. (At my mother's bedside, after the sixth birth, when Mom was thirty-eight years old, her husband's grandmother shared methods that she had used to space her four children.)

In the 1970s, despite technological advances, I conceived my own firstborn a few months earlier than intended due to a faulty contraceptive.

Moralistic attitudes, policies, and laws helped to maintain women's ignorance about their bodies in general and their lack of precise knowledge about controlling reproduction in particular, as represented in Helen's experience in the 1920s. Two generations later, even after wider dissemination of such information, a dearth of systematic research meant the absence of simple, effective, reliable contraception free from the unpleasant or dangerous side effects that plagued the pill, especially in its early days. Public birth control policy affects the intimate realities of women's lives: the political is personal.

The above stories (and there are more) explain in part my interest in the history of reproductive choices and the restriction of those choices. The current study focuses not on research or contraceptive methods per se but explores and analyzes the actions of women and men to create and sustain Ohio's first birth control clinic. The account lies within the much broader context of ongoing cultural ambiguities and tensions around sexuality in the United States. Disparate themes such as the power and reach of the law, the authority of physicians, the impact of voluntary action, the critical nature of networks, and the role of female agency in institution building and social change add texture to the tale.

Many, many people have supported me in bringing this book to fruition. I will not name all of you, but your help proved invaluable. A few individuals and organizations deserve special mention. Jane Kessler planted the seed that quickly blossomed into a fascination with the history of women's choices in America and the restrictions of those choices. Lois Scharf, Jan Reiff, Roberta Wollons, and Carl Ubbelohde encouraged that fascination. A fellowship funded by the Lilly Foundation at the Center for Philanthropy of Indiana University/Purdue University in Indianapolis piqued my interest in nonprofits and voluntarism. Special thanks to David Hammack for suggesting that opportunity and to Darlyne Bailey and others at the center for their perceptive comments. Other early funding sources included a Littleton-Griswold Research Award from the American Historical Association and travel grants from the Case Western Reserve University Alumni Fund. For financial support of a portion of this project, thanks to the American College of Obstetricians and Gynecologists and Ortho Pharmaceutical Corporation. My stint as an ACOG-Ortho History Fellow aided my transformation from student to scholar and opened my eyes to the wealth of fascinating untapped material in the history of women's health. Susan Rishworth, then the ACOG archivist, helped me set a research course and made my time at the ACOG history library most pleasant.

Cathy Gorn provided comfortable lodgings during those visits and welcome camaraderie. Conversations, both formal and informal, with Angus McLaren, Judith Leavitt, Johanna Schoen, Julianne Phillips, Peter Hall, James Reed, Regina Morantz Sanchez, and a host of other scholars enlightened and inspired me. Chris Link, Betsey Kaufman, and other Planned Parenthood of Greater Cleveland staff members enabled my obsession with the MHA story. Librarians in Cleveland and elsewhere provided excellent assistance. Special thanks to Elsie Findley, Mike Partington, and Sue Hanson at CWRU; John Grabowski, Michael McCormick, and Ann Sindelar at the Western Reserve Historical Society; Joanne Cornelius and others at the *Cleveland Press* Collection of Cleveland State University; the many helpful archivists at the Sophia Smith Collection of Smith College; Glen Jenkins and Jennifer Nieves at the Dittrick Medical History Center; Janet Huettner at the Center on Philanthropy; the friendly folks at the CWRU Archives and the Cleveland Public Library Photograph Collection; and John Bellamy and other former Cuyahoga

County Public Library colleagues. While this book was in its last stages, I sorely missed the earlier assistance of Sarah Snock and gratefully welcomed the help of Maren Miller and Emily Ryan.

Mike Grossberg offered welcome wisdom on legal points and theory as well as encouragement. The late David D. Van Tassel provided valuable editing opportunities along the way, and more encouraging words. Thanks to Rima Apple, Janet Golden, and Heather Lee Miller of The Ohio State University Press, who bolstered my confidence in this project, and to Andrea Tone for perceptive suggestions and thoughtful comments. Beth DiNatale Johnson, Patricia O. James, and my sister, Nicole Wilkinson Duran, also read every word of this work in some manifestation. Their sage commentary and their sense of fun and frolic, along with that of Susan T. Vitantonio, Kim Lenahan, Sister Mary Denis Maher, Paulette George Krieger, Janice Harclerode, Valerie Wojdat, my Meyer sisters, Joyce Howard, and Lisa Watts, in the face of my complaints and procrastination, kept me going . . . and going. Lynn Bravo Rosewater deserves special mention for teaching me about feminism, and about myself. The members of Women Historians of Greater Cleveland comprised a friendly and supportive audience; Gladys Haddad provided several opportunities to present my work-in-progress. Student assistants Marie Salupo, Molly Moreland, Maren Miller, and Katherine Nicholson put up with my air of distraction and always expressed an interest in my "other" work. Stacy Ingraham Smith did some tedious but necessary inputting. I'm grateful to all of you. Since I began this work, the constellation of my extended family has shifted dramatically. Upon the precious shoulders of those ancestors who have left this earth I gratefully stand, hands firmly clasped with the ones who remain. My late father, Malcolm Wilkinson, sparked a love of learning in all five of his children, bringing Shakespeare to the dinner table, for example, and offered, of course, his love.

Kudos to the most important men in my life, Carroll, Bryant, and Malcolm, on whom I can always count for distraction of some sort, often of the musical variety. Thanks for loving me in spite of my devotion to this project and for never suggesting that I give it up.

# Introduction

Women have attempted to control family size throughout history, employing an astonishing variety of methods and techniques to prevent or end unwanted pregnancies. Knowledge of contraception was often sketchy, of the "in the kitchen, under the table" variety, passed on from woman to woman. Some Roman Catholic women speculated that Protestants used tricks to prevent conception; women of the poorer classes often thought such information to be a secret of the wealthy. As one woman wrote to the United States Children's Bureau in 1928, "I think it unfair Dr.'s and Rich seek Birth Control and the poor can't seek nothing, only poverty and more babies." Yet in spite of the illicit nature of contraception, of wide variations in the general popular knowledge about the mechanics of reproduction, and of legal restrictions, the American fertility rate declined steadily beginning in the nineteenth century.[1]

Cultural variations, changing gender roles, and alterations within the family unit have affected how women and men perceive and use family limitation. Intimate realities often differ greatly from public policy.[2] Women created birth control clinics in the 1920s and 1930s as voluntary associations because of—and in spite of—discord between private practices and public regulation of sexuality, especially birth control.[3] The 1928 founding of the Maternal Health Association (MHA) of Cleveland, Ohio, by prominent white women demonstrates the power of women's voluntarism to influence public policy and private action as well as the limits of that voluntarism. The MHA and other birth control clinics of the 1920s and 1930s offered an innovative service to less privileged white and black women in Cleveland and across North America. These pioneer facilities stood on the edge of respectability and at the boundary of the law. Their stories shed light on the role of gender and class within a social movement. Exploring activity and policy at the level of local birth control clinics uncovers the ways in which national policies, laws, and ideologies played out within American cities and towns. This particular work adds the perspectives of clinic users as well as local leaders to the existing body of historical literature.

Like other community studies, this historical case study of one pioneer agency raises questions about the predominate values and tactics of a social movement. Did the same strategies get the same results in Denver as in Baltimore, in Cleveland as in New York City? Did a particular locale influence a clinic's direction and longevity? Did certain individuals or local groups modify national directives? How did national and state laws impact clinic activity in different regions of the country? Looking closely at local initiatives reminds us that individual acts can and do shape history. Within the context of broad social forces, cultural structures, and personal experiences, individual agency counts. The MHA lends itself to the principles of community study, with the understanding that "the records of a single community can change the way we look at the past."[4]

Founders and clients of early American birth control clinics helped to change policy, and their actions manifested the inconsistencies between rhetoric and reality in the area of reproduction. Due to the restrictive legal climate, MHA leaders and clients utilized extensive networks to provide and obtain birth control. The clinics and the clients employed traditional methods of female reform, such as quiet persuasion and private networking, in the area of maternal health and family well-being to legitimate a nontraditional end—women's control over reproduction. Certain themes recur within the Cleveland MHA narrative: quiet determination, mixed motives, organizational autonomy, and utilitarian strategies. These themes give texture to and modify the existing analysis of an important national movement. The disparate threads of this particular tale include a pregnant woman's suicide, "beneficent research," a bereaved inventor, ice skating galas, Lysol and Vaseline, Cleveland cooperation, better babies, clandestine train trips, and husbands both recalcitrant and supportive.

Weaving these threads and others into the fabric of history highlights the critical role of gender in voluntary activity, policy making, and state building. Biological differences between men and women as well as the biological and cultural mandates of those differences have altered and continue to alter history. The fact that women conceive, gestate, bear, and are expected to rear society's children affects women's choices, opportunities, and lifestyles, and makes them different from the choices, opportunities, and lifestyles of men. This is not an argument of biological determinism, of body as destiny. Rather, this reasoning recognizes the reality that, as Rosalind Petschesky asserts, "biology is a *capacity* as well as a limit."[5] Contradictory cultural directives complicate the relationship of a woman with her body, with procreation, and with motherhood. As Alexandra Todd notes, "On the one hand, women are defined in the lofty terms of perpetuators of the race—motherhood and apple pie; on the other hand, their very bodies and reproductive functions are denigrated as diseased and deviant." Anthropologist Emily Martin maintains that the very language of reproductive biology frames the female's role in the process in negative terms.[6] The history of gynecology in general and the birth control movement in particular starkly illuminates these inconsistent and damaging messages.

Deep-seated discontinuities became embedded in American law, politics, and language in the nineteenth century and continue to influence public polity and intimate reality two centuries later. From Puritan courting constraints, to the nineteenth-century medicalization of childbirth, to twentieth-century population control policies, to the technology of in vitro fertilization and cloning, outside forces have imposed legal, religious, scientific, and ideological conditions on sexuality in general and on women's bodies in particular.[7] Society's conflicting messages have created parallel conflicts within the individual woman, fragmenting woman's self and her body. The highly technical efforts of scientists to manipulate conception in the laboratory represent another instance of separating a woman from her bodily functions.[8] This fragmentation results in part from the fact that women exist with and within their bodies amid social restrictions and taboos around female bodily functions, amid blurred rules of what is acceptable and unacceptable in private and in public.

Over time women have reacted to oppressive social mores and confusion around sexual issues through active resistance. In some instances women instigated change, either individual or corporate, rather than passively accept victimization. The founders and clients of voluntary birth control clinics in the 1920s and 1930s exemplify such action. A unique collection of letters from early MHA clients to staff members offers a glimpse into the private motivations of women who sought help in controlling their fertility—and thus into their lives. Letter writers express concerns around a personal topic that is often absent from diaries or correspondence, adding their voices and experiences to our understanding of the private results of a social movement. Bringing such intimate experiences to the fore illuminates the "dynamism of consciousness and conflict" involved in controlling reproduction.[9] Based on a complex interaction of cultural factors and circumstances, reproductive choices involve more than personal decision making.

This case study provides a window through which to view women's experience and actions. Maternal Health Association clients and providers formed a network of relationships in their struggle for control over reproduction. Their interpersonal communications disclose a solidarity of interest and consideration for each other's well-being. Founders created the MHA in part to relieve women of the burden of poorly controlled childbearing, and satisfied clinic clients referred relatives and friends to the MHA out of the same motivation. These women, differing in class and ethnicity, shared a common biological bond of heterosexual femaleness. Each had experienced to some extent the cultural imperatives and strictures inherent in that femaleness. They shared the need to control fertility.

Yet each woman experienced life at the MHA in a different way, each has a different story to tell. This work attempts to uncover the local stories within the broad story of national voluntary action for birth control.[10] One scholar of the women's health movement notes that we too often tell "the stories of social movements" without paying attention to the experience of those who participated, both the leaders and the followers, those who became empowered through the movement. The agency of those who work for social change involves more than ideology and commitment. That agency at the same time reflects and embodies the breadth of their lived experience.[11] With multiple meanings and implications, experience at once embodies the collective and the individual. Collectively struggling towards an end such as reproductive control, individuals gave birth to a movement. Society shapes individual experience, and individual experiences both inform and comprise society.[12] By exploring the various stories within the story, this study illuminates the multi-faceted relationship between the personal and the political, a relationship complicated by questions of authority and control.

This case history studies the founding and early years of a long-lived birth control clinic created by upper-middle-class, white, urban women. Clients included black women, immigrant women, and rural women as well as Anglo-Saxon city dwellers. Staff did not note correspondents' race on the letters that the clinic saved. In the absence of case records, the ethnic origins of most MHA clients remain unknown.[13] These factors limit the results but challenge us to recognize difference nonetheless. While the historian will never be able to reconstruct each person's experience, a local study allows an interrogation of the birth control movement based on a variety of individual encounters.

"The Mothers, Mothers, Mothers," a large Cleveland *Plain Dealer* headline proclaimed in 1922. "There's no better friend to Motherhood," the article insisted, than the charitable work of the Community Fund of Cleveland. "Nobody has to argue about mothers," the full-page appeal continued. "Everybody knows the tenderness, the mystic, unreasoning faithfulness of a mother's love. Whatever else men believe in, all men believe in mothers!"[14]

Women structured the Cleveland Maternal Health Association under the powerful rubric of motherhood. Maternal Health Association founders and leaders resemble the maternalist reformers of the first two decades of the twentieth-century United States in their certainty about the value of women as the mothers of future citizens. Advocates across North America argued for birth control based, paradoxically, in part on the sanctity and importance of motherhood. They claimed that spacing one's children enabled a woman to be a healthier and better mother, to raise better babies as future citizens for a healthy state. After the first two decades of the twentieth century, few birth control leaders invoked women's right to control her own body, her own destiny. Like the maternalist reformers before them, these women envisioned and promoted their reform within a traditional family framework: a married couple with the male as breadwinner, the female as dependent caregiver to the household's other dependents. They assumed this construct even as the economic demands of the Great Depression modified family roles and sent more women out of the home and into wage labor. However, unlike many single reformers of the settlement house or child health movements, who remained single or lived in a community with other women, the majority of birth control advocates in the thirties, in Cleveland at least, lived within the traditional family framework. Among the first cadre of MHA board and staff members, only the executive secretary, a nurse, and one board member had never married. Most were married women with children.[15] They proclaimed the value of hearth and home based in part on their own lived experience.

And yet they chose to advocate a nontraditional service—fertility control—as women, for women. The leaders of the MHA chose to provide that service through an independent organization rather than a governmental or institutional agency. Kathleen McCarthy notes some common denominators that typify female philanthropy: "an abiding interest in helping women and children; a tendency to move into gaps overlooked by government and male donors and volunteers; and a desire to exercise power." The women who organized and promoted the MHA fit this prototype, utilizing and forging networks and friendships for change, entering territory neglected and as yet uncharted by male experts. But, following the example of extremists such as abolitionists and suffragists, these women took voluntarism and philanthropy in new and risky directions. Acting through voluntary associations to help other women control their fertility, they claimed some authority in the contested area of sexuality and reproduction. The present work looks through the lens of the voluntary sector to try to unearth how voluntary action and philanthropy shape state actions and are shaped by them. It attends to some of the holes in our knowledge of the history of women and voluntary action: Why did women commit to this cause? What factors shaped their actions and their strategic choices? How did women and men negotiate about reproduction and its control? What roles did men play in this movement? How did the women who patronized the new clinics view the new service?[16]

Planned Parenthood Federation of America president Gloria Feldt claims that behind every choice, there lies a story.[17] This work examines a few of those untold stories and opens the door for more telling.

## THE MATTER OF TIME

Birth control clinics like the MHA originated during a time of transition in the history of women's associations, after women gained suffrage and before large numbers entered the paid workforce during World War II.[18] The Cleveland MHA acted in that time period, and this story concentrates on the years of planning before the clinic opened (1920–1928) and its founding and first dozen years (1928–1940). During this era, the MHA preserved a fierce autonomy. It remained independent of national organizations that were active in the birth control movement but pursued influential and useful local attachments. Such a blend of independence and influence allowed the MHA to develop its own persona before joining the Planned Parenthood Federation of America in 1942.

During the 1920s and 1930s, birth control increasingly entered not only commercial, legal, and medical discourse but also public discussions and private conversations. Economic situations and worries about the family kept the subject before the public eye. Newspapers reported religious controversies, court cases, and social action in the arena of reproductive control. Magazines and novels took up the subject.[19] Some women discussed their plans for and methods of family limitation with relatives and friends, proving that "birth control" did become a household phrase in the early twentieth century, as historian Andrea Tone declares. Legal modifications in the 1930s opened the way for physicians to prescribe birth control and also spurred an increase in the manufacture and distribution of contraceptive devices in the popular market.[20]

Private action and professional influence each played a critical role in making contraception acceptable to the medical and social service communities. Attending only to the consequences of professionalization of birth control ignores the burgeoning voluntary activism within the movement.[21] Medical and social service professionals did become more involved in the movement for family limitation during the 1920s and 1930s, in part at the instigation of middle- and upper-class lay women who claimed the cause of birth control as their own. The enthusiasm of poor and working-class women for contraceptive services, as demonstrated by their clinic attendance and their support of the commercial market, invigorated the cause and further convinced professionals of the demand.

## DESIGN

This study explores how founders, funders, staff, and clients experienced birth control at the Maternal Health Association of Cleveland during its first decade rather than describing every clinic program in strict chronological order. Probing the background of American family limitation policy and providing a context for the study of voluntarism and birth control offer a base on which to analyze the clinic's legal and medical groundwork. Chapter 1 contends that unpredictable national and local legal climates, the radical nature of the cause, and medical and religious opposition necessitated the careful tactics that Maternal Health Association founders employed. Chapter 2 explicates the gendered nature of those tactics and examines the essential networks that formed a strong foundation for the new organization. Chapter 3 focuses on the first MHA boards and early staff, reveals the clinic's independent nature, and explores its class-based reliance on eugenics. This chapter introduces a key connection with the Brush Foundation, a local philanthropy, a close tie that made the MHA unique among early birth control clinics. Drawing heavily on client correspondence, chapter 4 investigates how clinic clients and their spouses, staff, and founders experienced birth control and the MHA during the clinic's early years. Expanding on the discussion of kin and social networks introduced in chapter 2, chapter 5 argues that these and other links of geography and reform stabilized the MHA, links not only among clinic founders but also among clients. This chapter further demonstrates how MHA leaders manipulated their connections—and the law—to sustain the venture. Chapter 6 describes how the close relationship with the Brush Foundation promoted research at the MHA and extended the association's influence far beyond Cleveland and Ohio.

❧

Maternal Health Association clients and founders expressed their identities as women, wives, and mothers by demanding and providing access to reliable birth control. In so doing they pulled the control of reproduction away from its radical roots and pushed it toward acceptability. Their actions sustained and vitalized the national movement and provided a model for other cities, states, and countries.

Let the tale begin.

# 1

## Radical Roots

"Where does this evil exist? Where are these traps set?" asked purity champion Anthony Comstock in 1884. "I reply, everywhere. Children of all grades of society, institutions of learning in all sections of the land, and the most select homes, are invaded by the evils of licentious literature." Comstock intoned the fears of other late-nineteenth-century American citizens, fears that a widespread indulgence "of secret vices" threatened to blot out the "moral purity" of young people and hence the nation.[1] According to purity advocates, those secret vices included contraception.

From the nineteenth century through the Progressive Era, legal and medical prohibitions and social taboos around contraception reflected and embodied larger cultural tensions in the United States. Such tensions propelled and became embedded in efforts to create local birth control clinics. Enthusiastic crusades against obscenity, on the one hand, and advocacy for access to effective family limitation methods, on the other, characterized each end of a broad spectrum of opinion and action. The context for the story of the distance between, and intersections of, reproductive policy and practice in the 1920s and 1930s includes historical factors such as laws, ideologies, and the attitudes of physicians, clergy, and other professionals.

### OBSCENE ARTICLES AND THEIR IMMORAL USE

Herbals, medical handbooks, and marriage guides provided some information about sexuality and contraception to Americans in the nineteenth century. To protect Victorian sensibilities and circumvent would-be censors, books that provided facts about reproduction and its control sported informative titles. These books included *Moral Physiology*, by Robert Dale Owen (1831), *Fruits of Philosophy*, by Charles Knowlton (1832), *Medical*

*Common Sense,* by Edward Bliss Foote (1858), and *Tokology,* by Alice B. Stockham (1884). Most of these texts survived throughout the century in several editions, indicating their widespread popularity despite censorship attempts.[2] In addition, advertisements, health lectures, and circulars sent to the betrothed and other women contained information—of varying degrees of accuracy—about preventing or correcting "menstrual irregularity" (a euphemism for pregnancy). Unfortunately, the douches and herbal preparations that were advertised and sold did not always prevent conception, cure irregularity, or end a pregnancy. Many were harmless but others caused discomfort, damage, or even death. Yet ads, circulars, books, and business records demonstrate that literate and interested citizens of the nineteenth century had access to family limitation information, preparations, and devices in some form.[3]

A burgeoning publishing industry offered nineteenth-century Americans access to other information about sexuality as well. Some of the widely circulated books and pamphlets sensationalized sex, and others simply presented factual information, information that many considered obscene. The borders between the prurient and the educational were fluid. Often the same people marketed both types of material; some publishers included pornography and contraceptive information in the same pamphlet.[4] Fearing the corrupting effect of explicit literature and pictures on the country's youth, states began to legislate against indecency in the 1820s and 1830s. Early obscenity legislation often focused on stopping the trade in abortifacients—devices, preparations, or information designed to induce abortion and end a pregnancy—assuming legal authority over what had been a private matter in previous years.[5] Congress first passed a general federal obscenity statute in 1842, mentioning only offensive pictorial representations. Legislators broadened the scope of these prohibitions throughout the century. By the 1880s federal and state laws banned obscenity in all forms, including information about the prevention of conception or abortion.[6]

Historians agree that increased legal regulation of such information in the nineteenth century represents a reaction on the part of political and moral leaders to the growing popular acceptance, public visibility, and commercialization of family limitation and abortion across the country. Legal expert Michael Grossberg contends that a shift occurred at this time in ideas about legitimate child spacing methods, with more women rejecting abortion, which they had accepted in an earlier day, in favor of other means of family limitation. Studying religious opposition to the regulation of reproduction generally, historian Angus McLaren asserts, "If stop signs imply the existence of traffic, the clergy's ongoing condemnations of abortion and contraception can at the very least be taken as evidence of the continued employment of such practices."[7] Early-twentieth-century studies of the intimate habits of white, American married women of the middle class reveal a wide range of attitudes toward sexuality and the common use of family limitation in some form.[8]

Over the course of the nineteenth century and into the twentieth, cultural and private attitudes changed toward sexuality in general and family limitation in particular. In earlier times the church or the community regulated sexual conduct with public punishment or banishment for those who committed moral offenses. Families exerted strict control over their young people, especially daughters. During the latter part of the nineteenth century, as the power of these regulatory systems eroded, especially among urban, middle-class white couples, sexuality increasingly became a private matter for individuals. At the same time, the press increasingly brought sex before the public eye. Novels, marriage guides, newspapers, the new women's magazines, and leaflets romanticized sexual love. Yet they also stressed proper dating conduct, abstinence before marriage, and moderation in sexual activity after matrimony to maintain one's reputation as well as physical health and well-being. While large families helped to sustain rural, labor-intensive farms, the same situation only exacerbated economic and social conditions in crowded industrialized cities and towns. Financial, personal, medical, and familial factors led many couples to attempt to limit family size. These diverse elements combined to distance sexual union from reproduction.[9]

Beginning in the early to mid-1800s, social purity advocates and policy makers worried about the growing separation of intercourse from procreation. Distancing the sexual act from its biological consequences offered women the potential of freedom from the sacred duty of motherhood. To some that portended the disintegration of the family. State legislatures passed laws between 1820 and 1860 that made it easier to end a marriage, and more American couples appeared in courtrooms to do just that. Divorce rates rose slowly but consistently throughout the century, "producing shivers and alarms in magazines and newspapers," according to one historian. By 1870 news articles warned of "divorce made easy" and pondered "the future of the family" in an era of changing marital expectations. The fact that women instigated divorce proceedings more often than men proved to many that women were shirking their traditional responsibilities and taking on new roles. Clergy, educators, writers, and congressmen attempted to ensure the future of monogamy and motherhood, and thus the nation.[10]

Privileged citizens worried about the effect on their sons and daughters of the "considerable number of neglected, destitute, and ignorant youth" on the streets of Cleveland and other cities, children who lived in a "filthy and poverty-ridden section breeding delinquency of all types and degree[s]."[11] Some of these young people turned to prostitution, gambling, or petty theft in order to survive. Clearly the mothers of these and other wayward youth did not perform their maternal task very well. Guides to child rearing emphasized the great responsibility of motherhood. Prescriptive articles on how to be a good mother appeared in women's magazines. For example, from 1837 to 1840 Clevelander Maria Herrick edited the *Mothers and Young Ladies Guide,* a magazine that instructed women on "Duties of Motherhood" and "How to Ruin a Son" as well as "Fashion" and "The Evils of Tight Lacing."[12] Especially among the middle and upper classes, anxiety over the future of babies, young people, the family, and "the race" increased as the century progressed.

Purity advocate Anthony Comstock embodied the paranoia of a newly industrialized, urbanized society in his crusade to rid New York City and the nation of obscene material. Backed by influential businessmen such as Samuel Colgate and organizations such as the Young Men's Christian Association (YMCA), Comstock emphasized the evils of abortion, prostitution, and pornography in his purification campaign. He argued against explicit material and information on the basis of protecting the country's youth. Using controversial methods such as entrapment, the vice hunter loudly proclaimed the numbers of the obscene rubber articles seized as a result of his efforts—60,300 by 1874. The fact that Comstock included contraceptive devices and literature in his attack signifies their close connection to obscenity in the public eye.[13] His manic efforts bordered on the ridiculous and would be laughable were it not for their serious and enduring effects.

Although the national nineteenth- and early-twentieth-century press focused on the flamboyant and boastful Comstock, local social purity advocates also attempted to purge their cities of vice during this era. Groups such as the Cleveland Purity Alliance, the Vice Commission of the Cleveland Baptist Brotherhood, the Cleveland Moral Education Society, and the Christian League for the Promotion of Purity joined other groups with broader reform agendas in the effort to reclaim Cleveland's "neglected children" from "a life of moral degradation." Maria Herrick, the Cleveland woman's magazine editor noted above, helped organize the city's Female Moral Reform Society in 1842. These organizations and their members focused on eliminating prostitution and juvenile crime and creating better conditions for children in and out of the home, as well as ridding the city of obscenity and pornography.[14]

Concerns such as these across the country, especially in America's cities, spurred Anthony Comstock to vigorously pursue and enforce national and state legislation against vice. He began his efforts in New York City, enforcing the state's new anti-obscenity law, passed in 1868, as a private citizen with a vengeance that caught the attention of the YMCA. That organization began to support Comstock's efforts through the Committee for the Suppression of Vice, created within the YMCA in 1872. The next year, Comstock succeeded in convincing Congress to severely restrict the expression of sexuality. In the closing hours of its session, the Forty-second Congress passed an act to suppress trade in obscene articles and material, strengthening a similar statute passed the year before. This ruling, dubbed the Comstock Law, transformed fears about the future of the family into doctrine in the United States.[15]

The Comstock Law prohibited contraception in the United States for almost a century, until 1971 (see figure 1). The law addressed the traffic in information intended "for the prevention of conception," abortion, or other obscene or immoral purposes. The act targeted the U.S. mail as a distribution network for objectionable and immoral materials. Federal tariff acts, including one passed in 1922 and another in 1930, reinforced the transportation restrictions. These statutes prevented the importation into the United States of any written material, drawing, or instrument "which is obscene or immoral, or any drug or medicine or any article whatever for the prevention of conception or for causing unlawful abortion." Although the U.S. Court of Appeals for the Second Circuit later interpreted the Comstock Law to permit physicians to purchase, import, and dispense contraception, the phrase "for the prevention of conception" remained on the books until 1971. The Comstock Law endures into the twenty-first century as the country's obscenity statute—and still prohibits the mailing of information about how or where to procure abortions.[16]

To define the elusive term "obscenity," U.S. judges cited Great Britain's *Queen v. Hicklin* decision of 1868: "[The] test of obscenity is this, whether the tendency of the matter charged as obscenity is to deprave and corrupt those whose minds are open to immoral influences, and into whose hands a publication of this sort might fall."[17] Comstock and other purity crusaders took advantage of this expansive interpretation and attacked science, art, and literature as well as pornography and information about contraceptives and abortion. Comstock enforced the new federal law as a specially commissioned agent of the U.S. Post Office. He also acted under the auspices and with the support of the New York Society for the Suppression of Vice (the successor of the YMCA committee), many of whose members appeared on New York's *Social Register.*[18] Anthony Comstock doggedly crusaded against what he viewed as obscene and immoral until his death in 1915. His actions and those of his supporters in other cities and towns seriously affected American policy toward sexuality, with results both immediate and long-term. A few New York City purveyors of vice, such as abortionists or distributors of "obscene material," committed suicide after being trapped and arrested by the vice hunter. While courts enforced the law only sporadically, many entrepreneurs lost lucrative businesses and, along with writers and activists, spent time in jail. Under the new restrictions, safe abortions and accurate information about sexuality and contraception became harder to acquire across the country. "The possibility of official reprisal, and the social opprobrium frequently associated with law-breaking," one historian says, often restrains "undesirable" behavior as effectively as criminal prosecution.[19] Over time, the law that Comstock so determinedly pursued irrevocably codified policy

---

**Federal Comstock Law:**
**An Act for the Suppression of Trade in, and Circulation of**
**Obscene Literature and Articles of Immoral Use, March 3, 1873.**

Sec. 2, amending Sec. 148 of "the act to revise, consolidate, and amend the statutes relating to the Post Office Department, approved June eighth, eighteen hundred and seventy-two."

BE IT ENACTED BY THE SENATE AND HOUSE OF REPRESENTATIVES OF THE UNITED STATES OF AMERICAN IN CONGRESS ASSEMBLED, . . .

SEC. 148 . . . THAT NO OBSCENE, LEWD, OR LASCIVIOUS BOOK, PAMPHLET, PICTURE, PAPER, PRINT, OR OTHER PUBLICATION OF AN INDECENT CHARACTER, OR ANY ARTICLE OR THING DESIGNED OR INTENDED FOR THE PREVENTION OF CONCEPTION OR PROCURING OF ABORTION, NOR ANY ARTICLE OR THING INTENDED OR ADAPTED FOR ANY INDECENT OR IMMORAL USE OR NATURE, NOR ANY WRITTEN OR PRINTED CARD, CIRCULAR, BOOK, PAMPHLET, ADVERTISEMENT OR NOTICE OF ANY KIND GIVING ANY INFORMATION, DIRECTLY OR INDIRECTLY, WHERE, OR HOW, OR OF WHOM, OR BY WHAT MEANS EITHER OF THE THINGS MENTIONED MAY BE OBTAINED OR MADE . . . SHALL BE CARRIED IN THE MAIL; AND ANY PERSON WHO SHALL KNOWINGLY DEPOSIT, OR CAUSE TO BE DEPOSITED, FOR MAILING OR DELIVERY, ANY OF THE HEREINBEFORE-MENTIONED ARTICLES OR THINGS, AND ANY PERSON WHO . . . SHALL TAKE, OR CAUSE TO BE TAKEN, FROM THE MAIL ANY SUCH LETTER OR PACKAGE, SHALL BE DEEMED GUILTY OF A MISDEMEANOR, AND, ON CONVICTION THEREOF, SHALL BE FINED NOT LESS THAN ONE HUNDRED DOLLARS NOR MORE THAN FIVE THOUSAND DOLLARS, OR IMPRISONED AT HARD LABOR NOT LESS THAN ONE YEAR NOR MORE THAN TEN YEARS, OR BOTH, AT THE DISCRETION OF THE JUDGE.

*Comstock Act, Chap. 258, 17 Stat. 598 (1873).*

---

FIGURE 1. Federal Comstock Law
An Act for the Suppression of Trade in and Circulation of Obscene Literature
and Articles of Immoral Use, March 3, 1873.

against the public expression of sexuality.[20] It set private conduct directly into the public and judicial realms.

## OHIO REGULATES OBSCENITY

After the passage of the 1873 obscenity statute, states passed "little" Comstock laws, some even stricter than their federal counterpart. The Comstock Law regulated that over which the federal government had jurisdiction: items sent in the U.S. mail, imported into the country, or transported across state lines (see sec. 3 of the Comstock Law for transportation restrictions). However, legal cases in the 1870s found that Congress had no power under this law "to make criminal the using of means to prevent conception."[21] That task was left to the states and localities. Ohio had passed an obscenity law in 1862. That statute banned the "advertisement, sale or gratuitous distribution of any drug, medicine, instrument or apparatus intended to prevent conception or procure abortion" as well as any "obscene notice." Having made abortion illegal almost thirty years earlier, the Ohio legislature strengthened that prohibition in the 1862 law and focused almost exclusively on information about contraception and abortion.[22]

State obscenity laws differed from the federal statute and from each other, demonstrating a striking discontinuity of policy toward contraception, abortion, and obscenity. The lack of a clear definition of objectionable material further confused the issue. The laws of Ohio and several other states specifically exempted medical colleges, medical textbooks, and physicians from criminal prosecution, provisions that never appeared in the federal Comstock Act.[23] Ohio legislators introduced these exceptions over the course of many revisions. The 1862 law specifically exempted "regularly chartered medical colleges" and "the publication of standard medical books" but did not mention physicians or druggists. Those exemptions nodded to the growing influence of professional "regular" medicine (as opposed to so-called irregular practices, including homeopathy and midwifery). The law held for almost fifteen years, until 1876.[24]

That year Ohio legislators broadened the reach of state obscenity regulation and expanded the law to six sections. With this legislation, state representatives repealed a more general state statute that had been passed in 1872 "to suppress and prohibit Obscene Publications." That act had described offending material as that which was "lewd and lascivious" but did not specifically target information about contraception or abortion. The state act of 1876 incorporated the provisions of both laws, 1862 and 1872, placing *all* obscene and immoral publications, images, and items under one ruling. The new statute added to the list of potentially illegal materials (described in 1862 as any "newspaper, circular, pamphlet, or book") the following: any "paper, drawing, lithograph, engraving, picture, daguerreotype, photograph, stereoscopic picture, model, cast, instrument, or article." A new section prohibited the transport or mailing of "any of the obscene, lewd, indecent or lascivious articles or things" previously mentioned, reinforcing the federal mandate. The ruling also made it a crime to possess objectionable printed material or objects and to pass on obscene information verbally to another person, compromising Ohioans' constitutional right of free speech.[25]

At the same time Ohio lawmakers of 1876 tightened regulations, they broadened the exemptions. The revised statute did *not* apply to the "practice of regular practitioners of medicine, or druggists in their legitimate business."[26] This exemption both recognized and furthered the increasing authority of organized medicine over matters of physiology in general and reproduction in particular, presaging the direction that the birth control movement would take fifty years later. This early deference to physicians in Ohio likely indicates the influence of "regularly chartered" schools of medicine in the state, such as the Cleveland Medical College, founded in 1843 to grant "a legitimate doctor of medicine degree," the Starling-Ohio Medical College (est. 1848) in Columbus, and the Charity Hospital Medical College (est. 1863) in Cleveland.[27] Legislators also allowed for "legitimate" pharmacists to sell contraception, attacking the brisk door-to-door and street corner trade in preventives of all sorts and perhaps recognizing popular perception of the Victorian pharmacist as an expert in health matters.[28]

State and federal laws differed, then, in their interpretations of who should hold the authority for providing information or articles that many considered obscene. While Ohio vested that power in medical professionals, the federal law withheld that power from those same professionals, prohibiting them from distributing contraceptives through the mail or via interstate commerce through the first two decades of the twentieth century. Tensions around the control of illicit sexual information, actions, and devices both evoked and evinced legal and moral confusion. This muddled question of authority led to a gap in medical service, a vacuum filled at first by the distributors of patent medicines and later by birth control clinics as well.[29]

One instance highlights the distance between advocacy and practice in the late-nineteenth-century social purity movement. In 1879 free-press defender Ezra Heywood brought public attention to a manufacturer's pamphlet describing the alleged contraceptive properties of Vaseline, a brand of petroleum jelly sold as a salve for burns and other conditions. The pamphlet claimed that Vaseline had another use: it would "destroy spermatozoa, without injury to the uterus or vagina." Samuel Colgate, a staunch supporter of Anthony Comstock, ran the soap business Colgate and Company, which held distribution rights for Vaseline. Apparently, this businessman's public opposition to obscenity as president of the New York Society for the Suppression of Vice did not prevent him from making a private profit with a product, based in part on its (unproven) reputation as a contraceptive. Heywood charged Colgate with hypocrisy and called attention to the class-based issues around the arrest and the prosecution of less well-known purveyors of vice. In response to the revelation about Colgate, Heywood and others dubbed the New York purity group the "Society for the Manufacture and Suppression of Vice."[30] Such discontinuities testify to the prevalence of family limitation in the private sphere as well as commercial venues, despite increasingly restrictive legislation.

By 1926, when free speech and birth control activist Mary Ware Dennett published *Birth Control Laws: Shall We Keep Them, Change Them, or Abolish Them?*, obscenity statutes restricted or banned contraceptive supplies and information in twenty-four states, the District of Columbia, and Puerto Rico. Many of those statutes remained on the books into the next century.[31] During the 1920s, Colorado, Indiana, and Wyoming, in addition to Ohio, exempted druggists from the legal repercussions of distributing family limitation information or supplies. Dennett noted that eleven states, including Ohio, considered *possession* of instructional materials or instruments for contraception a crime. Fourteen states specifically forbade anyone telling anyone else where or how to obtain birth control information or supplies. Connecticut actually prohibited the *use* of birth control, the only state to do so.[32]

However, a declining birth rate in the United States indicates that many citizens—along with druggists, some physicians, midwives, and mail-order entrepreneurs—regularly ignored these proscriptions. Arrests never accurately reflected the extent of either the sale or the use of contraceptives or abortifacients.[33]

By the 1920s the phrase "American family" was a European euphemism for a married couple with two children.[34] In 1933 President Herbert Hoover's research committee on social trends noted "the mild enforcement of restrictive laws [against birth control] by public authorities and the general disregard of them by individuals."[35] Despite legal restrictions and a lack of quality control of contraceptives, Americans had a worldwide reputation for limiting the size of their families well before the advent of birth control clinics.

The family size of professionals during this period embodies an ironic example of the unease between rhetoric and reality, between advocacy and action. Nineteenth- and early-twentieth-century physicians—along with attorneys, some of the very congressmen who voted for the Comstock Law, and other professionals—often had even smaller families than the population in general. In 1923 Rachel Yarros, a Chicago doctor and birth control advocate who had worked at the Hull House settlement, responded to another doctor's warnings about the dire consequences of contraception. Yarros noted sarcastically but accurately that, given the small size of many physicians' families, they must have been practicing birth control in their own relationships without "detriment to health, character or danger to civilization."[36] The methods employed to limit the number of one's progeny in this era included a variety of preparations and instruments.

## LEWD AND LASCIVIOUS DEVICES

Most contraceptive choices in the late nineteenth and early twentieth centuries did not require a visit to a physician. They included abstaining from sexual intercourse, also called continence; withdrawal of the penis before ejaculation, or coitus interruptus; having intercourse only during the "safe period" or "safe week" of the month, later known as the rhythm method; prolonged nursing of infants; vaginal suppositories, sponges, and douches (both homemade and commercially prepared); and condoms made of animal membrane or rubber. One creative and enterprising (if sarcastic) nineteenth-century company marketed a vaginal syringe for douching as the "Comstock Syringe." To correct the position of a tilted or otherwise "malformed" uterus, physicians often prescribed pessaries, devices designed to hold the womb in place. Pessaries came in an array of styles. Some were vaginal; others went into the uterus or cervix. The devices often prevented conception, if unintentionally. Cervical caps and diaphragms, called "womb veils" in the nineteenth century, were forms of the pessary used especially to prevent conception. Abortion and infanticide represented other more drastic means of controlling family size.[37]

The vulcanization of rubber in the 1850s greatly improved condoms and diaphragms, representing the first significant change in contraceptive technology in one hundred years. Before this process, temperature changes damaged rubber items of any sort, limiting their shelf life and their efficacy. Vulcanization created a more flexible and durable substance that resulted in thinner, stronger condoms, which could be manufactured more quickly and on a larger scale. Historian Andrea Tone notes that the revolutionary nature of this advance in technology and industry spurred Irish playwright George Bernard Shaw to call the rubber condom "the greatest invention of the nineteenth century."[38] Although the development of latex in the 1930s again improved the condom and its production rate, it would be years before the unregulated industry focused on product quality. The U.S. Food and Drug Administration did not begin formal testing of condoms until 1938. That same year a study confirmed what many couples already knew from hard experience: manufacturers had not tested three-quarters of the condoms then on the market before distributing them.[39]

The rubber diaphragm, also called an occlusive pessary, also benefited from vulcanization. The diaphragm prevents conception by providing a barrier between the vagina and the opening to the cervix, blocking the sperm's access to the ovum. While another method, the cervical cap, covers only the cervix, the diaphragm also covers the vaginal wall. Practitioners often preferred it over the cervical cap for this reason. In Holland beginning in the 1880s, doctors Johannes Rutgers and Aletta Jacobs popularized a type of diaphragm invented by German physician Wilhelm Peter Mensinga, one of Jacobs's mentors. Like the old pessaries but unlike cervical caps, the diaphragm had to be prescribed and fitted by a physician. Once trained in the technique, however, the woman could insert and remove the device at will in her own home. Its flexible nature and the addition of a spring to hold it in place made these processes much easier than with the older, more rigid models. Regular exams by a physician tracked any anatomical changes that would signal the need to prescribe a diaphragm of a different size. Birth control activists Margaret Sanger in America and Marie Stopes in Great Britain followed the Dutch example and recommended this form of contraception beginning in the 1910s and 1920s. The diaphragm became the method of choice prescribed by many, if not most, early American birth control clinics and some physicians. The Cleveland MHA used it almost exclusively. In spite of such marketing, though, the diaphragm never did reach a high level of popularity among American couples in general.[40]

The family limitation methods listed above worked to some extent, depending on several factors, including the quality of the device or preparation and whether or not the method was used correctly and consistently. While twenty-first-century experts do not consider douching a viable contraceptive in part because of its high rate of failure, historian Janet Brodie cautions that we cannot measure its effectiveness by contemporary standards. Physician and birth control advocate Regine Stix estimated in 1937 that using even the least effective family limitation procedure or device could cut the chances of pregnancy in half.[41] Yet through the 1940s, safety and unreliability remained a real problem for users of contraception. Since the manufacture and sale of birth control devices and preparations took place outside of the law, quality control did not exist. Women's magazines and newspapers touted preparations of all sorts intended to "cure" women's menstrual irregularity. Entrepreneurs and established businesses alike profited from the desire to limit family size and from the wide-open consumer market. Some firms unabashedly promoted the alleged contraceptive properties of common preparations, as in the example of the Colgate company's claims about Vaseline. The practices of the manufacturer of Lysol, the liquid cleaning and disinfecting agent, are an early-twentieth-century example of similar marketing.

Dear Sir:

I have been advised to write you in regard to how to use Lysol in femanine Hygiene so I will not become pregnant. I have One baby going on 8 months and am 6 months again we have been married 1 year this last Sept . . . Can't you help us?[42]

In the 1930s and 1940s, the manufacturer of Lysol advertised its household cleanser as, among its other uses, integral to "regular marriage hygiene" and essential to rid a woman of her fears that "some minor physical irregularity" might indicate "a major crisis." The Lysol manufacturer even included directions for preparing a vaginal douche. Although the recipe did not specify any potential spermicidal properties, many women employed this type of douche in the hope of preventing conception. The harsh substance produced side effects such as burning and inflammation, but some women continued to use it, believing in its contraceptive properties. A Cleveland physician remembered an incident at Margaret Sanger's New York birth control clinic. When one mother was asked how she got pregnant, she replied, "I just got darned sick of the smell of Lysol and so I didn't use it anymore."[43] Women included Lysol as well as Vaseline among their store of "preventives." One woman recalled the popular reasoning regarding the use of Vaseline: "They said a greased egg won't hatch."[44] Being able to purchase these consumer goods along with regular household items, without the embarrassment or extra expense of going to a pharmacist or physician, added to their popular appeal.

Relying on the safe period, or rhythm method, to prevent conception carried little potential for physical harm but failed especially often. For many years, it was based on an erroneous medical theory of the relationship between ovulation and fertility. Some posited the safe days to be in the middle of women's menstrual cycle, which in fact is usually the most fertile time. Medical research did not pinpoint the correct timing until the 1920s and still only dimly understood the hormonal process. Researchers continued to explore the optimum time for conception. Many more years passed before popular theory changed.[45]

## PERNICIOUS PRACTICES

In fact, the medical profession lagged far behind the public demand for family limitation. Some doctors quietly supported contraception, but most avoided venturing publicly into an area with obscene and illegal overtones. Early in the nineteenth century, physicians had successfully lobbied to criminalize abortion, cementing their expert role over lay midwives and abortionists but ignoring common custom and practice. An early draft of the federal Comstock Law actually exempted physicians and would have allowed them to provide contraceptive information.[46] Deleting that immunity in the final version of the law could indicate the continuing ambiguity about the role of the medical profession in reproductive control or last-minute concessions (or confusion) among legislators. The fact remains that few physicians clamored for the chance to enter the fray.[47]

General physicians of the nineteenth century received very little training in basic obstetrics or gynecology. Some American doctors even admitted to a lack of training in sexuality in general. At an 1898 medical symposium on "sexual hygiene," one physician commented that, while the public expected doctors to know "all about these things [sexual matters] . . . the text-books omit this department." The proceedings of this gathering, published as a "for doctors only" handbook, reflect many of the conflicts inherent in medical opposition to family limitation. The contributing physicians advised that, if a physician did learn about contraception and did offer it to his patients, perhaps he ought to be selective. Clearly, "the dragged-out woman on the verge of consumption" needed and deserved family limitation information. To protect women and their families from selfishness, however, the physician should withhold the same information from the "society belle who mistakenly thinks she does not want babies" or from other married women who simply did not want to be mothers.[48] The idea that a woman had a right to decide these questions for herself was unthinkable. Questions of race preservation, of class, and of gender tangled with science and moral duty—the duty both of women and of their physicians.

These questions continued to trouble the profession into the twentieth century. Canadian physician Elizabeth Bagshaw remembered that,
when she opened her practice in Canada in 1906, doctors "just didn't talk
about it [birth control]. . . . It was taboo, indecent. . . . We didn't know
much about it." Most medical schools in North America did not teach
techniques of contraception through the 1940s. General gynecological
textbooks avoided more than a cursory mention of the subject well into
the 1950s. Very few articles in the *American Journal of Obstetrics and Gynecology* (*AJOG*), the premier professional journal in the field, addressed
family limitation at all. Between 1914, when the term "birth control" was
coined, and 1940, *AJOG* published only twenty-six articles specifically
about contraception—an average of one out of an estimated total of forty
to fifty articles per year (excluding abstracts and book reviews). In contrast, during the same twenty-six-year period, *AJOG* carried sixty-five
articles about criminal abortion and more than a hundred on infant mortality.[49] Most physicians trained in the relatively new specialty of women's
gynecological health refused to even address contraception let alone recognize it as an integral component of their practice and their patients'
well-being.

Only two *AJOG* articles published between 1914 and 1919 focused on
contraception. However, the subject surfaced directly and implicitly in the
journal's burgeoning wartime discussion about infant and maternal mortality (a total of thirty-one articles between 1918 and 1919 alone). As in
previous decades, physicians argued against the "pernicious practices" of
birth control on grounds of morality and motherhood and added eugenic
and economic concerns. In October 1918 Dr. James Garber admonished
colleagues to "always bear in mind that the holiest names on earth are
Mother, Wife, Sister, Daughter." Garber claimed that mothers stand
"wrapped in filmy loveliness . . . just between us and Heaven," beckoning
physicians "to nobler aims, higher purposes, and loftier pursuits."[50] In a
time when some American women marched for suffrage and smashed
saloon windows for temperance, Garber evoked a sentimental Victorian
image. The wartime emphasis on the value of mothering in the early
twentieth century and fears of a diminishing population added to the
power of this representation. Through the 1930s, while a few physicians
provided contraception in their private practices, the profession in general
decried family limitation as immoral.[51]

In the 1920s and 1930s some Ohio citizens demonstrated a reluctance,
if not the same sort of repugnance, toward limiting one's family, as this letter illustrates.

October 193?
Ohio

Dear Miss Volk,

As yet my wife has nothing to report for she has not used it [the contraceptive]. She was upset by different things people had said about it. Her brother sort of caused most of the trouble by not believing in it. Given a few more week's and I believe she will be allright, Will have her write you then in regards to how she is getting along. Thanking you for your trouble.

I remain yours truly,

The woman described here by her husband had trouble dealing with the negative views toward birth control of the people close to her. Contributing to such public wariness about contraception, the American Medical Association (AMA) officially denounced birth control until 1937, when it belatedly acknowledged the practice as a legitimate medical concern. Professionalization of medicine and the tenacity of Victorian shame, especially regarding the female body, contributed to this reluctance. Many physicians linked birth control with midwives, irregular practitioners, unorthodox medicine, and quackery as well as immorality. Like many gynecologists and obstetricians, general practitioners proclaimed women's duty to *embrace* motherhood.[52]

Not all doctors shared these views, however. The Chicago Gynecological Society endorsed birth control in 1923. In a survey of New York physicians the next year, 80 percent of the fifty-one physicians who responded admitted that they suggested contraception to patients occasionally. The Section on Obstetrics, Gynecology and Abdominal Surgery of the AMA recommended liberalizing the Comstock Law in 1925. At its annual meeting in 1930, the Medical Women's National Association resolved that counseling patients about contraception was "a wholly proper medical function." As in the case of abortion, some physicians ignored the law, informed themselves about family limitation, and quietly recommended various methods to patients.[53] They acted without the support of the medical profession in general. To many if not most nineteenth- and early-twentieth-century American physicians, the use of contraception, especially the condom, implied promiscuity, even within marriage.

The condom's dual role of preventing pregnancy and venereal disease and its accompanying association with prostitution directly compromised the method's respectability. Concerns about sexually transmitted diseases led New York circuit court judge Frederick Crane in 1918 to allow physicians to distribute contraceptives (meaning condoms) specifically "for the cure and prevention of disease." The Crane decision continued to broaden physicians' authority over reproduction and set the precedent for physician prescription of the diaphragm. The ruling no doubt improved condom sales, but the method's reputation in general did not change significantly. In 1919, after America entered World War I, the United States military began distributing "rubbers" to soldiers and sailors overseas, attempting to slow an alarmingly high rate of venereal disease among the recruits. This action promoted a medical use for the condom but confirmed its disreputable association with a sexual disease. Many medical professionals refused to consider the rubber as legitimate. Court cases during the 1930s and 1940s sanctioned the condom as a disease prophylactic but warned against using it to "promote illicit sexual intercourse." That indecent image hinders condom sales, advertising, and use a century later.[54]

In the midst of such taboos, physicians generally ignored women's need for contraception. For health reasons, doctors sometimes advised women to avoid further pregnancies but did not usually offer the practical means to do so. Margaret Sanger of New York City insisted that one incident had convinced her to dedicate her life to birth control. In her work as a visiting nurse in 1912, Sanger cared for a patient, Sadie Sachs, who almost died from a self-induced abortion. During the doctor's final house call to Sachs after her recovery, he told the woman that she would not survive another pregnancy or abortion. Sanger claimed to have heard Sachs, the mother of three toddlers, ask how to prevent "getting that way again." The doctor allegedly offered an unrealistic suggestion: "Tell Jake to sleep on the roof." The woman then begged Sanger to tell her what she knew about contraception, which Sanger claimed was very little at the time. About a year later, with Sanger again at her bedside, Sachs died of another self-induced abortion. And Sanger committed herself to the cause (see figure 2). Historians and biographers have questioned the veracity of this conversion tale. Accurate or apocryphal, however, the story expresses the reality of some doctor-patient encounters and many women's lives.[55]

In her book *Motherhood in Bondage,* Sanger published a portion of the written requests that she received from people who were interested in—or desperate for—a reliable means of preventing conception. Thirty-one letters in the chapter "Doctor Warns—But Does Not Tell" graphically illustrate women's determined but futile attempts to obtain assistance

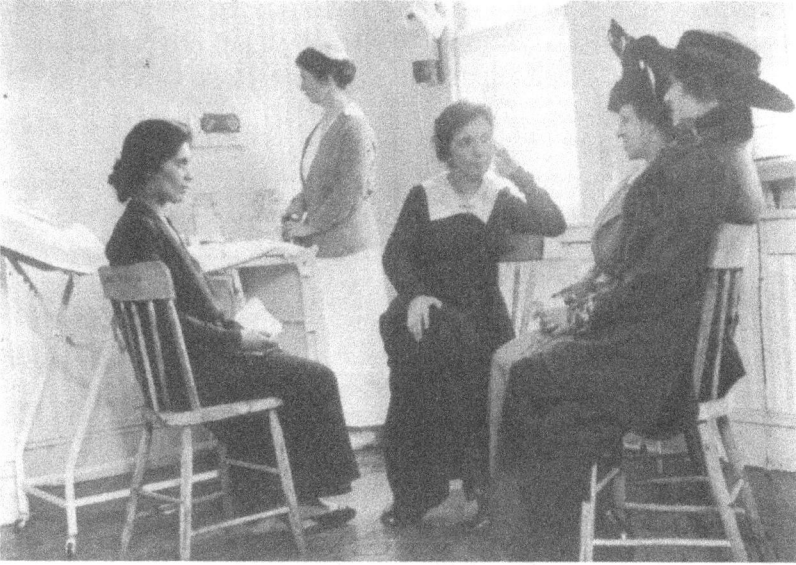

FIGURE 2. Margaret Sanger (center) in her Brownsville, New York, birth control clinic, 1916. The others are (left to right) Fania Mindell, Ethel Byrne (Sanger's sister, standing), and two clients. Cleveland Public Library, American Press Association.

from some physicians. Sanger may have modified some of the letters: statements about high fees for medical care, unfair laws, and the legislature often do not ring true, for instance. Perhaps many of the letter-writers had never even visited physicians. Taking those possibilities into account, the voices of overburdened mothers still convincingly reveal the distressing, sometimes tragic, results of the tension between rhetoric and reality in the area of reproductive policy.

The women represented in this chapter of Sanger's collection of correspondence were seriously ill. It is difficult to determine their social status. Since these women were literate and aware of Sanger as an information source, they were likely not among the country's poorest women, who would have depended on friends or relatives for information. The correspondents whom Sanger quoted suffered from tuberculosis, called "consumption," syphilis, heart trouble, or debilitating weakness resulting from too many pregnancies, difficult confinements, or problems during or after delivery.[56] Some women had borne many babies but had no living children. This woman represents one example:

> Have had four children, all dead at birth. . . . I am the short stout type and
> am very susceptible to pregnancy. My doctor only laughs when I tell him

> I'm pregnant again but what good does it do to go through with the whole
> affair when at the end I realize nothing but intense suffering and add one
> more death to the family list. If I am pregnant now, . . . I shall go on the
> table for an abortion.

Many women, like the writer above, gave themselves abortions or procured them to ease the situation temporarily. Others spoke of even more
drastic measures: "If I could tell you all the terrible things I have been
through with my babies and children, you would know why I would rather
die than have another one." Most women who wrote to Sanger reported
living in "constant fear" of conceiving another life, fear that damaged their
intimate relationships: "We are so young and suffering already for we are
afraid of intercourse . . . I love my husband and want him so, and, as for
him, poor kid, he's as nervous as the devil!"[57]

Mothers worried about the health of their children, living and unborn.
One woman explained, "I am not able to give them the care and attention
they should have. Neither am I able to give them the proper nourishing
food they require." Another mother said simply, "No one likes to see their
children not given half a chance."[58] Physicians had allegedly advised the
patients represented in this particular chapter of Sanger's book not to bear
more children. However, the women reported that, when asked about
"preventives," their doctors reacted with indignation, anger, name-calling,
evasion, or even jokes. A few medical professionals allegedly admitted to
not having the training to offer any contraceptive solutions other than
abstinence. Mothers responded angrily: "Doctors are men and have not
had a baby so they have no pity for a poor sick mother." Despair fueled
the rage. Women asked questions like, "Why do women have to suffer and
go through so much?" and "Must I go on like this always and my children
after me?"[59]

Healthier early-twentieth-century women also wanted to learn about
birth control, for reasons other than to improve their physical well-being.
Economic and personal factors along with increasing social pressures for
quality family life and the "well-born child" led couples to attempt to limit
their number of offspring. By the 1920s, the importance of heredity, a key
factor in eugenics, had modified public perceptions about the size and
quality of the optimum family.[60]

## FITTER FAMILIES

From the sterilization of the "unfit," to better baby contests, to prenatal
testing, to the Human Genome Project, scientists and the general public

have dreamed of and pursued the betterment of humans. The rhetoric and ideology of eugenics—selective breeding to improve population quality—drove this pursuit in North America throughout the last half of the nineteenth century, the entire twentieth century, and into the twenty-first. Physicians and statisticians quantified and standardized childhood measurements, legislators passed restrictive immigration laws, and physicians sterilized "less desirable" women and men, often without informed consent—all in the name of bettering the stock or the human race. Eugenic euphemisms commonly used in the early twentieth century included selective breeding, menace of the feeble-minded, human waste, careful mating, race suicide, unfit, and degenerates, and, on the opposite end of the spectrum, better babies, fitter families, well-born children, and mental and physical titans.

The term *eugenics*, coined in 1883, has become a catch-all term for wide-ranging doctrines with the common aim of bettering society by improving the inherited qualities of individuals. Cultural issues of class, race, and social control quickly entwined themselves with eugenic principles. The *Encyclopaedia of the Social Sciences* of 1930 defines eugenics as "the science and practise [*sic*] of improving hereditary characteristics in man." It explains: "Eugenics assumes that certain types of individuals are socially more desirable than others, and it proposes to improve future generations by increasing the proportion of individuals of desirable types through decreasing the rate of propagation of the inferior individuals (negative eugenics) and increasing that of superior individuals (positive eugenics)." The *Encyclopaedia* grossly understates the major controversial aspect of this social theory, noting that "it is mainly in deciding what individuals fall within the preferred groups that question and dissension [*sic*] arise."[61]

People have often utilized the same eugenic rhetoric to espouse opposing points of view. Rooted in nineteenth-century hereditarian philosophy and fueled by early-twentieth-century nativism, eugenics embodied arguments both for and against birth control. In 1905 President Theodore Roosevelt publicly characterized the American trend toward smaller families as a sign of moral disease that would destroy the white race, calling it race suicide. Public health advocate Helen MacMurchy of Toronto, Ontario, also employed the race suicide argument and decried birth control as unnatural.[62] On the other hand, founders of birth control clinics based their actions in part on the perceived eugenic *benefits*. The term encompassed all ideologies that aimed to better society by improving the inherited qualities of individuals, and therefore the family and the country. Cleveland birth certificates in 1916 pictured an infant and proclaimed, "A small one shall become a great nation" (see figure 3).

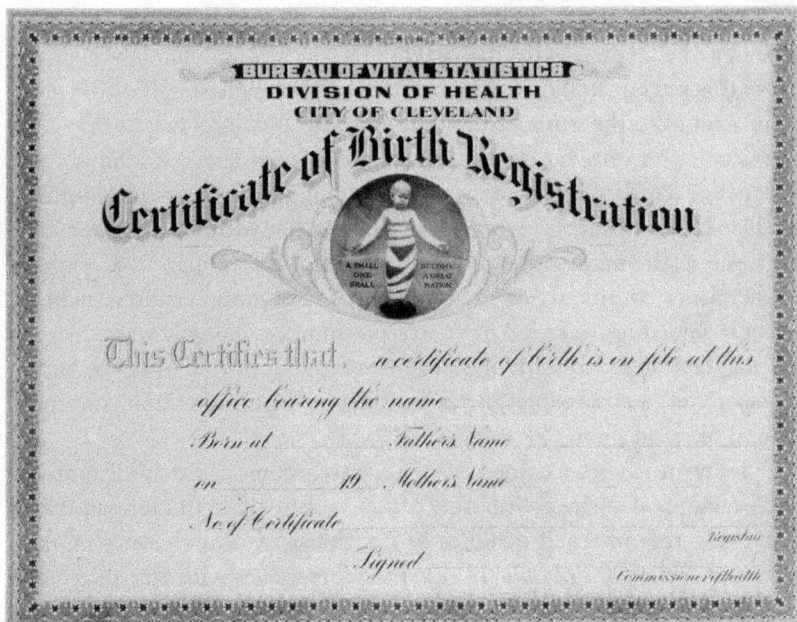

FIGURE 3. Birth certificate, city of Cleveland, 1916. The detail reads, "A small one shall become a great nation." *Cleveland Press* Collection, Cleveland State University, Heiser Company photo.

Some eugenicists of the 1920s and 1930s argued for birth control to improve population quality. Others pointed to the lower birth rate of the upper classes as compared to the proliferation of children among immigrants and the working class. They worried about the elite not reproducing themselves and the eventual disintegration of the white race.[63] The elitism of the eugenic philosophy permeated the American reform agenda of this era. Many academics and reformers saw the ideology as compatible with egalitarian social welfare goals. To most birth control activists and many eugenicists, the connection was obvious and unobjectionable before the Nazi atrocities of World War II. In 1938 eugenics proponent Lawrence K. Frank stated, "The two movements [eugenics and birth control] appear complementary, and each is more or less incomplete without the other because they have a common focus in the family and are directed to the same goals."[64]

The alleged beneficial potential of selective breeding—bolstering the ranks and quality of the upper classes as well as ridding society of the economic burdens of the poor and the unfit—attracted great interest.[65] Some leaders of races and ethnicities other than Anglo-Saxon Protestants also embraced eugenics, though the appeal was not as widespread and more subject to controversy. Black community and cultural leaders such as author and National Association for the Advancement of Colored People (NAACP) founder W. E. B. Du Bois and playwright and NAACP advocate Mary Powell Burrill took up the national cry for contraception on eugenic grounds, to ensure the survival of their race. Cincinnati celebrated National Negro Health Week in 1924 with a "Better Babies Contest."[66]

Eugenics appealed to science and logic, as did public health and other reforms. It depended on the Progressive "faith in the harmonious efficiency of scientific specialization," a central feature of early-twentieth-century business, medicine, and reform.[67] Professionals, academics, and the general public touted eugenic ideals, though in different languages and by different means. Most early-twentieth-century academic, medical, and social service associations maintained sections or committees on eugenics, mental or social hygiene, or race betterment (which often were interchangeable terms). At the 1929 Ohio Race Betterment symposium, Permelia Shields, president of the Cleveland League of Women Voters, carefully connected the whole agenda of the local League of Women Voters to racial betterment. She detailed the work of each of the league's departments and committees, including the Committee on Social Hygiene, as it related to improving the race. Nationally, the eugenic philosophy soon spread well beyond the science and social science communities and took on a patriotic bent, as this letter to Margaret Sanger indicates.

> We married for love only and we are happy, but poor, realizing that we are not in the circumstances to bring any children into the world until we have a few dollars saved, so that when we do have children we can give them the proper care and education they should have. My husband is one of twelve children and had to help bring his older brothers and sisters up, as the father only earned $13–$15 a week. . . . We both realize that it is not the proper thing to do for the children as well as for our country and therefore come to you for help.[68]

A desire for better babies coupled with a strong sense of economic responsibility for one's family, health concerns, and other personal considerations drove American couples to limit family size. Many couples actively sought a dependable method to do so.

Eugenicists, entrepreneurs, and charlatans abounded among nineteenth-century proponents of family limitation. Early in the next century, activists propelled the cause into the public eye. The political association with socialism added another dimension to the movement for birth control, one that many found suspect.

## RADICAL ROOTS

Cleveland was an industrial hub and a center for innovation and reform in organized charity in the nineteenth and early twentieth centuries. In an 1864 example of the city's philanthropic spirit, Cleveland women organized the Northern Ohio Sanitary Fair. The ambitious project raised over $78,000 in two weeks, with $10,000 profit to support Civil War soldiers. In the early twentieth century, ideas such as the community foundation, federated organizations of charities, and the community chest germinated in Cleveland and spread throughout North America. Founding private organizations to solve public problems represented a typical reaction during this era of distrust of the state.[69] A high level of tension between private and public plagued Cleveland and resulted in a fever pitch of organized charitable activity in the city.

Since the turn of the century, the city of Cleveland had almost tripled in size, with a population of 900,429 in 1930. The Midwestern port was the sixth largest city in the United States by 1930 and the largest in Ohio. An influx of immigrants accounted for much of the twentieth-century growth: over 60 percent of Clevelanders in 1930 were either foreign born or of foreign-born parentage. Industrial opportunities in the city also attracted people of color. With the Great Migration from southern states, the city's black population quadrupled between 1910 and 1920, and then doubled from 1920 to 1930. Blacks accounted for 8 percent of the city's residents by 1930.[70] The new demographics reflected population shifts common in other U.S. cities during the early twentieth century. The dramatic transformations did not go unnoticed.

White American-born citizens reacted to the changing population with nativism typical of the era. They worried about the future of the "race," the possibility of increased mental deficiency, and the alleged high birth rates of their new neighbors. Other concerns included the sharp changes brought about by industrialization and urbanization coupled with the loss of the "best" young men in World War I and with the loss of life during the flu epidemic of 1918–1919. In addition, the New (more independent) Woman, high rates of infant and maternal mortality, a declining birth rate among middle and upper classes, and an increased divorce rate threatened the status quo. Such circumstances and fears about the population and the family set the stage for a keen interest in birth control.[71]

Cleveland's reputation in the early twentieth century as a progressive, reform-minded city, protective of free speech, made it a preferred stop for radicals on cross-country tours.[72] In the decade before Clevelanders created the city's first birth control clinic, national activists lectured in the city and spurred supporters to organize a state birth control group. In April of 1916 Margaret Sanger took her first speaking tour across the United States. She spoke in eighteen cities in three months, selecting locations where sympathetic organizations or at least a known interest in family limitation already existed.[73] On Easter Sunday, sponsored by social workers, Sanger delivered her first Cleveland speech. Later that day she spoke to "400 men and women" at another location in Cleveland. An unidentified "radical" group sponsored this speech. According to the *Cleveland News*, Sanger "made a strong plea for national clinics where poor women should be taught sex hygiene and birth control." An MHA history declares that, after Sanger's Cleveland talk, "radicals . . . paraded down Euclid Avenue handing out printed birth control propaganda."[74]

Local newspaper accounts do not confirm (or perhaps chose not to report) this parade. Nor did they quote from Sanger's speech. However, in Chicago on the same tour, Sanger called for "WOMAN'S LIBERTY, for the freedom OF HER OWN BODY, for her release from the domination and control, of CHURCH AND STATE," and for "special scientific advice on birth control" from "DOCTORS AND NURSES," as "the proper authorities."[75] Existing evidence proves that Sanger delivered a similar message in Cleveland with the dynamism that became her trademark. She inspired her audience to action. A local Congregational pastor, the Rev. David Rhys Williams, "convinced by the cogency of [Sanger's] arguments," advocated "Woman Suffrage and Birth Control" in a public statement published the next month in local papers.[76]

Another Clevelander, social worker Frederick Blossom, offered his assistance to Sanger as a result of her Cleveland appearance. He obtained an unofficial speaking engagement for her at the National Conference of Social Workers in Indianapolis. In August of 1916, Blossom took a leave from his position as business manager at the Associated Charities of Cleveland, a relief organization, to devote his time to the presidency of the new Ohio Birth Control League. In December of that year he left Ohio to help Sanger establish an office for her newly created New York Birth Control League. Blossom, an active socialist, edited the first two issues of the *Birth Control Review* in 1917 before a dispute with Sanger led to his hasty departure. Blossom physically emptied the office and the coffers of the New York organization that he had helped to create. When Sanger reported the theft to the police, Blossom secured a resolution from a committee of the Socialist Party, denouncing her. The rift effectively distanced Sanger from some of her early radical supporters. However, this radical legacy remained attached to both Sanger and the birth control movement for decades.[77] The negative associations around Blossom's actions and

Sanger's response surely influenced Cleveland MHA founders to separate their enterprise from the earlier birth control efforts in the city.

A local arrest during the same year exemplified the unpredictability of the enforcement of obscenity law even in a city of liberal reputation. When anarchist Emma Goldman spoke in Cleveland on December 12, 1916, about "The Educational and Sexual Dwarfing of the Child," fellow activist Ben Reitman and volunteers from the audience distributed birth control pamphlets. Police arrested only Reitman, and the jury later found him guilty of distributing what Judge Dan Cull called "filthy propaganda." Judge Cull pronounced the maximum sentence: six months in jail and a fine of a thousand dollars plus court costs. This sentence was six times longer than the one Sanger had received earlier that year in New York City for distributing actual contraceptives in addition to literature. So-called progressive Cleveland had pronounced one of the longest sentences that Reitman ever served for his activism.[78] This case graphically illustrates the convoluted nature of obscenity law and its erratic enforcement. Cultural tensions and inconsistency characterized policy toward sexuality not only in conservative, rural areas but also in more open-minded, urban locations.

Despite this volatile and unpredictable climate, organizing for birth control continued in Cleveland. The first issue of the national periodical *Birth Control Review* (February 1917) listed eight Cleveland residents, in addition to Blossom, as officers of the Birth Control League of Ohio. The *Review* reported that the Ohio league had formed on June 23, 1916, "at a gathering of three or four hundred interested persons." In the *Review* the Ohio league presented its two-fold purpose: "First-The modification of existing laws in such a manner as to allow physicians, nurses and other competent persons to give information concerning methods of preventing conception. Second-The extension, under proper auspices, of the practice of family limitation as a means of reducing poverty, immorality, crime, physical and mental defectiveness and other human ills."[79] The first of these goals indicates a general lack of understanding about the state's legal restrictions. Ohio obscenity law in fact already allowed physicians (though not nurses or "other competent persons") to provide birth control.[80] In its second goal, the Birth Control League of Ohio approached the problem more broadly: contraception represented one way to improve society and attack social ills.

This agenda exemplified the tenets of most public advocacy of birth control in North America in the early twentieth century and set the stage for its medicalization. By emphasizing the role of doctors and nurses, activists such as Margaret Sanger shaped the control of reproduction as a problem to be addressed in the medical realm. The *Birth Control Review* article about the Ohio Birth Control League further claimed that the group had published twenty thousand copies of a pamphlet, conducted weekly study classes and a men's group, held monthly meetings and public events, and informed physicians about the provisions of Ohio law. The league asserted that "one large hospital" and "several public dispensaries" in Cleveland already provided birth control instruction.[81] While the evidence for these particular family limitation efforts has not yet surfaced, clearly some Clevelanders listened, discussed, and supported birth control as a socialist reform in the early 1900s. Outside speakers and local advocates placed the illicit topic of contraception on the city's public, political, and professional agendas. And, along with the rest of the nation, some Cleveland citizens privately employed some type of family limitation.

## FALLING BIRTH RATE

The birth rate declined in spite of legal and medical prohibitions. In 1850 the average U.S. white woman bore fewer than six children, and the average African American woman eight; by 1900 white women bore fewer than four children, and African American women bore fewer than six. In 1920 the national fertility rate was more similar for both races than it had ever been: black women, 3.64, white women, 3.17. In seventy years, black women's fertility rate dropped more than 50 percent; for white women the decline was almost as dramatic.[82] In the Cleveland area, family size reflected the national trend. The census of 1850 recorded an average family size of 5.46 persons for the residents of Cuyahoga County (which includes metropolitan Cleveland and several suburbs). While the number of households in the county rose through the next hundred years, the size of those households dropped consistently: to 4.65 in 1900, 4.32 in 1920, 4.01 in 1930, and 3.62 in 1940.[83]

The birth rate decreased despite many "modern" conditions conducive to higher fertility: more marriages in 1920 than in 1900, at slightly younger ages for both men and women; safer childbirth for both mothers and infants; a longer life span for mothers, babies, and children; and an increased likelihood of couples having private bedrooms.[84] Historians disagree about the explanation of this drop. Angus McLaren convincingly contends that the younger ages at which women ceased to bear children, from the mid-1800s to the end of World War I, proves that couples used contraceptive devices as opposed to the less effective natural methods of abstinence, withdrawal, or extended breastfeeding. Janet Brodie, on the other hand, suggests that, with a broadening knowledge of family limitation, couples varied and combined natural and artificial techniques and devices until they achieved the desired results. Respondents to researcher Clelia Mosher's survey of forty-five women in the nineteenth century employed a variety of approaches to space the births of their children, confirming Brodie's hypothesis, albeit on a small scale.[85]

Letters to Margaret Sanger written in the early twentieth century clearly delineate the use of various means of family limitation. The couples represented in these letters often did not achieve the desired results, however. One couple reported that, having unsuccessfully tried abstinence, they attempted to time intercourse to avoid ovulation. However, the woman unfortunately discovered that she was "one of those women who have no safe period." She further admitted that "the simple contraptions I have used have all failed." Many women described circumstances similar to another mother, who reported, "I have tried dozens of preventives my neighbors advised only to find myself pregnant again."[86]

Obviously, many Americans utilized family limitation before the advent of clinics or modern devices. Statistics from the first birth control clinics suggest that 80 percent to 90 percent of their clients had previously practiced some form of contraception.[87] Angus McLaren admits in his history of contraception that, over time, there were many different statistical fertility transitions among classes and regions worldwide. However, he insists that "the fertility decline [in general] was indeed remarkable and took place in the absence of major improvements in contraception and in the face of the avowed public hostility of the medical profession, the churches and the state. Clearly, enormous restraint and determination were exercised by millions of ordinary men and women. What counted was their desire and motivation; it overcame any inadequacy of means."[88] When laywomen organized birth control clinics in the 1920s and 1930s, they institutionalized this private desire and motivation. Their actions and women's positive response to this new service propelled public discourse about child spacing in the context of legal confusion and the silent antagonism of the medical profession.

Medical and legal policy intersected with local factors and ideologies to affect the formation and success of birth control clinics in Cleveland and elsewhere. Many women and men chose to limit their families independently of laws, public policy, cultural and moral perceptions, or the proclamations of national leaders. Some women and men chose to provide clinical contraception in that same restrictive climate. The information about the context of those choices, the personal reasons behind them, the

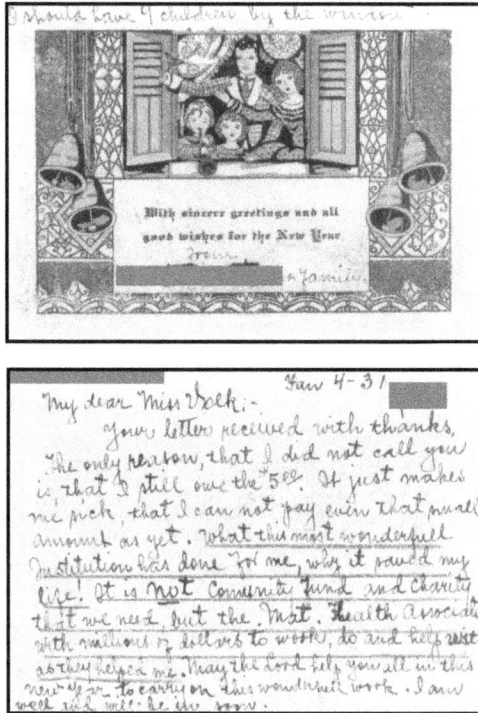

FIGURE 4. Postcard from MHA client, January 4, 1931. The text along the top
of the front of the postcard reads, "I should have 9 children by the window."
PPGC, box 6, Western Reserve Historical Society.

choices themselves, and the actions taken as a result of those choices help
to explain the movement's success. These decisions and actions challenged
moralistic rhetoric and policy.

Jan. 4, 1931
My dear Miss Volk:-

Your letter received with thanks. The only reason that I did not call you is
that I still owe the $5. It just makes me sick, that I can not pay even that
small amount as yet. What this most wonderful Institution has done for
me, why it saved my life! It is not community fund and charity that we
need, but the Mat[ernal] Health Association with millions of dollars to
work, do and help with as they helped me. [See figure 4]

Just how Cleveland women founded "this wonderful Institution," with far
less than "millions of dollars," is the subject of the next chapter.

# 2

## Nagging and Networking

Maternal Health Association founders carefully, quietly, and privately laid the groundwork for an independent birth control clinic in Cleveland between 1921 and 1928. The long preparation time resulted from suspicion of earlier radical activity, the unpredictable legal climate, medical opposition, and, naturally, unforeseen circumstances. The women countered local resistance with traditionally feminine tactics. To garner legal, social, medical, and financial support for their innovative and, at times, suspect service, they massaged familial and social networks. When the MHA opened, it represented not only seven years of preparation but also a culmination of local and national influences and personalities. This chapter describes the commitment of young Cleveland mothers to the birth control cause, their cross-generational and gendered recruitment tactics, and the deliberate way in which they built the base for a pioneer health service.

### COMMITMENT

Like Margaret Sanger, MHA founders Dorothy Hamilton Brush and Hortense Oliver Shepard would later recount a specific incident that led them to dedicate their energies to advocating birth control. According to Shepard and Brush, in the spring of 1920 the *Cleveland Plain Dealer* reported that a woman—pregnant for the tenth time—had purposefully stepped off the East Ninth Street pier into Lake Erie and drowned. Brush and Shepard allegedly knew the suicide victim, a "repeat patient" at the 35th Street prenatal clinic of Maternity Hospital, where the two volunteered as part of their Junior League obligations. A clinic physician had confirmed the woman's pregnancy the week before her suicide. The distraught mother allegedly cried, "My husband is crippled and can't support

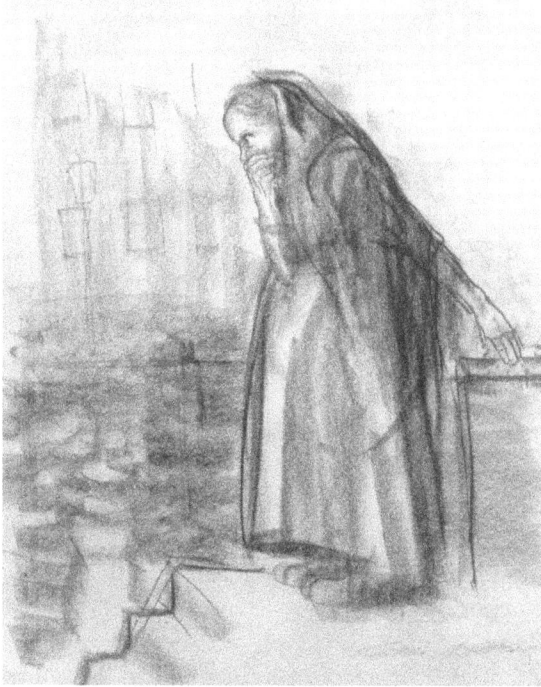

FIGURE 5. Käthe Kollwitz, *Pregnant Woman Contemplating Suicide,* c. 1926. Black chalk or charcoal, 64.3x49.7 cm. © The Cleveland Museum of Art, 2002. Gift of The Print Club of Cleveland in honor of Leona E. Prasse, 1962.291.a.

the nine we have now! I'm still washing diapers for the last two! I'm so tired!" Apparently, the Cleveland doctor advised this woman to deliver the baby in a hospital rather than at home, due to her poor health, but did not explain how to prevent future pregnancies. The volunteers had heard this mother and others like her desperately question clinic physicians about preventing conception, to no avail.[1] Whether out of ignorance or because of legal, religious, or moral scruples, these medical professionals would not provide the needed information. Mothers the world over experienced the burdens of frequent childbearing, and a few reacted in the same way as this Cleveland woman, inspiring Käthe Kollwitz, a German artist working in the 1920s, to depict the situation in *Pregnant Woman Contemplating Suicide* (figure 5).

The Clevelanders' story continues that, in response to this tragedy and to similar situations encountered at the prenatal facility, Brush and Shepard began imparting what little birth control information they knew to the dispensary patients who asked. Brush later recalled that, as young wives and mothers, "We did have sketchy information provided before we married by our mothers—our husbands could buy condoms to protect us, or, if they didn't want to, we might use germacidal [*sic*] douches. . . . We knew very well such measures were not fool-proof as we told them [the prenatal clinic clients]." According to Brush, a doctor at the clinic warned the two young women, "Just don't tell me what you are doing, as birth control is against the law." However, the chairperson of clinic volunteers soon instructed Brush and Shepard to stop providing the information— allegedly a Roman Catholic nurse had reported the subterfuge to the city government. Dorothy Brush left the dispensary in protest. Hortense Shepard remained but soon found herself "separated" from her volunteer position there.[2]

In November 1921 another incident greatly influenced the tempo and direction that the MHA founders would take. Juliet Barrett Rublee, a friend and ardent supporter of Margaret Sanger, invited four Clevelanders to attend the first American Birth Control Conference in New York City. Rublee was the cousin of Dorothy Brush's husband, Charles Francis Brush Jr., and later became an officer in the American Birth Control League (ABCL).[3] Dorothy Brush, Shepard, and their mothers, Jane Adams Hamilton and May Lockwood Oliver, went to New York City and attended the three-day meeting. Alice Butler, a doctor from Cleveland, lectured in the first session, titled "Individual Woman's Need of Birth Control." Other speakers and attendees from around the world discussed the possibilities and consequences of providing accessible, safe contraception.[4]

On November 13, a friend of Sanger's, Harold Cox, a British editor and former member of Parliament, was to help Sanger lead the discussion at a public meeting in New York's Town Hall. The conference program listed the title of this event as "Birth Control—Is It Moral?" With other conference participants, the Cleveland women arrived at Town Hall to find the doors blocked by police. Margaret Sanger soon emerged, escorted by police officers. Rublee and the Clevelanders followed Sanger and the crowd down Broadway to the police station. The authorities first charged Sanger and another participant with disorderly conduct but later released them for lack of evidence. A precinct captain, supposedly acting on orders from Roman Catholic archbishop Patrick Hayes, had blocked the public meeting and ordered Sanger's arrest. While he never took responsibility for the police action, Archbishop Hayes declared his opposition within the week: "The laws of God and man, science, public policy, human experience are all condemnatory of birth control as preached by a few irresponsible individuals."[5] The Cleveland women experienced firsthand the depth of hostility toward birth control and its use as well as any public dis-

cussion of the topic. Although this encounter made them wary, it heightened rather than quenched their growing interest.

Gender issues provided one impetus for creating the Maternal Health
Association. Along with Margaret Sanger and other leaders, clinic
founders believed that, for many women, effective child spacing was an
unknown or unavailable luxury. Although drugstores, barbershops, and
mail-order companies did a brisk business in contraceptive goods
throughout the early twentieth century, the most effective commercial
method, the condom, depended on a man's cooperation. Emma Goldman
and Margaret Sanger, among other activists, sought to expand women's
access to dependable family limitation. Existing national service organizations such as the U.S. Children's Bureau and local medical facilities such
as Cleveland's 35th Street Dispensary ignored women's need for reliable
control over reproduction as did many physicians in their private practices. Clearly, as the first MHA annual report stated, "a gap existed in the
circle of agencies promoting the health and welfare of the family."[6]
Dorothy Brush and Hortense Shepard proceeded to gather the forces
necessary to fill that gap, to widen the opportunity for more Cleveland
women to obtain safe and reliable birth control. They soon became as
determined as the opposition.

The clinical birth control movement of the 1920s and 1930s focused
almost solely on serving women. Movement leaders and birth control
clinics across North America advocated, popularized, and perfected the
use of the diaphragm.[7] Although diaphragm use in the United States
between 1930 and 1960 remained low in comparison to other contraceptives, by emphasizing this particular method, pioneer birth control clinics
affected matters other than family size. Offering diaphragms rather than
condoms, the clinics put control over reproduction into women's hands.
At the same time, they set family limitation firmly in the woman's sphere.
Contraception became a woman's, a mother's, responsibility, a responsibility that required medical supervision.[8] Maternal Health Association
physicians occasionally addressed the issue directly, stating, for example,
"Of course, the problem of contraception is man's problem as well as
woman's, but he is not concerned so vitally as is woman. It is the woman
that bears the penalties in disease, injury and death as well as the mental
torture that is involved. Woman has a right to know how she can intelli-
gently, not crudely and dangerously—control her sex life." Framing birth
control as a woman's concern and a medical matter determined the direction of later biological research into reproduction and its control.[9] It also
attracted some women to the movement in the 1920s and 1930s and
underlay their deep commitment.

Brush later claimed that, even before the MHA opened, she had focused on birth control as her sole cause. She remembered that she began resigning from other activities, "believing a person can serve best in one straight line." On another occasion, Brush elaborated bluntly, "All through these years I had served on several charitable boards. I grew convinced that most case-loads could be materially lightened if only the bung of birth control could be plugged into the barrel of misery. I resolved to devote all my own 'charity' toward that one end alone."[10] Brush and her friends laid the foundation for the MHA and enlisted the assistance of other Clevelanders who came to share this devotion.

## CLIMATE OF OPINION

Between 1914 and 1921, the leadership of the larger movement for birth control in the United States shifted its associations from anarchism and socialism to health reform. Sanger's socialist ties frayed as she focused on providing contraception as a goal in itself rather than a small piece of a broader agenda to change society. Modifying her original argument of the right of women to space their children, Sanger repositioned the cause within the mainstream debate about reversing the perceived disintegration of home and family. She and other national advocates such as Mary Ware Dennett, Robert Latou Dickinson, and Clarence Gamble found support in the coffers and energies of middle- and upper-class women across the country. These supporters included older activists who had just completed a successful drive for women's suffrage and younger women who had watched their relatives win that struggle.[11]

As organizers, funders, physicians, social workers, volunteers, and clients, women acted in birth control clinics as both conscious and unconscious agents for change. Since the nineteenth century, American women had advocated for social causes, focusing especially on issues affecting women, children, and the family, such as temperance, suffrage, and infant and child health.[12] Women joined the movement for the control of conception in part as an extension of this concern and in part because of the continuing disinterest of many male professionals in reproductive matters. That disinterest left the doors of opportunity wide open.

With their practice options already limited by gender bias, women physicians, for example, pioneered in a new field: the control of reproduction. Women led the effort national and internationally. While some men supported birth control clinics as clinicians, managers, medical or legal advisers, or funders, women staffed many if not most North American clinics as volunteers, physicians, nurses, and social workers. One survey completed in the 1970s indicates that women instigated and helped to run most of the fifty clinics founded between 1920 and 1940 in the United States that later became Planned Parenthood affiliates. Some of these local personalities, such as Gladys Gaylord, executive secretary for the MHA, and MHA founders Roslyn Campbell Weir and Dorothy Brush, contributed to national and international birth control organizations. Working-class women who gratefully patronized the clinics and personally recruited other clients also propelled the movement.[13]

During the 1920s, support and advocacy for privately run birth control clinics spread across the United States. Middle- and upper-class women, especially, took action. Inspired by Sanger's charismatic lectures and motivated by a combination of eugenic nativism, gender solidarity, and concern for the family, they organized their communities and educated them about clinical contraception. Women formed birth control leagues in Detroit (1922), Syracuse (1924), Wilkes-Barre (1926), and Newark (1927), for example. They opened clinics in these cities and other locations, such as Chicago (1923), Los Angeles (1925), and Reading, Pennsylvania (1927).[14] These groups and facilities organized along the lines of Sanger's clinic in New York and those founded by Marie Stopes in London.[15]

Other North Americans of the era attempted to encourage child spacing in very different venues, however. For instance, Lydia DeVilbiss and Alfred Kaufman distributed simple items such as the vaginal sponge or the condom door-to-door during the 1930s. DeVilbiss worked in Miami, Florida, and Kaufman in Kitchener, Ontario, Canada. During the same decade, manufacturers of contraceptives also marketed their goods door-to-door and through the mail (albeit illegally) as well as in pharmacies, barbershops, and department stores. DeVilbiss, Kaufman, and others recommended sterilization as well as family limitation devices or preparations, but most birth control clinics in the United States did not offer that choice during this era.[16] The clinical birth control movement that later evolved into Planned Parenthood did not choose the large scale service options promoted by Kaufman and DeVilbiss. A loose federation of small private facilities emerged across North America instead. Usually staffed by a single nurse and doctor and funded and managed by volunteers, the clinics provided one-on-one medical service.

The founders of Cleveland's Maternal Health Association cautiously waited to open such a clinic, a wait that turned into seven years. Shepard, Brush, and others feared that even social prominence might not shield them from birth control's religious, legal, or medical opponents or its left-wing reputation. Police had raided Sanger's Brownsville, New York, clinic in 1916 and arrested Sanger, her sister, and another clinic worker. All three spent time in prison for distributing birth control.[17] But the law did not represent the only barrier to starting a contraceptive service. Along with the rest of the country, Cleveland suffered from post-war distrust of socialist causes. The bloody 1919 May Day riots in Cleveland, among the most violent such demonstrations in the country that year, vividly proved the depth of the city's "red fear." In June 1919 the Cleveland mayor's house was bombed, an act that was attributed to radicals. The incident escalated the city's anxiety.[18] Though Sanger had practically abandoned her socialist connections and anarchist ideals by 1920, those connections affected the birth control movement for decades. Clinic organizers across the country in the 1920s, in cities such as Denver, for example, warily eschewed the movement's radical roots. Denver founders "took pains to avoid the radical connotations attached to the birth control movement on the East Coast."[19] The New York Town Hall incident made clear the strength of Roman Catholic opposition to contraception. Clevelanders hoped to avoid such confrontations. Like the women of Denver, MHA founders shunned the left-wing character of early birth control activities as well as its popular association with free-love attitudes and practices.

It is unclear which—if any—of the founders or supporters of birth control clinics in Cleveland in the 1920s attended the speeches in the city during the previous decade or participated in the Ohio Birth Control League. In her autobiography, Margaret Sanger claimed that she had first met Dorothy Brush in 1916. But in her own recollections, Brush placed the meeting later, in 1921.[20] None of the Clevelanders listed in the *Birth Control Review* as active in the Ohio Birth Control League in 1916 worked in the local movement's later phase. They do not appear in Maternal Health Association accounts of preliminary discussions about birth control in Cleveland or among the MHA membership. MHA founders clearly separated their venture from the earlier, more radical activism. These actions, combined with Blossom's socialist ties and shady activity, Reitman's highly publicized Cleveland arrest, trial, and sentencing, and movement leaders' anarchist connections and propaganda techniques affected the way the public viewed contraception. According to one MHA founder, these factors "created a climate among influential conservative people . . . which militated against" the idea of a birth control clinic in Cleveland.[21]

As a researcher observed a decade after the founding of the Maternal Health Association of Cleveland, "The [Maternal Health] Committee took all of this into account when laying their plans. They proposed, by careful education, to change the climate of opinion," to prepare Cleveland for a new look at a new service.[22] Following Sanger's model and working at the beginning of a national trend, this city's birth control clinic would emphasize the welfare of the child and the family rather than a woman's right to control her fertility.

Brush and Shepard returned to Cleveland from the 1921 New York conference inspired by the wide range of professionals concerned about birth control but intimidated by the depth of the hostility to the cause. Statements from two Cleveland social workers in the 1930s indicate some of the prevailing opposing arguments: "One has to guard against marriage becoming merely childless mating," and "[Birth control] is race suicide, medically disastrous and economically unsound. . . . The moral by-products are: It has a bad influence on the moral life of youth and destroys the sacredness of the marriage bond."[23] Proponents of contraception also faced significant religious opposition locally and nationally. Roman Catholics outnumbered Protestants and Jews in Cleveland at the turn of the century. The number of Catholic parishes in the city increased in the first half of the twentieth century, from 65 in 1908 to 90 in 1947.[24] Catholics influenced local, state, and national public policy as judges and legislators, as well as priests and bishops. Clevelander Martin L. Sweeney, for example, opposed birth control (and Prohibition). An attorney and an active Roman Catholic, Sweeney served in the Ohio legislature (1913–1914), on the Cleveland municipal court bench (1923–1931), and as a member of the U.S. Congress (1931–1942). At a 1932 federal hearing he argued against a bill to allow the importation of contraceptive devices, citing the American Academy of Medicine's opposition to contraception. Sweeney invoked motherhood and patriotism, characterizing birth control as a "vicious doctrine which, if not restrained, would destroy the Nation itself" and arguing that it would "lower the dignity of motherhood" and "bring ruin and destruction to the inhabitants of the greatest Republic on earth." Sweeney proclaimed the Catholic stance on the subject: "Interference with the natural laws of God [by preventing conception] invite [*sic*] disaster."[25] In such a tension-filled atmosphere, Brush and Shepard set out to broaden the support base for contraceptive services in Cleveland. They lobbied in personal discussions within the area's social, legal, and medical communities to prepare the city for a birth control clinic.

## GENERATIONS AND GENDER

The women first recruited relatives. "We quickly secured the enthusiasm of our young husbands," Dorothy Brush remembered. In fact, Charles Brush Jr. was listed with his wife as a patron of the first Ohio conference on birth control, held in Columbus on November 21, 1922. Jerome Fisher, a young attorney with the Cleveland firm of Thompson, Hine and Flory, was one of the five presenters at that event, giving a talk on "The Ohio State Laws Concerning Birth Control." The program for the event also named Fisher and his wife, Katherine Bingham Fisher, as patrons, along with Hortense Shepard and her husband, Brooks. Clevelanders made up at least a third of the list of the state conference supporters.[26]

The search for backing crossed generational as well as gender lines: Shepard and Brush approached older women already established in the city's social agencies. An MHA history noted that, in their late twenties, the two women felt "too young and unknown to enlist community support." As Brush later reasoned, "To whom should we turn for help? Why, naturally, to our mothers!" Shepard's mother, May Lockwood Oliver, served various local organizations such as Associated Charities and the Traveler's Aid Society. Brush's mother, Jane "Jennie" Adams Hamilton, led many activities at Calvary Presbyterian Church and supported the 1922 Columbus birth control conference.[27] After hearing the story of the young dispensary patient's suicide (and presumably other persuasive arguments), the older women agreed to try to "interest their friends."[28] Founders had tied together the first strands of what would become a strong intergenerational and cross-gender web.

Including men in the preliminary planning and on MHA boards represented an important gender strategy, conscious or not, typical of women's groups of the time. Historians have noted a "devaluation of women's culture in general and of separate female institutions in particular" in the United States in the 1920s. Between 1870 and 1940 many American women's organizations incorporated men into management, if not the day-to-day work. Men broadened the power base and widened the sphere of influence for women's organizations. In Cleveland specifically, men had participated in women's causes since at least the turn of the century. For example, around 1910 Cleveland civic leaders organized the Men's Equal Suffrage League to support the fight for woman suffrage. According to the *Birth Control Review* report in 1917, the early Ohio Birth Control League had a men's service. Cleveland had gained fame for pioneering the popular "scientific philanthropy," organized along the parameters of business and industry. The local and national concentration on efficient voluntarism and a growing disdain for women-only groups in the United States probably influenced MHA founders to include men in their venture.[29] They chose select men of influence and high community standing.

In their quest for credibility, Shepard and Brush appealed to three couples, all related to the Brush family circle: William Weir, M.D., and Roslyn Campbell Weir; Roger Perkins, M.D., and Edna Brush Perkins; and Jerome and Katherine Fisher. Roslyn Weir was the grandniece of Charles Francis Brush Sr., Edna Perkins was his daughter, and Jerry Fisher worked for Thompson, Hine and Flory, the law firm that Charles Brush Sr. used. The Weirs and Perkinses were "12 to 14 years older" than the Brushes (Dorothy and Charles Jr.), Shepards, and Fishers (see figure 6).[30] Family networks formed the basis for many enterprises across North America. In Cleveland, for instance, family bonds existed between and among the residents of fancy Euclid Avenue. In the mid- to late nineteenth century, many of Cleveland's elite, including Charles F. Brush Sr., lived on the avenue, nicknamed "Millionaire's Row." Relatives built or purchased homes near their families on the broad, tree-lined parkway. Together they worked, played, and participated in cultural activities, business ventures, and reform causes.[31]

## BRUSH
## FAMILY CONNECTIONS

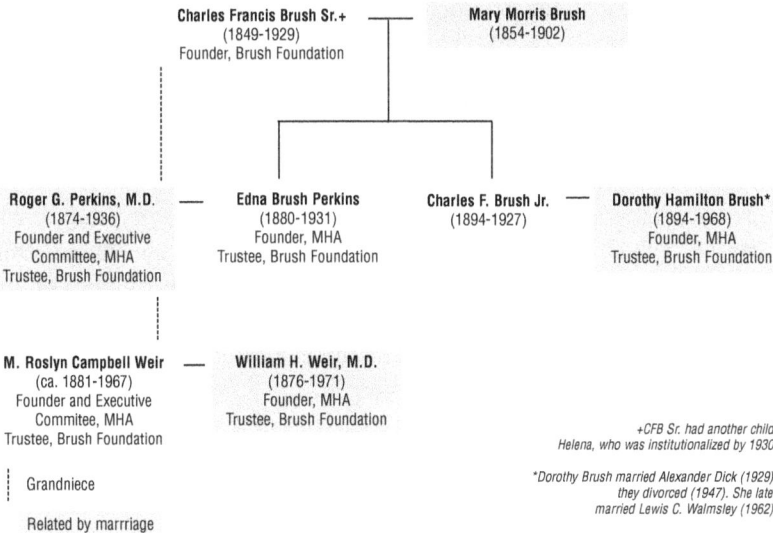

**Charles Francis Brush Sr.+**
(1849-1929)
Founder, Brush Foundation
— **Mary Morris Brush**
(1854-1902)

**Roger G. Perkins, M.D.**
(1874-1936)
Founder and Executive Committee, MHA
Trustee, Brush Foundation
— **Edna Brush Perkins**
(1880-1931)
Founder, MHA
Trustee, Brush Foundation

**Charles F. Brush Jr.**
(1894-1927)
— **Dorothy Hamilton Brush***
(1894-1968)
Founder, MHA
Trustee, Brush Foundation

**M. Roslyn Campbell Weir**
(ca. 1881-1967)
Founder and Executive Commitee, MHA
Trustee, Brush Foundation
— **William H. Weir, M.D.**
(1876-1971)
Founder, MHA
Trustee, Brush Foundation

Grandniece

Related by marrriage

+*CFB Sr. had another child, Helena, who was institutionalized by 1930.*

**Dorothy Brush married Alexander Dick (1929); they divorced (1947). She later married Lewis C. Walmsley (1962).*

FIGURE 6. Brush Family Connections

Familial and social networks sustained the national and local suffrage movement. Suffrage activism often led to advocacy for family limitation in Cleveland and elsewhere. On the East Coast, Katherine Houghton Hepburn, the mother of the actor and film star, joined the Connecticut Women's Suffrage Association (CWSA) in 1905 along with friend and neighbor Josephine Day Bennett. Hepburn created the Hartford Equal Franchise League. Two older CWSA colleagues, Anne Webb Porritt and Bennett's mother, Katherine Beach Day, provided significant financial support for suffrage. Only one year after the passage of the Nineteenth Amendment, these three women attended the same national birth control conference in New York City that attracted the Cleveland women. Hepburn, Bennett, and Porritt took major roles in the new American Birth Control League and later in the Connecticut Birth Control League (CBCL). By 1933 Porritt served on the CBCL board, her daughter-in-law was treasurer, and Sallie Pease, another of Hepburn's friends, chaired the new Hartford County group.[32] Suffrage activism had brought these women together, and they extended their advocacy to include access to reliable contraception. Networking for a cause invigorated and sustained much voluntary activism, especially among women.[33]

In the birth control movement, family networks assumed heightened importance. Contraception's shady reputation and shaky legal standing necessitated that clinic founders solidify a firm, private support base before venturing outward. The women who originated the MHA remained sensitive to the intimate character of this particular issue. Opposition from powerful relatives could doom the effort in its fledgling stages. The women first broached their ideas at home. They secured crucial familial support before entering the public realm. MHA founders and their families lunched and talked with friends about establishing birth control services in the city. Other prominent Clevelanders, including Julia McCune Flory, Frances Southworth Goff, Mabel Breckenridge Wason, and Lenore Schwab Black, sympathized and expressed tentative interest but would not further commit themselves. Resolutely and stubbornly, Brush and Shepard periodically brought the intergenerational group together with their familial backers to discuss the matter until they had formed an ad hoc committee.[34] They expanded and strengthened their web of support.

The older women in this group (in their mid-thirties to late forties) together had created and held offices in many of the same local voluntary social service agencies. Some also advocated for other national causes, as was the case in Connecticut. Edna Perkins and Roslyn Weir had actively worked for suffrage. Perkins had chaired the Woman's Suffrage Party of

Cleveland and orated nationally on woman's right to vote. Frances Goff had lent her name to that cause. Goff, Wason, Black, and Oliver chaired many committees of Associated Charities, where they also served as trustees. Associated Charities was a large, multifaceted social service organization and a predecessor of the Welfare Federation of Cleveland (and its successor, the Family Services Association). Perkins, Goff, and Black had attended the National Conference of Charities and Corrections, held in Cleveland in 1912. In 1926 Black and Goff served as first and second vice president, respectively, of the Women's City Club of Cleveland (WCC), in which they held charter membership, along with Perkins and Flory. Various other social, cultural, and political causes also attracted the attentions, energies, and money of these women.

Edna Perkins officiated on the boards of the Anti-Tuberculosis Association, the Consumers' Customers' League, and the Welfare Federation. Julia Flory served as a trustee for the Cleveland Day Nursery and Free Kindergarten Association and helped found the Cleveland Playhouse. Her husband, Walter, was a partner in the established Cleveland law firm of Thompson, Hine and Flory. A Vassar College graduate (class of 1886), Frances Goff was a trustee of The Cleveland Foundation, the pioneer community trust founded by her husband, Frederick, president of Cleveland Trust Bank. In earlier years, Mabel Wason, another Vassar graduate (class of 1896), had presided over the Day Nursery Association and participated in the women's committee of the Ohio branch of the Council of National Defense. Married to the president of Lindner's, one of Cleveland's leading department stores, Lenore Black belonged to the board of the Rainbow Hospital for Crippled and Convalescent Children (formerly Babies Dispensary and Hospital).[35] Such credentials indicate that Brush and Shepard purposefully chose for their endeavor community leaders with wide-ranging interests. While family ties abounded in the MHA, a broader, more complex matrix of commitment and voluntarism also linked the participants.

These and other potential supporters voiced concern that their respective organizations might suffer from association with the cause of birth control. Before the clinic even opened, MHA founders decided to avoid "any action which could bring harm to other community agencies." They were convinced that "a community so unusually united and dedicated to many kinds of social improvement should not be split by controversy." Cleveland was known by the 1920s as a national leader in organizing federations of civic organizations such as the Community Chest, the Jewish Welfare Federation, and Catholic Charities. The common phrase "the Cleveland approach" referred to the city's reputation for efficiently centralizing philanthropy and reform. Nonprofit charitable agencies worked independently in the city yet maintained close relationships with each other. One outside observer, R. L. Duffus, wrote in the *New Republic* about "community patriotism" and much "ballyhooing for cooperation" in Cleveland. He claimed that "Cleveland would cooperate even if it had to be genteelly clubbed into doing it." In 1927 James E. Cutler, the founder and first dean of the School of Applied Social Sciences (SASS) at Western Reserve University, described the relationship between the social science school and community agencies as "Cleveland cooperation."[36] Associated Charities provides a good example of the power of the federation model in Cleveland.

Since its establishment in 1900, Associated Charities had tried to systematize access to Cleveland's reform community. The group first maintained a card file of charitable agencies. In 1905, with Mabel Wason (later an MHA trustee) heading the publication committee, Associated Charities printed a "classified and descriptive directory of the philanthropic, educational, and religious resources of Cleveland." True to the standard of Cleveland cooperation, the preface stated, "No modern charity lives to itself alone." The directory's very existence modeled and embodied the ideal of efficient charity to which many new city agencies, including the Maternal Health Association, later aspired. With the Committee on Benevolent Associations of the Chamber of Commerce, Associated Charities attempted to streamline charitable functions in Cleveland, evaluating the financial and management practices of existing groups.[37]

These watchdog organizations and others closely attended to the formation of new Cleveland service organizations as well. For example, Western Reserve University's 1916 creation of the School of Applied Social Sciences to train social workers rested on detailed research into community and professional needs and meticulous scrutiny of the services already in place.[38] Working compatibly with other agencies from the beginning, MHA founders utilized rather than threatened this cooperative ideology. In a similar vein, they employed other tactics and legal maneuvers to avoid controversy and help establish birth control as a legitimate personal and social concern.

## INTERPRETING THE LAW

The planning committee decided to address Ohio's regulation of birth control because of what they saw as general confusion about the state law's provisions regarding physicians. On March 13, 1922, Jerome Fisher wrote a clarification of Ohio's obscenity law in the form of a legal opinion.

Fisher practiced law with Thompson, Hine and Flory, the firm that Charles Brush Sr. used and in which Julia Flory's husband was a partner. Amos Burt Thompson, head of the firm (and the brother-in-law of MHA committee member May Oliver), signed the legal opinion drafted by Fisher. The document asserted that Ohio doctors could legally advise their patients about birth control provided that they did not use any "secret nostrums" or send materials through the mail (see figure 7). As noted in chapter 1, the Ohio obscenity law already exempted physicians and pharmacists but was apparently highly misunderstood and unevenly enforced. Since the federal Comstock Act did *not* exempt physicians or druggists, confusion reigned. In the legal opinion, Fisher articulated and emphasized the lawful place of physicians with regard to birth control in Ohio. The *Ohio State Medical Journal* published his statement a few years later.[39] Such strong legal backing provided a firm basis for the Maternal Health Association—without challenging or modifying federal or state statutes.

The legal opinion structured MHA policy and marked the boundaries of its legal and illegal activity. It clearly illustrated that clinic founders accepted the necessity of the control of birth control by a physician as opposed to a nurse or layperson, although debate about this service venue does not exist in the organization's historical record. Placing contraception under medical auspices played an important strategic role in the struggle to attain legitimacy for birth control methods and information as

---

**Legal Opinion**

Composed for the Maternal Health Association
Jerome Fisher, Thompson, Hine and Flory, 1922

EXAMINATION OF THE GENERAL CODE MAKES IT CLEAR THAT A PHYSICIAN IS PRIVILEGED TO GIVE SUCH INFORMATION, TREATMENT, OR MATERIAL, ALTHOUGH IT IS ILLEGAL FOR A LAYMAN TO DO SO. FURTHERMORE, IT IS NOT NECESSARY THAT THERE BE ANY DISEASE-REASON, BUT THE PHYSICIAN MAY GIVE THIS HELP TO ANYONE WHO CONSULTS HIM. THE OHIO STATUTES EXPRESSLY PROVIDE THAT "REGULAR PRACTITIONERS OF MEDICINE" ARE NOT COVERED BY THE LAWS AGAINST CONTRACEPTION (GENERAL CODE 13037). THERE IS ONLY ONE EXCEPTION TO THIS, AND THAT IS THAT NOT EVEN A PHYSICIAN MAY DISTRIBUTE A "SECRET DRUG OR NOSTRUM." IT IS THEREFORE DESIRABLE THAT ANY PREPARATION FOR THIS PURPOSE, CARRY ITS FORMULA ON ITS CONTAINER.

THE ONLY JURISDICTION OF THE FEDERAL LAWS, IS AS TO USE OF THE MAILS, AND INTERSTATE COMMERCE. NOT EVEN A PHYSICIAN CAN LEGALLY USE THE MAILS, OR COMMON CARRIERS IN INTERSTATE COMMERCE, FOR THE CONVEYANCE OF CONTRACEPTIVE INFORMATION OR MATERIAL.[40]

FIGURE 7. Legal Opinion, 1922

well as in the effort to ensure the safety of those methods and accuracy of that information. Treating birth control as a medical concern distanced it from herbal or pharmaceutical contraceptive preparations (which often got confused with abortifacients) as well as from the condom (which carried a disreputable association with venereal diseases). Organized at a time when the commercialization of contraception led many couples to corner drugstores rather than doctor's offices, the clinical birth control movement took a different route. Advocates such as Sanger and her followers in Cleveland chose this course as the most practical one, courting the support of the medical profession to stay within the law. They perceived a need to earn respectability for contraception, and organized under medical supervision as a means to that end.

Historical surveys and primary sources indicate that most early U.S. clinics employed physicians to dispense birth control. Most if not all clinics also dealt with legal issues. In 1917 Chicago's fledgling birth control organization, the Parents' Committee, asked the state attorney general about the legality of a clinic in Illinois. The official replied that Illinois law did not prohibit a physician from giving contraceptive advice. However, when the committee tried to obtain a license in 1923 for its new birth control clinic, the Chicago Department of Health refused, describing the effort as "against the public interest." The group won a suit for the license later that year but lost on appeal. Abandoning the legal route, the Chicago committee opened a center for birth control in the medical offices of Dr. Rachel Yarros rather than in a separate clinic. Sanger's Birth Control Clinical Research Bureau in New York City operated in the same way, under the private practices of first Dr. Dorothy Bocker and then Dr. Hannah Stone, for the same reasons. Some facilities, including the Maternal Consultation Center in Rochester, New York, had legal advisers; other maintained legal funds. Between 1917 and 1940, the Birth Control League of Massachusetts (BCLM) repeatedly asked judges and attorneys to interpret the state law and published those opinions in the *New England Journal of Medicine* and in BCLM literature. The BCLM opened a clinic in Brookline in June 1932, but arrests and unfavorable verdicts doomed contraceptive services there for forty more years. For the Cleveland MHA, acting in a less oppressive atmosphere, publishing an interpretation of obscenity law by a prominent law firm cemented a firm foundation for action.[41]

While Fisher and his colleagues secured the legal base for the dissemination of contraceptive information and devices in Cleveland, Brush and Shepard educated potential supporters—family, friends, and acquaintances. They raised money and invited Anne Kennedy of New York City, a field worker for the American Birth Control League, to speak to small groups in Cleveland. Kennedy stayed at the home of Lenore and Morris Black, on East Eighty-ninth Street. She lectured there and in the Oliver home on Magnolia Drive without publicity from the national organization. A fledgling organization itself, the ABCL adapted to whatever reasonable demands might expedite the organization of local groups.[42]

Using their influence, the Cleveland women helped to secure a pro–birth control speaker for the regular program of the Women's City Club (WCC) of Cleveland. In 1916 Edna Perkins, Julia Flory, Helen Chase Bassett, and Lenore Black (all charter members of the MHA) had helped create the WCC in Cleveland, a women's forum for the open discussion of "community problems." Another MHA charter board member, Mary Dunning Thwing, served as the first president of the WCC. Members not only debated issues but also endorsed legislation. By 1922 the WCC had six thousand members and a "club house" located on East Thirteenth Street. Placing the topic of birth control before these informed and involved women removed it from radicalism and set it alongside other crucial and more respectable issues of the day. Once more, MHA founders worked the system, using their connections to WCC founders and board members to push their agenda.[43]

On May 25, 1922, Edith Houghton Hooker of Baltimore, a member of the American Birth Control League national board of directors, spoke to an overflow crowd of about three hundred women at Cleveland's WCC. This particular lecture, limited to WCC members only, caused some anxiety among local birth control committee members. Katherine Fisher later recalled her husband saying that morning, "There may be trouble. I think I'll plan to be there." The attorney stood in the back of the room, but apparently problems did not materialize.[44]

Having prepared the way using their families and social networks, established a firm legal ground, and connected with the national movement, Shepard, Brush, and the other members of the ad hoc committee moved ahead. They created a formal birth control organization, as yet unnamed, late the next winter, on February 23, 1923, at a meeting held at the WCC. The constitution included an explicit statement of the association's compliance with the law. The founding officers were as follows: president, Mabel Wason; first vice president, Lenore Black; second vice president, Roslyn Weir; secretary, Katherine Fisher; and treasurer, Madeleine Almy Mather. Maternal Health Association records give no explanation or background for the choice of officers. Dorothy Brush had a toddler and a newborn in 1923, which might well account for her absence among the official leaders.[45]

## "AND WHAT ARE YOU DOING FOR B.C.?"

In addition to securing support from their families and the social service and legal arenas, the birth control planning committee members sought advice and approval from Cleveland's medical professionals and the public health community. Like other clinics across the country, the MHA organized with medical support. While the profession still officially opposed contraception as a medical matter, some physicians quietly took up the cause. Maternal Health Association founders consulted doctors William Weir and Roger Perkins about local birth control services throughout the clinic's planning stages. The Weirs and Perkinses traditionally spent Sunday evenings at Brush family gatherings, either at the Charles F. Brush Sr. mansion on Euclid Avenue or at the Weir residence on Richmond Road, which was then "out in the country." Weir was a gynecologist and Perkins a bacteriologist who served as chief of the Bureau of Laboratories for the City Division of Health. Both men taught at the Western Reserve University School of Medicine—Weir, gynecology, and Perkins, preventive medicine. The two physicians consistently supported the MHA, serving on the first Medical Advisory Board. The close involvement of these medical professionals in designing the Maternal Health Association's organization and services must account in part for the clinic's compliance with the model of medical control.[46]

In October 1923 Cleveland birth control committee members met with Weir, Fisher, and four other medical leaders: the director of the Cuyahoga County Health Department, and the superintendent, the director, and the social service director of Lakeside Hospital. The group discussed various approaches to providing birth control in Cleveland.[47] On the advice of these physicians and administrators, MHA founders initially decided to incorporate contraceptive services into an existing hospital outpatient clinic rather than create a separate facility.

Early-twentieth-century medical professionals generally preferred hospital-run dispensaries to freestanding clinics. Having only recently expanded their authority over childbirth, midwives, and the purveyors of patent medicines, physicians distrusted health care facilities managed by nonprofessionals, especially laywomen. Although independent dispensaries provided training opportunities for young medical students, they also competed with local practitioners and hospital clinics for business, offering free or low-cost services. Private dispensaries closed in the late nineteenth and early twentieth centuries as larger medical institutions expanded. New York City doctors and hospitals, for example, assumed control over small, lay-run neighborhood clinics in the 1890s by means of government regulation.[48] Throughout the 1920s Robert L. Dickinson, a New York City obstetrician/gynecologist and researcher who advocated for birth control, attempted unsuccessfully to convince Margaret Sanger to put her Clinical Research Bureau under hospital auspices.[49] Midwestern cities experienced a similar trend.

A Cleveland effort to slow the alarming rate of infant mortality offers one example. In 1899, before the widespread testing of milk for bacteria, Edith Dickman began providing safe milk to poor Cleveland mothers, charging a nominal fee or no fee at all. The daughter of an Ohio supreme court justice, Dickman organized the Milk Fund as a private charity. In 1904 a Cleveland pediatrician and the Visiting Nurse Association collaborated with the Milk Fund to open a babies' dispensary at the Friendly Inn, a settlement house. Two years later the group incorporated the facility as Babies Dispensary and Hospital. The dispensary moved in 1907 to East Thirty-fifth Street, close to Maternity Hospital. Within five years of the Milk Fund's founding, the medical establishment had taken over its services. Created as a lay organization by a woman who was neither a doctor nor a nurse, the fund had quickly proven to the medical profession the value and efficacy of providing safe milk for infants. A charitable effort had instituted a valuable service. Voluntary action rather than medical inspiration launched this reform in Cleveland.[50]

The centralization of the city's health care under hospital control continued through the 1920s. In 1926 Lakeside Hospital and its related institution, Western Reserve University, united both Babies Dispensary and Maternity Hospital under Lakeside's and Western Reserve's auspices.[51] Other hospitals subsumed clinic services under their outpatient divisions.[52] Organized medicine diminished the number of Cleveland's freestanding clinics. Maternal Health Association founders apparently agreed with the medical advice to locate Cleveland's new contraceptive service within an existing facility. With services, equipment, and clientele already in place, baby clinics or hospitals (like the one pictured in figure 8) seemed the ideal vehicles to distribute birth control.[53]

According to MHA histories, the planning committee approached administrators of Lakeside, Mt. Sinai, and Maternity (later called Mac-Donald) Hospitals with the idea of operating a contraceptive clinic, to no avail. Some hospital officials sympathized, others opposed the plan, but all feared that providing contraception would threaten existing institutions and services. Apparently the highly touted philosophy of Cleveland cooperation did not extend to birth control clinics.[54]

Minutes of the management committee of Lakeside Hospital from 1928 to 1930 tell a slightly different tale, albeit an incomplete one. These

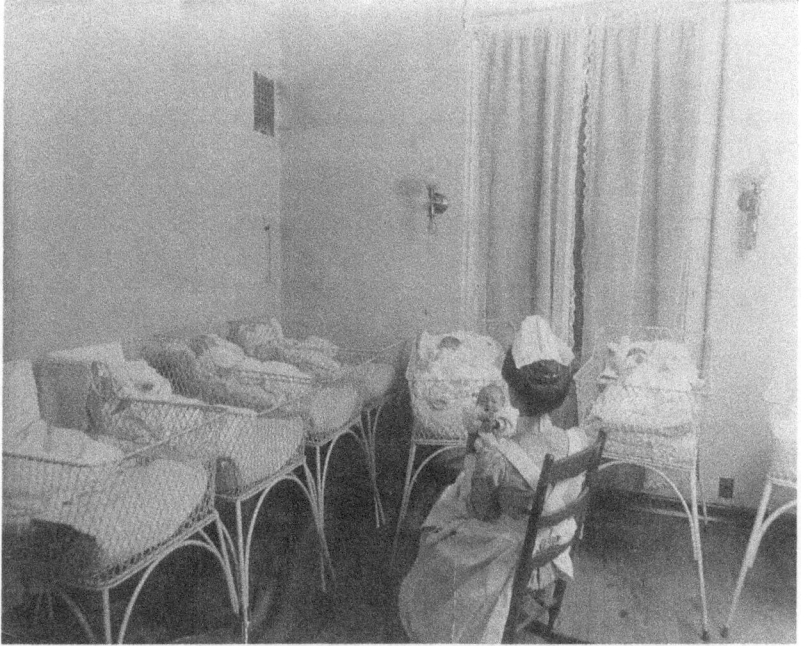

FIGURE 8.  Free Maternity Ward at St. Luke's Hospital (Methodist), Cleveland, Ohio, 1912.
*Cleveland Press* Collection, Cleveland State University.

documents state that Lenore Black and Hortense Shepard did approach
the director of administration at Lakeside on behalf of the MHA. What
differs between the Lakeside and MHA accounts is the timing and the
hospital's response. The hospital minutes indicate that, in October 1928,
a few months after the MHA had already opened its doors as an independent organization, Black and Shepard proposed "the establishment of
a [weekly] birth control clinic at Lakeside Hospital," with the Maternal
Health Clinic to supply the nurse and the doctor. According to Lakeside
minutes for October 30, 1928: "He [the hospital director] stated that the
staff had already approved of the establishment of such a clinic. It was
moved and seconded that a birth control clinic be established in the gynecological division of the outpatient department of Lakeside Hospital."[55]

Maternal Health Association records do not mention such an agreement. Furthermore, it is not clear whether the plans ever moved beyond
the question of who would pay for clinic supplies—the MHA or the hospital. Almost one year later, in August of 1929, with costs still an issue, the
Lakeside Management Committee minutes again reported, "It was
moved and seconded and carried that the birth control clinic at Lakeside
Hospital should be put into operation." The November 5 minutes stated,

though, that "concerning the birth control clinic, no meetings of the advisory committee had been held." Discussion at that meeting still centered on who would belong to the advisory committee itself.[56] Since the subject does not appear again in Lakeside's minutes, the hospital plan seems never to have come to fruition.

Lakeside and other hospitals refused to incorporate birth control into pre-existing programs in the 1920s despite the medical profession's distrust of independent dispensaries. This resistance casts doubt on the Ohio Birth Control League's earlier claim that Cleveland hospitals offered such services in 1917. City health officials apparently would not provide contraception in a public facility because they feared legal reprisal and opposition from Cleveland's substantial Roman Catholic community.[57] The Catholic diocese ran one of the city's major hospitals in the 1920s, St. Vincent's, in addition to other smaller, community-centered facilities such as St. John, St. Alexis, and St. Ann's.[58] Fears of Roman Catholic opposition to providing contraception in a hospital or public clinic had a factual basis, proven elsewhere later, in the 1930s and 1940s. Catholic leaders in Cincinnati, Albany, and St. Louis did pressure officials to close birth control clinics or at least remove them from public institutions.[59] While the MHA escaped such prosecution in Cleveland, founders still fought social, legal, moral, and religious stigmas.

In a speech during the 1930s to supporters of a newly organized birth control clinic in Rochester, New York, Dorothy Brush described and advocated a method that she and other founders used to counter resistance and garner medical support for birth control, calling it "an organized campaign of nagging." She explained:

> You don't have to raise money to nag—you don't have to learn how either. And I promise you it is very effective. We did it in Cleveland and now we have one of the finest and most active clinics in the country. What's more we have an advisory board of doctors whose names glitter like diamonds. We did it all by nagging. If we went to have a treatment for a cold, we said, 'And what are you doing for B.C.?' And if we went to have a baby! Well, our obstetricians were our best converts. They were only too thankful to tell us how not to have babies to get rid of us. It was the only way they could.[60]

Although Brush probably exaggerated her nagging efforts for the sake of oral argument, the fact remains that she and other women activists and organizers utilized a variety of means to achieve their goal. Women had already tested the age-old tactic of nagging and proven it effective in other realms. For example, in 1832 orator Maria Stewart had advised women,

"Sue for your rights and privileges. Know the reason you cannot attain them. Weary men with your importunities."[61] Maternal Health Association founders conformed to legal directives and to gender role expectations in some areas. They turned to traditional feminine resources to achieve their the nontraditional end: reproductive control.

## ACCIDENTS OF HISTORY

The time was right to offer birth control services to women in Cleveland and elsewhere. Economic and cultural factors primed Americans to seek and welcome such services. Rapid and extensive industrialization, the changing face of America's population, and economic slumps represented "accidents of history" that provided an opportunity for a new interpretation of contraception.[62] During the first decades of the twentieth century, as Cleveland developed into a modern industrialized city, its problems increased along with its size and financial base. While the developing suburbs attracted some former downtown residents, many people from a variety of ethnic backgrounds lived close to center city, often in overcrowded or unsanitary conditions.[63] In a 1919 parade in Cleveland, Associated Charities promoted its work as conserving family life through "home savers" such as "spiritual development, education, work-play, and health." The organization employed the image of a mother with a toddler and a babe in arms being assisted by an angelic figure (see figure 9). Poor families in Cleveland needed an angel—between 1922 and 1933, the city offered no public relief services. When Associated Charities compiled the problems of the 7,245 Cleveland families whom it aided in 1927, unemployment topped the list. Rural county residents did not fare any better. Since the area already suffered from economic woes, the Great Depression hit fast and hard. By April 1930 Cleveland's unemployed totaled an estimated forty-one thousand; the number increased dramatically to a hundred thousand by the next January. Ten times the number of Clevelanders applied to Associated Charities for assistance in 1932 as had only two years earlier. In 1935 some sort of relief supported one Cleveland family out of three. The city's citizens together lost an estimated $1.2 billion in wages and salaries between 1928 and 1937.[64] Such a drastic shift in living conditions for many Clevelanders contributed both to the support for and the success of the Maternal Health Association during its first decade. Changing cultural expectations in the areas of motherhood, marriage, and the family also set the stage for a new look at birth control.

Newspapers and magazines as well as published manuals proclaimed the value of paying close attention to the mechanics of motherhood.

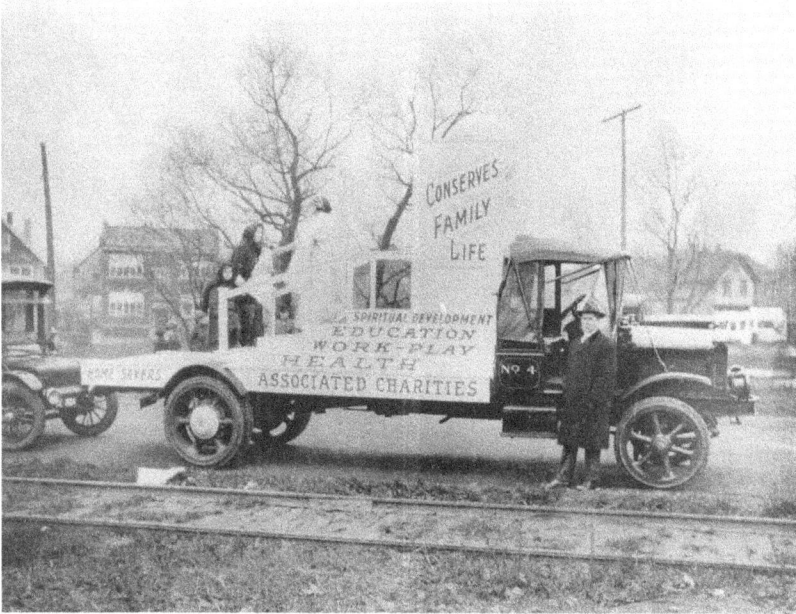

FIGURE 9. Associated Charities float in the 1919 Community Fund parade in Cleveland. *Cleveland Press* Collection, Cleveland State University.

Articles stressed the importance of systematizing child care, replacing popular wisdom or motherly intuition with science. Visiting nurses and other professionals demonstrated "modern" child care techniques, such as feeding babies from a bottle rather than breastfeeding (see figure 10).[65] More than four hundred communities across the United States celebrated Better Baby Week in March 1916, reacting in part to the country's high infant morality rates. In Cleveland the Federation of Women's Clubs sponsored the educational effort. The *Cleveland Plain Dealer* Sunday magazine ran a long article the month before the event titled "How to Make Your Baby a Better Baby." While advising mothers on the optimum baby wardrobe and other matters, the writer insisted, "Mothers must also be made to realize the deadliness of dirt." Seeing dirt as the enemy, this author equated motherhood with patriotism: "Mothers begin to realize their duty to Country as Well as to Child," a headline read.[66] Articles like this in local papers and in national magazines such as the *Woman's Home Companion,* which maintained a Better Babies Bureau, spread the word. Outside of American city limits, agricultural publications and displays at county fairs extolled the value of "maternal efficiency."[67] The cultural message rang clear in cities and in rural areas: the serious business of

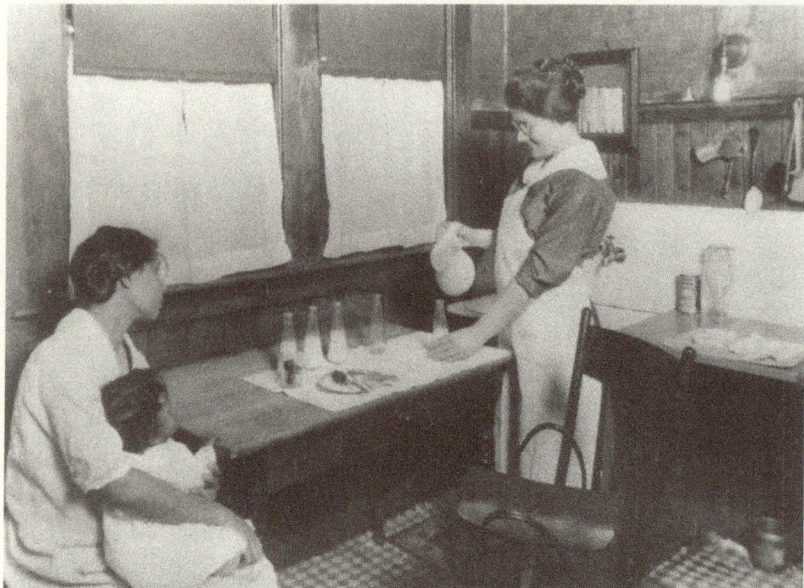

FIGURE 10.   Visiting nurse instructing Cleveland mother how to prepare formula, ca. 1915.
*Cleveland Press* Collection, Cleveland State University.

scientific, modern motherhood required careful attention and contributed to the well-being of the nation. Bearing and raising children remained at the heart of womanhood and was the central function of marriage. Yet popular expectations and descriptions of marriage also underwent changes in the early twentieth century.[68]

By the 1920s, the ideal of a "companionate marriage" involved building a strong financial base and nurturing an intimate relationship before assuming the tasks of bearing and raising children. In her 1926 book *Happiness in Marriage,* Margaret Sanger advised couples to maintain an equitable yet romantic relationship and delay childbearing until they had secured a comfortable economic state. Sanger frankly discussed the value and mechanics of satisfactory "sex communion" for both wife and husband. Though this particular book did not sell well, others of its type, such as *The Ideal Marriage* by Th. H. Van de Velde (also published in 1926), became best-sellers. The books escaped censorship, indicating in part a new popular acceptance of the need to plan one's family, the perceived benefits of guidance in the bedroom, and the value of sexual intimacy to the marital relationship.[69]

These idealistic concepts of marriage and motherhood in addition to personal and economic circumstances fueled women's desire to learn about and take advantage of safe, reliable ways to postpone or space their pregnancies. Correspondence to the U.S. Children's Bureau and to Margaret Sanger in the first two decades of the twentieth century and later letters to the Maternal Health Association of Cleveland and other clinics reveal a keen interest in and great need for this information. American couples pursued the dream of better babies and fitter families, but many struggled in the face of economic pressures and health concerns. Women and men matter-of-factly requested advice about how to delay parenthood. One MHA client explained:

> Even though we've suffered misfortunes in other ways, we have been able to set aside a reasonable sum each week and when the time comes to have our family we have overcome fear of financial difficulty and a much greater fear of responsibility. . . .
>
> . . . and though we both work hard, we have a future which we will not only be ready for but happy to share.

One woman, grateful for the help she had received at the MHA, described a quite different state of affairs among her friends.

East of Cleveland, Ohio

July 1937

My Dear Miss Alger
. . . Nine of the girls of our group were married around the same time as we were. Four of them are already mothers—and 2 more expect babies within a few months. Not more than 3 could really afford to have them so you see we both thank you very much for your instructions and as a nurse I certainly wish more young brides knew about the Maternal Health Association.

Yours truly,

Like the four mothers and two mothers-to-be mentioned in this particular letter, many other Cleveland women had not succeeded in spacing their children or delaying parenthood. Whether out of a lack of knowledge or effective birth control, or both, these couples often had several children within a few years of their wedding days. They described desperate situations in their correspondence. Mothers spoke of deteriorating well-being due to the exigencies of frequent childbearing and caring for many children. Many wished to protect their families from the ill health they saw around them, in homes such as this one: "All last fall and winter and part of the spring we have been under quarantine, then my sister's little girl got the whooping cough and the measles and she was under quarantine. . . . Can you advise me?" Another family experienced similar health problems, compounded by housing troubles:

> Our two oldest children and myself were very ill at the same time and then we were obliged to move. We weren't successful at finding a place with no objections to children. My mother is allowing us to stay with her until we do find a house.
> Now my little baby has just been very ill and for the past two weeks my time has been devoted to him.

In numerous families, too many children stretched already lean budgets to the breaking point. For people who could barely make ends meet, going to a physician for prenatal or infant care or childbirth—or birth control, if they could find someone who was sympathetic and knowledgeable— was out of the question. Situations like these existed in both cities and rural areas around the country. In 1918 an Idaho woman wrote to the U.S. Children's Bureau:

> We have 4 small children and my Husband is only making 1.35 a day, and every thing is so high it takes all he makes to keep our babys in cloth[e]s and food, as we have ev[e]ry thing we put in our mouths to buy. I am looking for the stork about the 19 of april, and all I can do is to get a few outing [flannel] slips and a few Di[a]pers. So hear is what I would like for yous to answer if you can: how am I going to get 35 dollar to have a doctor, for he will not come for less.[70]

This letter graphically depicts the economic discrepancies between the income of many American families and the cost of a medical visit or even a contraceptive from the drugstore. One mother of eight remembered the hard choices that she made in raising seven of her children to adulthood between 1929 and 1970 in rural Ohio: "When we had an extra fifty cents, we put it towards clothes or food rather than buying one of those things [a condom]."[71] Having internalized cultural messages about ideal marriages and healthy children, parents, including mothers like this one, agonized over their inability to provide even the most fundamental care for their many progeny. Some sought help by corresponding with virtual strangers such as Margaret Sanger and anonymous private or government agencies. On the eve of and throughout the Great Depression, couples searched for an effective form of relief from uncontrolled childbearing, relief that, most importantly, would allow them to care for their children properly.

Cleveland, Ohio
Sept. 1, 1938

Dear Miss Alger

. . . to be frank with you, we have had so much trouble in moving and the cost was great that every cent we have we have to save for food. For the reason that where whe are living now we are paing much more rent than before, and could not find anything chiper in account of the children that no one wish to have them in there houses, and this really makes life a strugel.

The method you have given me works very successful, and I feel that I'm very much in debt with you for what you have done for us. My husband feels much better in healt since he do not have to use the method we were using before. I'm realy in need of suply, but soon has I can save a few cents I will call to see you.

Again I'm thanking [you] very much.

Sincerely yours,

Birth control clinics like the MHA succeeded in part because of the public's eager willingness to accept the services that the clinics provided. The timing was right.[72]

Local and national personalities, ideologies, issues, and critical timing influenced the preparations for a birth control clinic in Cleveland. Two young, upper-class women, new mothers themselves, empathized with the plight of less-privileged women who desperately sought effective contraception and who were exhausted from bearing child after child. Convinced that existing medical institutions denied these mothers vital information, the Clevelanders determined to use their power and privilege for change.

MHA founders employed extreme caution in order to remove their effort as much as possible from previous activism and from moral and social stigmas. They sought assistance among older family members and social contacts and built a firm foundation on the city's reform base. During the long planning process, they informed themselves and their new supporters about the birth control cause, attended conferences, and imported speakers from the national movement. Using tactics well known to women and to female voluntarism, founders discreetly but tenaciously laid a solid footing across generational and gender lines. Rather than agitating for change in marches or other public acts, they quietly worked within existing constraints and stretched them to fit a new service. With single-minded, private proselytizing among members of the city's medical, legal, and social service establishments, Dorothy Brush, Hortense Shepard, Katherine Fisher, and their supporters set the stage for opening the Cleveland Maternal Health Association.

# 3

## Heir Conditioning

Among the first fifty birth control clinics in North America, the Cleveland Maternal Health Association acted on the cutting edge of the movement. The MHA did not formally affiliate with national birth control groups in its first decade, yet it emulated them in purpose, structure, and philosophy. Organizers assiduously avoided controversy, choosing caution over innovation. A bereaved inventor, eugenic ideals, private philanthropy, and family, professional, and social networks—the interlocking relationships among these disparate elements maintained and legitimized the venture. Women created the Maternal Health Association as a woman's voluntary association. Boards of laypeople (women and men) and physicians (men) governed the organization, female professionals staffed it, and female volunteers managed it. Local foundation money, private donations, and fees supported the endeavor.

### PROTECTING MATERNAL HEALTH

Expense topped the list of considerations in creating a freestanding birth control clinic. Maternal Health Association founders acted prudently in finance as in other matters, looking toward the clinic's long-term survival. In early discussions, before the committee had abandoned the idea of utilizing existing hospital facilities, Charles Brush Jr. had offered start-up money. Planning committee members estimated that five thousand dollars would be needed for the first year of service. After Brush died suddenly in 1927, his widow, Dorothy, promised half of the funds necessary to open the clinic, in her husband's memory, if the committee could raise the other half. With this financial impetus and based on the careful preparation of the last seven years, the time seemed right to begin an independent birth control clinic in Cleveland, Ohio.[1]

The Maternal Health Association formally chose its name in February 1928, specifically avoiding the potentially inflammatory term "birth control." Most other North American clinics that organized during the 1920s and 1930s used similar titles, such as the Maternal Health Center in Santa Fe, New Mexico, and the Maternal Health Clinic of Denver, Colorado. A few bravely chose more directly descriptive names, including the Birth Control Society of Hamilton (Ontario, Canada) and the Arkansas Eugenics Association in Little Rock. The Minnesota Birth Control League of Minneapolis began in 1930 with the more innocent title Motherhood Protection League but boldly changed its name the next year. The Baltimore Birth Control Clinic admitted, "It might be more politic under certain conditions to use other names and thereby get approval for the undertaking." Thirty-seven out of fifty-seven birth control centers responding to a national questionnaire referred to mothers or maternal health in their names.[2] The Cleveland MHA maintained an emphasis on motherhood, keeping the appellation Maternal Health Association for years, even after affiliating with the national Planned Parenthood Federation of America in 1942.[3]

In focusing on the health of mothers, birth control clinics built on Judge Frederick Crane's 1918 legal decision. Referring to New York state codes that permitted a physician to prescribe contraception to prevent the spread of disease (meaning specifically venereal disease), Crane stated that the law was broad enough "to protect the physician who in good faith gives such help or advice to a married person to cure or prevent disease"— making it clear that in future cases, "disease" could be interpreted in any way that fit within the *Webster's International Dictionary* definition.[4] In states like Ohio, which exempted doctors from obscenity provisions, the decision paved the way for clinics to provide contraception to prevent or assuage a variety of medical conditions, as long as the facilities served only married persons (Crane's specification, not the Ohio law's) and worked under the direction of physicians. Emphasizing the health of mothers in their nomenclature kept birth control providers, often organized in the voluntary sector, within this medical and cultural parameter. In 1923 gynecologist, medical researcher, and child spacing advocate Robert L. Dickinson offered a precedent for clinics like the MHA by calling his professional research organization the Committee on Maternal Health.[5] The Cleveland MHA and other clinics associated themselves with mothers and their health rather than contraception per se to earn and keep the respect of the medical and social service communities and the general public, and to stay within the law.

## Birth Control in Cleveland and the United States:
## Local and National Developments before 1942

| | |
|---|---|
| 1834 | Ohio law bans abortion |
| 1862 | Ohio law bans obscenity, includes contraception and abortion |
| 1873 | Federal Comstock Law bans obscenity, contraception, abortion |
| 1876 | Ohio expands obscenity law but exempts doctors, druggists |
| 1914 | First use of the term "birth control" nationally |
| 1915 | Mary Ware Dennett founds National Birth Control League (NBCL) |
| 1916 | Margaret Sanger speaks in Cleveland |
| 1916 | Ohio Birth Control League organized, Cleveland |
| 1916 | M. Sanger opens birth control clinic in New York City |
| 1916 | M. Sanger and two others arrested and jailed, New York City, for birth control work |
| 1916–17 | Activist Ben Reitman arrested and jailed, Cleveland, for distributing pamphlets on birth control |
| 1918 | Crane decision, physician may dispense birth control to prevent disease |
| 1919 | M. W. Dennett founds Voluntary Parenthood League (VPL) |
| 1921 | First American Birth Control Conference, New York City |
| 1921 | M. Sanger founds American Birth Control League (ABCL) |
| 1922 | Interpretation of Ohio Obscenity law, Cleveland |
| 1923 | MHA founding meeting at the Women's City Club, Cleveland |
| 1923 | M. Sanger founds Birth Control Clinical Research Bureau (BCCRB), New York City |
| 1923 | Robert L. Dickinson founds Committee on Maternal Health (CMH), New York City |
| 1928 | Maternal Health Association of Cleveland opens |
| 1928 | Brush Foundation created for race betterment, Cleveland |
| 1929 | Police raid Sanger's Clinical Research Bureau |
| 1929 | Margaret Sanger speaks, City Club of Cleveland |
| 1930 | *Youngs Rubber Corp. v. C.I. Lee & Co.*, U.S. circuit court of appeals, sets parameters for business in condoms |
| 1930 | Papal encyclical condemns birth control for Roman Catholics |
| 1936 | *U.S. v. One Package*, U.S. circuit court of appeals, allows importation of contraceptives by physicians |
| 1937 | American Medical Association condones birth control |
| 1939 | BCCRB and ABCL merge into Birth Control Federation of American (BCFA) |
| 1942 | Planned Parenthood Federation of America (PPFA) created |
| 1942 | Cleveland MHA joins PPFA |

FIGURE 11. Birth control in Cleveland and the United States:
local and national developments before 1942[6]

The first MHA annual report declared this philosophy in the clinic's goal statement: "The purpose of the Maternal Health Association is to aid and support physicians in medical service and advice to married women for the protection of the health and strength of such women and their children, especially to the end that children shall be begotten only under conditions which make possible a heritage of mental and physical health."[7] This declaration stressed the improvement of maternal health and the importance of genetic heritage to the health of children. The MHA did not propose legal change or broad social reform, as did the Ohio Birth Control League of the previous decade. The new clinic chose a less controversial path but stretched moral codes and legal ambiguities for its own purposes. Keeping its distance from the national movement played a key role in the clinic's development.

## LOCAL AUTONOMY

The Cleveland MHA organized separately from the two national birth control organizations that existed at the time (see figure 11). Founders consciously decided "to remain independent of both the National [American] Birth Control League [ABCL] and The Voluntary Parenthood League [VPL]." All but one annual report during the clinic's first decade clearly stated that the MHA was "not affiliated with any national organization." By 1940 the association had joined the National Conference of Social Work and the National Association for Public Health Nursing and had helped to create the Maternal Health Association of Ohio. However, the MHA's annual report for 1940 explicitly established the local organization's continuing separation from national groups that specifically advocated birth control: "Our Association is not affiliated with the Birth Control Federation of America [the successor of the ABCL]."[8] MHA leaders repeatedly proclaimed the clinic's autonomy.

Concern for finances and reputation likely influenced this decision. The ABCL required member clinics to contribute one-fourth of their membership fees to national coffers. Dependent on private donations for its existence, like most pioneer birth control facilities, the MHA did not stand on solid ground financially during its first decade. For example, between 1931 and 1932 the clinic spent half of its income of $20,518 on salaries and almost one-fourth for rent, maintenance, and equipment. At the end of that fiscal year, the balance on hand totaled just over $1300.[9] Without institutional backing, money was tight. The MHA had no extra dollars to send to a national organization. The clinic's need for private funds provided a strong motive to avoid controversy.

Local leaders also wished to further remove the Cleveland MHA from the notoriety and activities of national birth control groups. Sanger's socialist and confrontational reputation and Voluntary Parenthood League activist Mary Ware Dennett's legislative agenda posed threats to the fledgling group in Cleveland. One outside observer concluded in 1938 that the MHA did not affiliate with national groups in its formative years "since considerable time and effort is spent by the National Organizations in propaganda and legislative reform. These goals do not coincide with the aims and the purposes of the Cleveland Organization which from its beginning has aligned itself with preventive health and family welfare." Indeed, the ABCL executive secretary noted in 1923 that Cleveland MHA founders "opposed the Federal work being anything but secondary in the B.C. program" and instead placed top priority on local efforts. Maternal Health Association executive secretary Gladys Gaylord explained the distinction between the MHA and national groups in 1940: "Fundamental differences of procedure and of ideals have kept us apart. We have believed in building our organization slowly and quietly. . . . We have neither dramatized or advertised our services." Gaylord denied that finances played a role in the separation but cited a lack of "strong leadership" in national programs as well as unacceptable "publicity and advertising methods." An early annual report describes the MHA as "a conservative and scientific demonstration under the direction of a carefully selected board and with specially trained women physicians."[10] To preserve its respectability and not endanger its local reputation, the Cleveland facility rejected any national activist role.[11]

With such a local emphasis, the MHA stayed out of the organizational confusion that characterized the national birth control movement during the late 1920s and through the 1930s. The ABCL claimed that Sanger's tactics and militant legacy impeded fund-raising. In 1928 Sanger herself broke with the ABCL to form the Clinical Research Bureau (later the Birth Control Clinical Research Bureau [BCCRB]). The splintered national organizations worked independently, alongside Dickinson's Committee on Maternal Health. In 1937 the ABCL and BCCRB united as the Birth Control Federation of America. A 1930 study of birth control clinics suggested that Sanger redirected BCCRB publicity efforts from propaganda to research in order to obtain credibility. The study claimed that to win physician support, Sanger purposely rejected "non-medical activities" such as the public activism that characterized her earlier efforts.[12] Cleveland organizers objected to the promotional efforts of national birth control organizations for similar reasons. The medical profession as a whole discounted the ABCL and its successors. The close

relationship between the Cleveland MHA and its medical board surely
affected the decision not to affiliate.

Fearful of local reprisals, MHA staff expressed concern in 1938 that
"the extent and type of their [BCFA's] publicity continue to cause opposition from religious and racial groups." One MHA history stated a similar rationale for not seeking the formal support of the local medical society: "No attempt was made to gain clinic sponsorship by the Academy of
Medicine [of Cleveland] . . . [because] the cooperation of Protestants and
Roman Catholics was greatly needed at that time for other Academy programs." Quite possibly MHA leaders acquiesced to the Academy of Medicine's wishes in this matter. In any case, the clinic needed to win and preserve the trust of local physicians and other groups in order to survive.
Motivated by a combination of such financial and political considerations,
the MHA sustained this official autonomy until 1942, when it affiliated
with the Planned Parenthood Federation of America, the successor to the
ABCL and the BCFA.[13]

The Cleveland MHA's actual separation from the national movement
extended only so far, however. Design and services clearly followed the
medical style of Sanger's model—a physician-directed clinic staffed by
professional nurses and advised by a board of physicians. The MHA recommended the birth control method preferred at Sanger's clinic, the
diaphragm. Ideologies and procedures in Cleveland also imitated those of
other existing facilities. The MHA utilized printed material and speakers
supplied by the ABCL and its successors. The association sought advice
from national leaders and brought these people to Cleveland for consultation. The MHA carefully gathered and proudly supplied research data
for national surveys. Clinic officers and other Cleveland MHA board
members attended national birth control conferences. They participated
on committees and contributed to strategy sessions about the larger
effort.[14] Consistent with its other utilitarian strategies, MHA's unaffiliated
status allowed clinic leaders to take advantage of the ABCL's resources if
they chose to do so without compromising the local clinic's reputation or
autonomy. The Cleveland group even turned to the national organization
for advice on where to place the new clinic.

## AVOIDING PUBLIC AGITATION

The MHA planning committee invited ABCL's Anne Kennedy to Cleveland a second time to assist in fund-raising and in selecting a location. The
committee chose to place the MHA downtown in the Osborn building, a
center for other medical offices (see figure 12). Prominent gynecologist

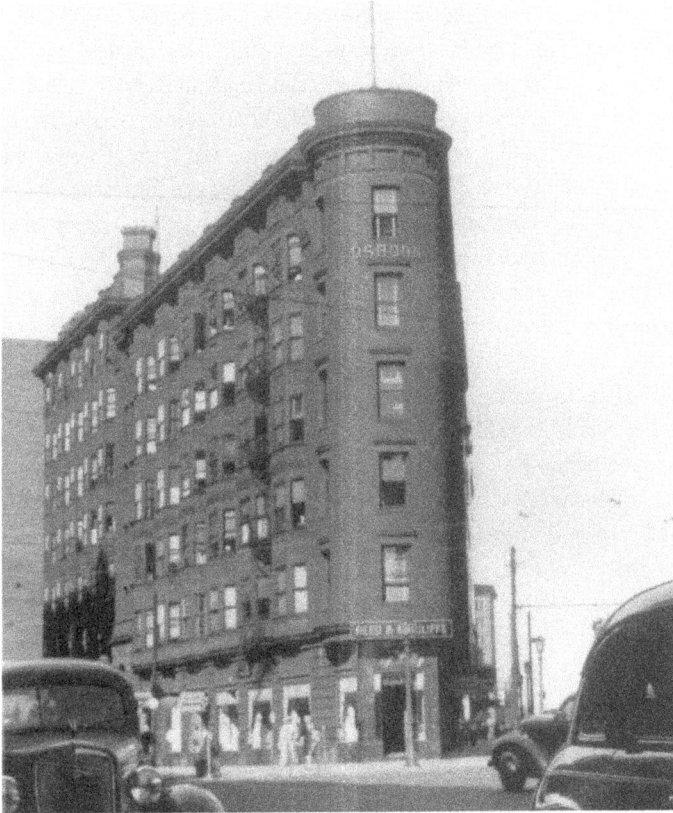

FIGURE 12. Osborn building, Huron and Prospect Streets in Cleveland, 1930s–1940s, where the MHA offices were located from 1928 to 1939. Cleveland Public Library.

William Weir, who served on the clinic's founding committee and its Medical Advisory Board, maintained his own practice there.[15] Situating the MHA amid legitimate medical professionals approximated the original plan to locate the venture within the sphere of medical practice rather than social service or public health. Since hospitals and public dispensaries had refused to incorporate MHA services, few options remained.

Some American birth control clinics began in medical facilities such as hospitals or doctor's offices, but others organized in less likely locales. A clinic in Denver, Colorado (later part of Planned Parenthood of the Rocky Mountains), opened in a church basement; one in Sioux City, Iowa, first operated from City Hall. The Birth Control Committee of Kalamazoo, Michigan, worked out of the Civic League for its first thirteen years, and the Tucson Birth Control Clinic met in a small house.[16] In the first decades of the clinical birth control movement in North America, variety prevailed in terms of office space. The Cleveland Maternal Health Association established itself, and later its branch clinics, in separate, institutional spaces rather than in churches, the headquarters of other reform organizations, or private homes.[17] The site both reflected and determined the path that the MHA would take, setting its work directly in the milieu of medical professionals. While the choice conveyed a message of permanence and added an aura of respectability, the association maintained through the 1930s that the arrangement was temporary. The freestanding MHA clinic was a demonstration meant to sway public opinion and medical authorities in favor of placing contraceptive services in a hospital dispensary.[18]

Until that time, the physical environment of the Osborn building helped the MHA establish legitimacy as a health agency. Working out of a private medical office allowed the clinic more freedom and independence than might have been available in a hospital or dispensary. The building offered a convenient location near streetcar stops, nine blocks east and one block south of Public Square, the city center. (Public Square became a transportation hub for commuter and passenger trains with the completion of the Cleveland Union Terminal in 1929.) In the days before self-service elevators, Osborn's elevator operators worked at night, which aided the MHA in holding evening clinic hours. Local historians later noted an "inconspicuous" side entrance as an appealing feature. The building sits on a triangle between two streets—and one street away from the busiest portions of Euclid Avenue, where shoppers would have congregated. Maternal Health Association leaders wanted to help clients preserve their anonymity or, at the very least, modesty, as well as maintain a low profile as an institution.[19] With all of these positive attributes, however, the clinic's choice of a site presented one major drawback. Placing the clinic downtown, in a commercial district rather than in a residential neighborhood, distanced it from the city's poorest residents, those who lacked a means of transportation or the time to make the trip. While no evidence exists as to arguments against placing the clinic in the Osborn building, the decision limited access to the MHA in favor of promoting legitimacy.

In matters of public relations, MHA founders took no chances. They employed quiet persuasion, used their civic influence, and manipulated private social contacts to safeguard the clinic. To prevent unfriendly articles in the press and "avoid public agitation," two MHA executive committee members visited each of the editors of Cleveland's three largest newspapers, the *Plain Dealer*, the *Press*, and the *News*. They explained the services and policies planned for the MHA and requested *no publicity* for the clinic's debut. According to histories written later, all three editors initially agreed to "hold up any news stories but explained that some 'unto-ward incident' might conceivably make news that they could not keep from the papers." To ward off any such incident, attorney Jerry Fisher himself explained to local law enforcement officials "the clinic's intention to operate within the law."[20]

By beginning quietly, the MHA assumed and furthered a pattern established elsewhere. In New York City a few years earlier, different advisers had cautioned both Robert L. Dickinson and Margaret Sanger to proceed with discretion in establishing birth control clinics in order to avoid antagonism. Dickinson proceeded so cautiously in 1923 that he only attracted nine patients in the first three months! Likewise, the Buffalo, New York, Maternal Health Clinic waited six long weeks after opening for its first clients to appear. The low profile was designed to avoid attacks from a potentially hostile medical profession, the Roman Catholic Church, or other sources of opposition.[21]

The pall on publicity in Cleveland was short-lived, however. On May 28, 1928, barely two months after the clinic opened, the *Cleveland Press* featured a brief article on the MHA titled "Clinic Aids in Solving Child Birth Problems." Apparently written without the organization's approval, the article still conservatively stressed the medical and legal propriety of clinic services. It never actually mentioned birth control; the rest of its headline read "Solving Child Birth Problems . . . Under Physicians Super-vision, to Mothers and Children." This vague wording could have de-scribed a prenatal or infant care facility. The negative repercussions that founders had feared from publicity did not ensue. Maternal Health Asso-ciation trustee Brooks Shepard expressed his relief in a letter to Dorothy Brush a few days later: "It's too bad that the *Press* felt it had to write up the Clinic. I felt, though, that if they had to . . . they could scarcely have done it with more restraint. There seems to have been no serious attack as a result of it, thus far, and a few more months will make our position enor-mously stronger to resist."[22]

During the clinic's first decade, publicity in local newspapers followed this pattern. Articles about fund-raising activities appeared on the society pages. The *Bystander*, a monthly that chronicled Cleveland's social scene, featured lively descriptions of MHA social events and pictured the promi-nent women involved as officers or volunteers. The stories named the MHA but never directly revealed the group's purpose—nor did they men-tion birth control. A 1936 *Cleveland Press* editorial, for example, cited the problem of caring for the many babies "being born into this troubled world" and commended the Cleveland Maternal Health Association for making a necessary "contribution to general human improvement." The writer says that "enlightened parents" should consider "the phenomenon of child-birth" as "a serious business" to alleviate physical, economic, and social problems in the family. Finally, the editorial describes the increase in MHA clinic attendance as "encouraging." However, the article concludes without any reference to the birth control services that the clinic offered.[23] Apparently, the MHA encouraged such obfuscation.

With such a wary attitude, MHA organizers and trustees must have feared public reaction to Margaret Sanger's speech about the national birth control movement at the all-male City Club of Cleveland in 1929. Despite her moderation over the past decade, Sanger represented the type of agitation and attention—propaganda—that MHA founders and trustees scrupulously shunned. This trip to Cleveland took place only a few months after police had raided Sanger's Birth Control Clinical Research Bureau, arrested clinic staff, and seized medical records. Reports of that raid had appeared in national newspapers. The *Cleveland Plain Dealer* covered Sanger's local City Club lecture on the front page of Sunday's edition, December 17, 1929.[24]

The paper reported that John J. Thomas, M.D., Cleveland City Club president—who also chaired the MHA Medical Advisory Board—had to restore order following Sanger's speech. Supporters loudly proposed a motion to endorse her efforts to legalize birth control distribution, but Thomas refused to recognize that motion. In his role as president, Thomas upheld the City Club's characteristically neutral position. The club staunchly stood by the principle of free speech and avoided advocating particular issues.[25] In spite of many close ties between the MHA and the City Club, the club avoided taking a stand. This group of liberal citizens supported a quietly run, autonomous local birth control clinic but would not publicly endorse the national movement. Making distinctions such as these in the area of reproductive policy reflected the larger cultural distinctions between local action and national policy, between private practice and public advocacy. Such vacillation only added to the general confusion around reproductive issues.

In part because of its deliberate distance from the national birth control effort, the MHA developed singular attributes, including a relationship with the Brush Foundation. The close connection with a local, private philanthropic entity represents a key link in the MHA support system. The MHA's predilection for independence from other groups adds special import to this particular alliance. While determined to remain separate from the national ABCL, the Cleveland Maternal Health Association nourished this particular local connection. Clinic leaders used the Brush Foundation and the foundation's patron, Western Reserve University, to achieve credibility. In turn, the Brush Foundation tie shaped MHA philosophy, and later, its services.

## INTIMATE CONNECTIONS

In 1928 Cleveland inventor and wealthy philanthropist Charles Francis Brush Sr. created the Brush Foundation "to improve the human stock" as a memorial to his only son and namesake, who had died suddenly the year before. In the late nineteenth century Brush Sr. lit Cleveland and cities around the world with his improved electric arc light. He began his foun-

---

### The Brush Foundation:
### an excerpt from the Deed of Gift of Charles Francis Brush

Whereas, my beloved son Charles Francis Brush Jr. who died on May twenty-ninth, 1927, was devoting his life to scientific research for the advancement of human knowledge; and

Whereas, in my opinion the most urgent problem confronting the world today is the rapid increase of population which threatens to overcrowd the earth in the not distant future, with resultant shortage of food and lower standards of living, which must certainly lead to grave economic disturbances, famines and wars and threaten civilization itself; and

Whereas, beneficent scientific research has contributed toward the prolongation of life and the preservation of the weak and the unfit who under former conditions could not have survived nor added descendants to the race; and

Whereas, I believe that scientific knowledge cannot safely be used for these humane objects, unless it be used at the same time to improve the quality and reasonably limit the numbers of those who are born into the world;

Now, therefore, out of my belief that such restriction of the increase of population and the betterment of the human stock are fundamental to the well-being of humanity, I have established a foundation for the benefit of mankind and as a Memorial to my beloved son Charles Frances Brush, Jr.

The income of this trust shall be used by the Board of Managers to finance efforts contributing to the betterment of the human stock and toward the regulation of the increase of population, to the end that children shall be begotten only under conditions which make possible a heritage of mental and physical health, and a favorable environment. These purposes include the furtherance of scientific research in the field of eugenics and in regulation of the increase of population; the education of the people to the importance of the betterment of the stock and to the economic and social evils which result from too great increase of population; and any activities which shall serve the intent set forth in this instrument and its preamble.

Charles F. Brush[26]

---

FIGURE 13. The Brush Foundation: an excerpt from the Deed of Gift of Charles Francis Brush.

dation with five hundred thousand dollars and directed that the income be used to check "the increase in population" as well as to improve population quality. The benefactor acted independently of his daughter-in-law's birth control clinic activities. Although Dorothy Brush, his son's widow, had helped found the Cleveland Maternal Health Association in the same year, the two organizations were legally separate entities. Personal correspondence indicates that Charles Sr. surprised Dorothy with this particular memorial. With characteristic effusiveness, she described the foundation as "epoch-making," "the most thrilling thing that has ever happened."[27]

Unlike the MHA's quiet beginnings, Brush announced his new fund with great fanfare. He enthusiastically informed Dorothy Brush a few weeks later that he had "about two bushels of newspaper clippings . . . and several barrels of letters" about the foundation. Local and national newspapers hailed the Brush Foundation as the "Eugenic Dawn," a "munificent gift to human welfare," "a foundation so sensible that we marvel no one thought of it sooner."[28]

From the pulpit of the Pilgrim Congregational Church in Cleveland, the Rev. Dr. Dan Bradley commended Brush and "scored those who protest against Brush's actions." Some did protest, including Roman Catholic bishop Joseph Schrembs of the Diocese of Cleveland. The bishop objected to the use of the phrase "human stock," complaining that "we are being classed with the animals on the farm."[29] In general, though, Clevelanders applauded this addition to the city's growing philanthropic community. A letter from *Cleveland Press* advice columnist Mrs. Maxwell indicates high regard for the MHA and the new foundation, and underscores their close connection in the public eye.

Dear Friend:

The Maternal Health Clinic, Osborne [*sic*] Building, Room 311, will help you in your dilemma. This is maintained by the Charles Brush Foundation, and a group of out-standing citizens of the city. It is sponsored by the best of our people so you need have no reticence or qualms about going there. You do have to go in person, where able people tell you these things you've despaired of ever knowing. I apologise for taking so long in answering you. I needed to obtain the exact location. Their telephone number is Cherry 2252.

Yours truly,
[Mrs. Maxwell][30]

The bond between the clinic and the foundation ran deeper than appearances or reputation. The Brush Foundation funded and staffed a portion of the MHA's activities. Its six founding trustees also served on the first MHA Board of Trustees (see figures 14 and 15).[31] Although the two organizations remained legally separate, their statements of purpose reveal a close tie. One identical phrase appears in both declarations: "to the end that children shall be begotten only under conditions which make possible a heritage of mental and physical health." The purposes of both the Brush Foundation and the MHA stressed the eugenic benefits of birth control to future children and, by extension, to families, rather than to women in particular.[32] While the MHA provided one-on-one service to mothers, the organization also embodied and promoted popular eugenic principles.

Placing its philanthropic mission squarely within this trend of social thought, the Brush Foundation emphasized scientific research within the context of the well-born child, a key concept of eugenics. The foundation sought to put population betterment "upon a scientific basis, which, by the very forcefulness of demonstrated fact, shall appeal to all who have the Nation's progress at heart." It aimed to "improve the quality and reasonably limit the numbers of those who are born."[33]

The link with the Brush Foundation focused MHA philosophy on the scientific determination of fitness and the greater good of population quality. The MHA acted as a demonstration center for the Brush Foundation not only in the particular area of contraception for individuals but also for the larger goal of improving the population. Clinic founders had articulated this philosophy in their statement of purpose. T. Wingate Todd, a doctor who presided over the Brush Foundation board, introduced the MHA's 1929 annual report by stressing eugenic goals: "Conservation of the birth-rate, preventive medicine, and enlightened motherhood are the three successive stages of organized Community endeavor for the promotion of National Physique and Intelligence." The Brush Foundation's emphasis on race betterment clearly influenced MHA rhetoric. The association's intimate relationship with the Brush Foundation intensified its dependence on popular eugenic philosophy. The connection added the "promotion of National Physique and Intelligence" to the clinic's focus on improving the health of women and children.[34] Along with some other eugenicists and birth control advocates of the time, clinic and foundation leaders did not see a conflict between these ideals.

Discord and confusion characterized the complex relationship between the larger movements for eugenics and for birth control in the early twentieth century. In order to legitimize the cause, Margaret Sanger and other birth control advocates chose what they needed from the philosophy of eugenicists. Historian Carole McCann points out that the scientific terminology of eugenics (substituting "pregnancy wastage" for miscarriage or abortion, or "exposure to the risk of pregnancy" for intercourse, for example) removed family limitation from explicit sexual language and especially aided in promoting contraception as reputable. Eugenics as science refuted claims that controlling reproduction was unnatural and offered solid reasons for collecting data about sexual functions. Sanger also tempered eugenic premises with the feminism of voluntary motherhood as well as economic arguments: women had a racial duty to bear and rear children, but only as many as her health and family finances allowed. For Sanger, for the Brush Foundation, and for the MHA, providing accessible contraception represented the first step to racial betterment. On the other hand, many leaders of the movement for eugenics such as Paul Popenoe opposed birth control as inhibiting racial progress. Popenoe and others contended that with a broader dissemination of knowledge about contraception, society's "superior" groups would produce even fewer children while the "'reckless and improvident'" would continue to ignore or misuse birth control. Such a pattern threatened racial deterioration.[35]

In the midst of these conflicting messages, some early-twentieth-century citizens saw immigration and migration, racial mixing, and the coupling of "degenerates" as threatening future financial security as well as racial purity. The child development activities and information offered by the U.S. Children's Bureau in the 1910s and 1920s led to and reflected an increasing emphasis on the quality of one's progeny and home life. Better baby and fittest family contests at state and county fairs emerged by the 1920s as a popular expression of experts' drive to reduce the high rate of infant mortality in America and enhance the population as a whole.[36] The letter below reflects both the wide-ranging effect of this ideology on the general public and the resentment that its class-based nature sometimes engendered.

> Talk about better babys, when a mother must be like some cow or mare when a babys come. If she lives, all wright, and if not, Just the same. The nearest one [doctor] . . . is 1 mile and a _ and my oldest child is 9 years old. My husband only comes home onest a week, that is on saterday. I have my own wood to cut by myself so how can there be better babys when they must come in to this world like a calf or colt I would like to know.[37]

This mother, effectively a single parent, graphically articulates her lack of access to health care and the inability even to care properly for herself, let

alone her children, a common situation in poverty-ridden urban neighborhoods as well as rural areas during the Great Depression. She was
acquainted with the philosophy of better babies but did not have the
means to implement that philosophy in her own family.

Gladys Gaylord, MHA executive secretary from 1929 to 1948,
claimed that the Cleveland MHA "persistently promoted a program for
better children." In a 1938 article for the *Journal of Contraception* entitled
"Eugenic Value of a Maternal Health Center," Gaylord detailed the allure
of scientific efficiency for the birth control movement. She described the
clinic "as a practical demonstration that family life may be built up and
enriched through a wise use of this new tool of medicine—the spacing of
pregnancies."[38] Gaylord clearly expressed the prevailing belief that applying science to a biological function would enhance the family. This interpretation of eugenics and race betterment had become embedded in talk
about preserving the family system, apparently even in a few private bedrooms, as the following letter demonstrates.

> [My] husband and I have reconsidered our budget on the basis of his last
> pay and decided the time is right for "heir conditioning." I am pregnant at
> the present time and expecting confinement in the Fall. Thank you for . . .
> the service of the Maternal Health Association. I may be calling on you at
> a considerably later date.

The Brush Foundation supported "heir conditioning" by promoting contraception as integral to a heritage of mental and physical health. Following the model of such foundations as the Rockefeller in other areas of
social welfare, the Brush Foundation included demonstration projects,
such as a new birth control clinic, in its efforts. In 1929 the foundation
funded the Maternal Health Association as one of its first two under-
takings.[39]

## FINANCIAL CONNECTIONS

The Maternal Health Association depended entirely on private donations
for its first few months. The clinic opened in March 1928 with a balance
of $3,671.03 and received almost that amount, $3,132, in contributions
the first year. Although early records are unclear, the bulk of the opening
balance must have been Dorothy Brush's gift in her husband's memory.
Presumably the year's income also included charges to the 385 women
served by the clinic. These sliding scale fees ranged from thirty-five cents
to ten dollars per visit.[40]

### Founding Board Members:
### The Maternal Health Association of Cleveland and
### The Brush Foundation

*Maternal Health Association of Cleveland Board of Trustees, 1928*

Edgar E. and Elizabeth Carlton Adams
Elizabeth Leopold (Mrs. Newton D.) Baker
Helen Chase (Mrs. Edward S.) Bassett
Lenore Schwab (Mrs. Morris A.) Black, *2nd Vice Chairman*
Rev. Dr. Ferdinand Q. Blanchard
Roberta Holden (Mrs. Benjamin) Bole
Francis Payne (Mrs. Chester C.) Bolton, *Honorary Chairman*
Dorothy Hamilton Brush, *1st Vice Chairman*
Julia Cobb (Mrs. Benedict) Crowell
Flora Morris (Mrs. S. Homer) Everett
Jerome C., *Exec. Committee,* and Katherine Bingham Fisher, *Secretary*
Walter L. and Julia McCune Flory, *Exec. Committee*
Ella White (Mrs. Horatio) Ford
Frances Southworth (Mrs. Frederick H.) Goff, *Treasurer, Exec. Committee*
Caroline Brewer (Mrs. William S.) Goff
Virginia Bonnell (Mrs. Merwin C.) Harvey
Kate Hanna Ireland (Mrs. Perry W.) Harvey
Rev. Joel B. Hayden
Helen Schwab (Mrs. Max) Hellman
Theodore P. and Barbara Goss Herrick
Bertha Beitman (Mrs. Siegmund) Herzog
Mary Sterling (Mrs. Charles) Hitchcock
Margaret Allen (Mrs. R. Livingston) Ireland
Arthur and Gertrude Fuller Judson
Raymond and Charlotte Seaver Kelsey
Lucia McCurdy (Mrs. Malcolm) McBride
Rev. Dr. Thomas S. McWilliams
Cliffe Johnson (Mrs. Walter B.) Merriam
Herman and Florence Marks Moss
Helene North (Mrs. Carl) Narten
F. May Lockwood (Mrs. John G.) Oliver, *Exec. Committee*
Roger G., *Exec. Committee,* and Edna Brush Perkins
Alexander C. and Marjorie Woods Robinson III
Charles Baldwin Sawyer
Brooks and Hortense Oliver Shepard, *Chairman*
Rabbi Abba Hillel Silver
Mary Dunning (Mrs. Charles) Thwing
Delia White (Mrs. Herman L.) Vail
Thomas, *Asst. Treasurer,* and Lucile Andrews Veach, *Exec. Committee*
Mabel Breckenridge (Mrs. Charles W.) Wason, *Exec. Committee*
John T. and Estelle Cook Webster

FIGURE 14. Founding board members: The Maternal Health Association of Cleveland and
The Brush Foundation.

---

### Founding Board Members:
### The Maternal Health Association of Cleveland and
### The Brush Foundation (cont'd.)

William H. and Roslyn Campbell Weir, *Exec. Committee*
Delia Holden (Mrs. Windsor T.) White
Virginia Wing

*MHA Medical Advisory Board, 1928*

J. J. Thomas, M.D., *Chairman*
A. S. Maschke, M.D.
J. C. Placak, M.D.
Vernon C. Rowland, M.D.
Roy Scott, M.D.

*The Brush Foundation, 1928*
*First Board of Managers*
(Appointed for Life by the Founder)

T. Wingate Todd, M.D., *President*          Edna Brush Perkins
Dorothy Hamilton Brush                       M. Roslyn Campbell Weir
Jerome C. Fisher                             William H. Weir, M.D.
Joel B. Hayden, D.D.

---

FIGURE 14. (CONT'D.) Founding board members: The Maternal Health Association of Cleveland and The Brush Foundation.

Founders, trustees, and volunteers "begged or borrowed" or donated most of the furnishings for the clinic's "three small rooms" in the Osborn building. Striving for a homey atmosphere, they painted the walls and room dividers, and made curtains. In the first year, the MHA spent $584 on equipment, including a sterilizer, examining table, and typewriter—all secondhand. Transportation, including home visits by MHA nurses, cost $75. The MHA paid out most of the $4,615.45 in expenses that year for rent ($744) and salaries ($3,232.45) to the professional medical staff. In April 1929, the clinic ended its first year with a balance of $2212.48. Service during the summer months quickly depleted that surplus.[41] That year the Brush Foundation began a long-standing practice of contributing to the clinic's financial stability.

Monetary records for the MHA and the early years of the Brush Foundation are sketchy at best. Sources suggest that the MHA never relied solely on Brush Foundation funding. According to existing reports,

# Selected Maternal Health Association Trustees

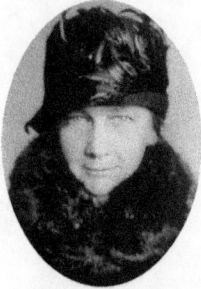

Dorothy Hamilton Brush*
Planned Parenthood of Greater
Cleveland [1950s]

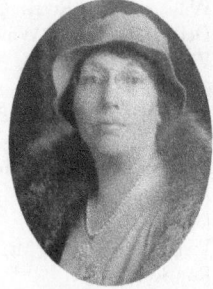

Lucia McCurdy McBride*
© Standiford Studio, 1928
Cleveland Press Collection

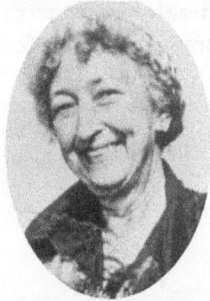

Bertha Beitman Herzog*
Ben Strauss photo, 1928
Cleveland Press Collection

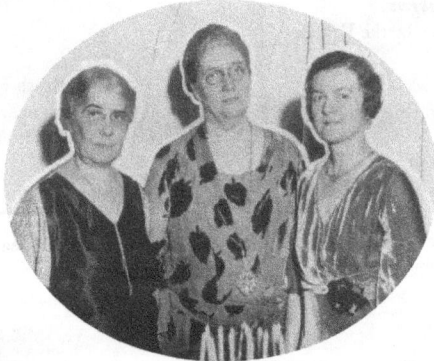

(From left) Lenore Schwab Black*,
Elizabeth Baker McGean,
Margaret Hamilton Bates
Cleveland Public Library, 1932

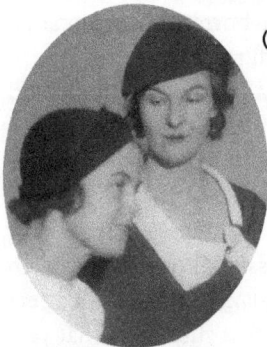

Martha Darden Zeising (left),
Elizabeth Leopold Baker*
Cleveland Press Collection, 1933

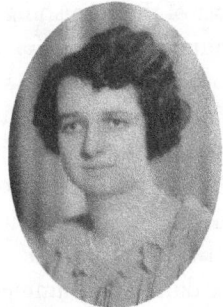

Delia White Vail*
George M. Edmondson photo, 1927
Cleveland Press Collection

FIGURE 15. Selected Maternal Health Association Trustees.

# Selected Maternal Health Association Trustees (cont'd.)

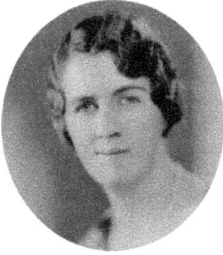

**Gertrude York White**
Trout-ware photo [1925]
*Cleveland Press* Collection

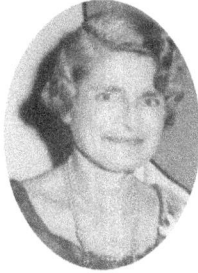

**Katherine King White**
*Cleveland Press* Collection, 1930

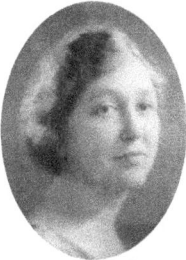

**Roberta Holden Bole***
Frank Reed photo, 1964
*Cleveland Press* Collection

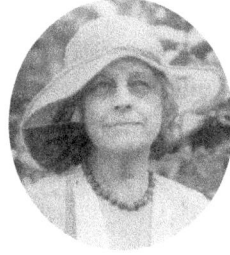

**Hazel Petty Hayden**
Bachrach photo 1927
*Cleveland Press* Collection

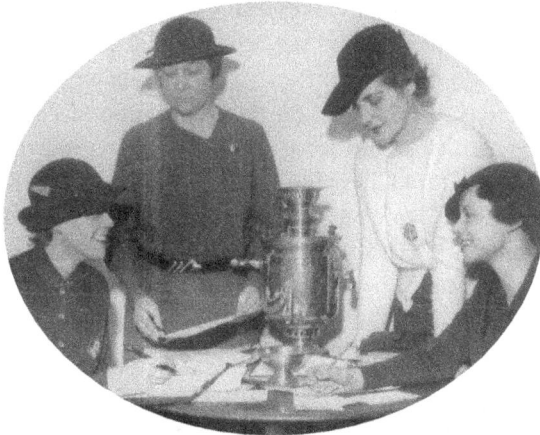

**M. Virginia
Stearns White**
Ben Strauss photo, 1929
*Cleveland Press* Collection

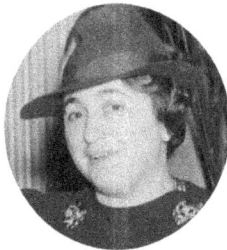

**Virginia Horkeimer Silver**
James Meli photo 1940
*Cleveland Press* Collection

**(Above, from left) Helen Chisholm Halle,
Constance Calkins Curtiss, Mary Stanton Macomber,
Eleanor Cottrell Hatch**
Cleveland *Press* Collection, 1935

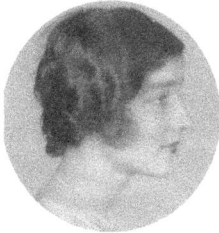

* Founding board member

FIGURE 15. (CONT'D.)  Selected Maternal Health Association Trustees.

the foundation provided almost 50 percent of the dollars spent in the clinic's first two years, a little more than 25 percent after four years, and less than 15 percent after seven years. This proportion then stabilized at under 15 percent. From 1935 to 1940, Brush Foundation dollars accounted for an average of 13 percent of MHA's budget. The foundation followed the common philanthropic pattern of offering start-up funds to a new venture and then cutting back as the project became self-sufficient.[42] The partial rather than full support also signals the separate missions of the two endeavors. While MHA rhetoric touted a broad eugenic agenda and attempted to legitimize contraception on the local level, it directed its services primarily toward women. The foundation, on the other hand, promoted the ideal and practice of scientific birth control as a solution to a social problem and did not provide direct care. For the Brush Foundation, the MHA and its clients served as a demonstration, a means of changing public opinion. Private contributions and income from fund-raising events provided the rest of the MHA's budget.[43]

Dependent on some Brush Foundation support, the MHA remained separate from another local funding source, the Cleveland Community Fund (CCF), also called the Community Chest. The CCF continued the very fruitful fund drives begun by the Cleveland War Council in 1918. The Victory Chest Drive that year raised six million dollars. In 1919 the first Community Fund appeal garnered four million dollars from 148,234 donors, dollars that the CCF then divided among participating organizations. These annual appeals significantly boosted the treasuries of member charitable and service agencies and eventually evolved into United Appeal and then United Way Services. The MHA did not participate in the coordinated effort, however. Early association reports state, "The clinic cannot be included in the Community Fund for reasons which the Association recognize[s] and respect[s]."[44] The MHA focused on winning acceptance from other health and social service agencies and remained wary of potential religious opposition. A historical account of the MHA explains that "an application [to the Community Fund] might have caused Roman Catholic opposition (as it did years later in New York) and hurt the Fund. The Association preferred to take on the responsibility of a separate annual fund-raising campaign."[45]

Caution and characteristic independence kept the MHA out of the Community Fund for many years, in spite of the fact that many clinic trustees also served that organization. A similar relationship existed in other cities between birth control clinics and community chests or equivalent groups. In both Indianapolis and Albany, the Council of Social Agencies, comparable to the Community Fund, denied membership to contraceptive clinics until the 1950s and 1960s, respectively. In April 1951, the Cleveland MHA still did not belong to the Cleveland Community Fund. The clinic's newsletter that month published what it called "an interpretation of the Board's attitude" toward the situation: "The Maternal Health Association recognizes that its program is a controversial one. Its leadership does not wish to indulge in religious or political controversy that might be a wedge in splitting the community, but hopes to win community support through its educational program and individual service."[46] As in the case of Sanger's 1929 Cleveland City Club speech, MHA board members chose not to use their influence within another local organization to gain visibility for the clinic. They carefully avoided conflict with other groups in the local social service system and did not battle for territory. The association's desire to establish its authority and stay removed from potential adversaries and controversy limited its fiduciary sources. But the same factors provided excellent reasons to court Brush Foundation aid.

The Brush Foundation influenced the birth control clinic in many critical areas. In 1937 foundation president T. Wingate Todd referred to the "intimate relationship" between the MHA and the foundation.[47] The link to the Brush Foundation validated MHA activities and added respectability. Promoting birth control as a scientific solution to social problems, the foundation provided an aura of academic correctness for the clinic, which offered a service at the edge of legality and social and scientific propriety. The close ties between the boards of the organizations and the alliance with renowned scientist Charles F. Brush Sr. marked the MHA as a legitimate social agency in the Progressive reform tradition.

## "THE BEST OF OUR PEOPLE"

Clinic founders established two governing boards for the MHA, one of trustees and one of physicians. According to institutional histories, the MHA board of trustees and its executive committee provided "moral and financial support" and met annually at first "to receive a report and to discuss any new policies necessary in the conduct of the Clinic."[48] The Medical Advisory Staff (later called the Medical Advisory Board) "set professional standards and assumed responsibility for their maintenance" and served as a liaison between laypersons (trustees and volunteers) and medical professionals. In theory, at least, these governing bodies worked in tandem. An MHA history stated that "while the Medical Advisory Board acts in an advisory capacity only, the Board of Trustees has never formulated any policy without the sanction of the Medical Advisory Board."[49]

The 1940–41 MHA annual report gives a more realistic picture of the roles of the two boards. That report states that while the Medical Advisory Board "directs all medical policies," the board of trustees "meets monthly . . . to raise the budget and govern all functions (except medical) of the Association."[50] Many MHA medical board members and trustees had served on the original ad hoc planning committee for the MHA. Five MHA trustees belonged to the family of Charles Brush Sr.: Dorothy Brush, his son's widow; Edna Brush Perkins, his daughter, and her husband, Roger; and Roslyn Campbell Weir, Brush Sr.'s grandniece, and her husband, William (see figure 6, chapter 2).

Only seven people served on the Brush Foundation board, considerably fewer than on the first MHA board of trustees, which numbered fifty-seven individuals and represented forty-four families. Charles Brush picked four family members to serve as his first foundation trustees: Edna Perkins, William and Roslyn Weir, and Dorothy Brush (see figures 14 and 15). The other three Brush board members represented professionals close to the family circle: the Rev. Joel Hayden, Jerome Fisher, and T. Wingate Todd, board president. Todd, an anatomist, worked closely with Dr. Roger Perkins on the Western Reserve University Medical School faculty.[51] All of the foundation board members except Todd and Hayden also served on the first MHA board; three of the six, Dorothy Brush, Roslyn Weir, and Jerry Fisher, held MHA Executive Committee positions. By 1931 both Hayden and Todd had also joined the MHA board, completing the interconnection.[52]

Founders of both the Brush Foundation and the MHA used the social status of board members to help protect the fledgling organizations from attack or prosecution. The 1927 *Social Register* for Cleveland lists thirty-one of the forty-four families involved on the first MHA board. All but one of the Brush board members appear in the same list. Among the male MHA trustees known to have graduated from college (more than 10 percent), degrees were most often from Western Reserve, Yale, and Harvard Universities. The few women trustees known to have pursued study after high school attended finishing schools on the East Coast or prestigious women's colleges such as Vassar or Smith. At least one-fifth of the MHA board members could claim a family link to a mansion on fashionable Euclid Avenue. As *Cleveland Press* columnist Maxwell wrote, the MHA and the Brush Foundation involved only "the best of our people," "outstanding citizens."[53]

Social standing did not guarantee freedom from criminal prosecution, however. In other cities during this time, authorities arrested birth control clinic founders and volunteers of similar social status. In St. Louis in 1929 and in Salem and Boston, Massachusetts, in 1937, newspapers featured photographs of society women jailed for their actions in birth control clinics. The women who created a birth control clinic in Des Moines, Iowa, in 1934 later remembered that "under the Iowa Code, this group was illegal and remained so for many years. The joke was that everything was going to be signed by four members so that they would have a foursome for bridge if they went to jail."[54] While these clinic leaders mocked the idea of arrest, the precarious legal situation dictated that providing birth control in the 1930s was indeed risky business.

At least one local marketer felt the effects of the Comstock Law during this era. Cleveland police arrested John Paganelli in 1932 for displaying birth control items in the window of his drugstore, the Mall Drug Company at St. Clair Avenue and East Sixth Street downtown, only a few blocks from the Osborn building. In addition to the Ohio law, Cleveland regulated obscene exhibits, depictions, and publications in the municipal code.[55] The court fined Paganelli and sentenced him to thirty days in the workhouse.[56] Cleveland advocates rightly worried about the clinic's legal standing. By joining with the Brush Foundation, MHA founders deflected local critics. Attacking the MHA meant attacking its powerful patrons, especially the Brush Foundation and its related institutions, such as Western Reserve University (WRU).

During the presidency of Charles Thwing (1891–1921), WRU acquired a national reputation and six new schools for graduate study. By the late 1920s the school represented academic prestige to citizens of the Midwest in general and Clevelanders in particular.[57] The Brush Foundation and the MHA each shared close connections with WRU. By March 1929 the foundation operated out of rent-free office space in the WRU School of Medicine. The university supplied facilities and personnel for the Brush Inquiry into child development.[58] Charles Brush Sr. served as a trustee of WRU (1901–1929) and of Adelbert College (1908–1929), the men's undergraduate school. Of the six Brush Foundation board members, at least four had ties to the university, one directly and three through family members.[59] These close connections to WRU were replicated in the MHA. Thirty-one of the fifty-seven members of the first MHA board had direct links to Western Reserve. For example, MHA founder Mary Dunning Thwing was married to WRU president Charles Thwing and served on the advisory committee of Flora Stone Mather College, a women's college within the university. Eight other original MHA board members belonged to the Mather College advisory committee; many held offices.[60] All of the twenty physicians who served on the MHA board of trustees or the Medical Advisory Board taught or had previously taught at the WRU School of Medicine. Seven had graduated from the same.[61] In August 1939, the Maternal Health Association moved its offices from the Osborn building to new headquarters on Adelbert Road at the WRU campus. The university provided the office and clinic space "at a nominal rate," according to one historical account.[62]

That MHA history, written in 1957, confirms an important strategy behind the unofficial but close alliance between the voluntary health facility and the university: "The proximity to Western Reserve University's School of Medicine and University Hospitals was invaluable for prestige and expansion."[63] While eschewing direct affiliation with national groups that might damage its conservative reputation, MHA leaders manipulated local philanthropic and academic connections to the same ends, to ensure respectability, stability, and growth. The organizers had these very concerns in mind when choosing the birth control clinic's staff. Once again they utilized local influence but turned to Sanger's clinic for training.

## SYMPATHETIC STAFF

The MHA preferred a background in public health for its early nursing staff. The clinic emphasized the need to be able to work with a variety of agencies and with the family as a unit. Staff members should "already have the respect of their community" and be "outstanding" in their chosen field but also be "balanced personalities." Other qualities played an important role, according to an MHA lecturer: "Our women and men physicians and public health nurses on the staff are chosen because of their interest in and feeling for people." Three experienced professionals advised MHA organizers about choosing the clinic's first nurse: Marion Howell, the director of the nursing school at Western Reserve University; Elizabeth Folckemer, executive secretary of the local Visiting Nurse Association; and Hanna Buchanan, the director of the Children's Fresh Air Camp and Hospital. This group recommended Rosina Volk, a public health nursing graduate of WRU (1910), because of her experience locally and overseas. Volk held memberships in local, state, and national nursing organizations, adding professional contributions to her qualifications.[64] (See fig. 16.)

The Medical Advisory Board just as carefully selected Ruth Robishaw as the clinic's first physician. First in both her class at the WRU School of Medicine (1923) and the state medical boards, Robishaw had trained as a dermatologist but obtained public health experience in a local health clinic. The fact that Robishaw chose to work in gynecology, outside of her specialty, may have reflected an interest in the birth control cause. Her flexibility certainly reflected the limited employment opportunities for women

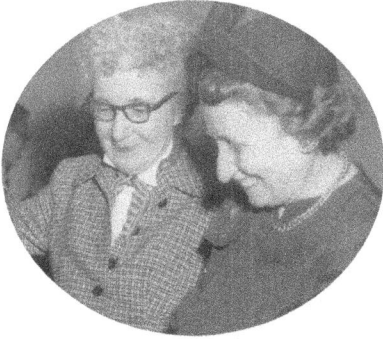

Edith Hammill, M.D. (left)
and Sarah Marcus, M.D.
MHA Physicians
Glenn Zahn photo, 1951
*Cleveland Press* Collection

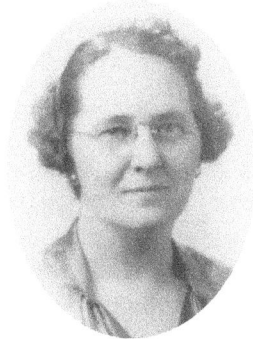

Gladys Gaylord
MHA Executive Secretary
Halle Bros. photo, 1938
PPGC, box 4
Western Reserve Historical Society

## Early staff members: the Cleveland Maternal Health Association and the Brush Foundation

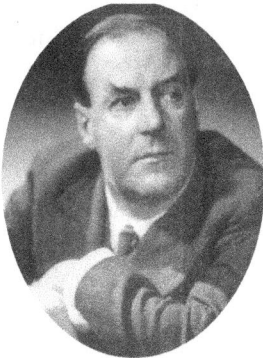

T. Wingate Todd, M.D.
President, Brush Foundation
Geoffrey Landesman photo, 1938
*Cleveland Press* Collection

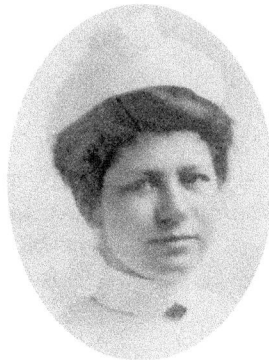

Rosina Volk, R.N.
MHA Nurse
Case Western Reserve University
Archives, 1910

FIGURE 16. Early staff members: The Cleveland Maternal Health Association
and The Brush Foundation.

physicians in the early twentieth century. Excluded from operating rooms and from intern and residency positions at many hospitals, qualified women physicians usually took on a variety of tasks in many fields, some of them on a volunteer basis, in order to build a private practice.[65]

By April 1930, the MHA had hired a second staff physician, Sarah Marcus. Marcus later claimed that she approached the MHA after working south of Cleveland with a physician who actively promoted birth control in his private practice. She remembered that this man provided his patients with the stem pessary and supplemented that method with contraceptive suppositories that he and his wife manufactured in their kitchen. Marcus came to the MHA with an obvious interest in and experience with providing birth control to women.[66] (See fig. 16.)

Facing a precarious employment situation on account of their gender, medical staff members further endangered their careers by working for birth control. Robishaw and Marcus each lost other professional posts due to their MHA affiliation. Conflicting information exists about the nature of the job that Robishaw was forced to relinquish. One source claims that she had to give up a teaching position at St. John's Hospital, and another says that it was an appointment with the city's Children's Bureau. Marcus recalled that a Lutheran hospital on the west side of town fired her because she was "that woman connected with Planned Parenthood." Physicians at birth control clinics in other cities experienced similar rejections. The problem endured for at least twenty years in Cleveland. In 1948 St. John's Hospital asked three MHA physicians to sever their connections with the birth control clinic. When they refused, the hospital removed them from its staff.[67] Despite this career risk and the minimal financial remuneration offered for MHA work, both Marcus and Robishaw remained with the clinic well into the 1940s and served on the MHA Medical Advisory Board for another two decades.[68] Evidently the birth control cause inspired them as well as the founders. Gender played a role in this commitment. Marcus insisted that women doctors had a special responsibility to help other women control their fertility. She maintained that, in addition to not being very interested in birth control, male physicians could not fit diaphragms as well as their female counterparts. Marcus asserted, "It's a field that a woman physician and only a woman physician does properly."[69]

Since neither medical school nor nursing school curriculum included instruction about contraception in the 1920s, the MHA sent Robishaw and Volk to Sanger's Birth Control Clinical Research Bureau (BCCRB) in New York City for training. The clinic later sent Marcus and Leona V. Glover, M.D., to the BCCRB for the same purpose.[70] Other physicians

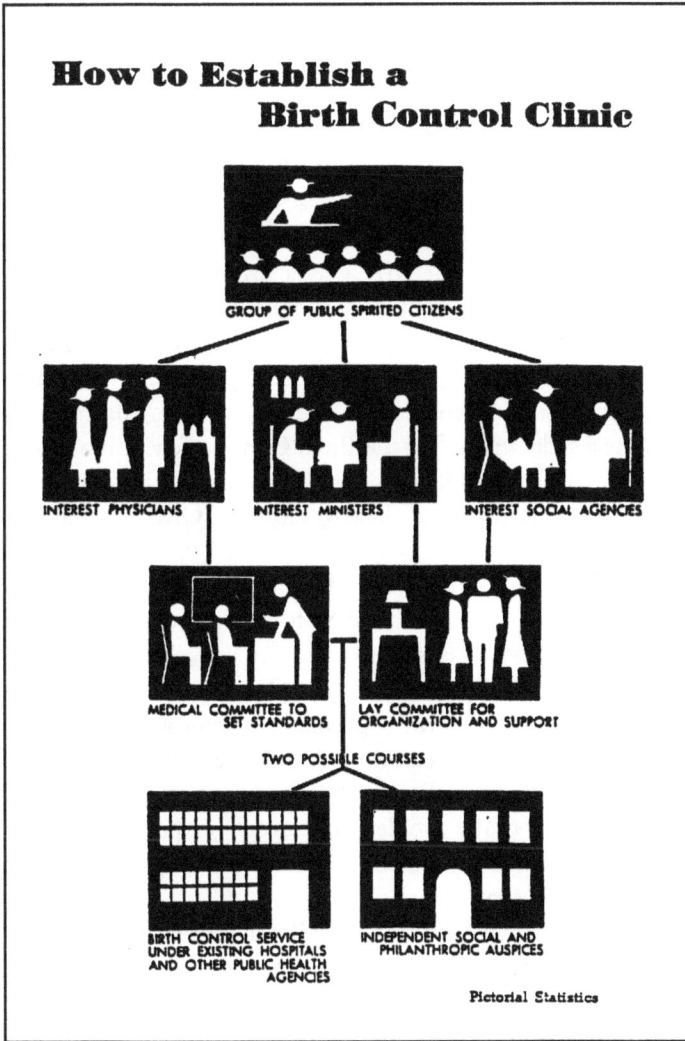

FIGURE 17.  How to establish a birth control clinic. Cover of booklet for BCCRB, M. Sanger, director. PPFA, Sophia Smith Collection, Smith College.

served on the MHA's medical staff during its first decade, the majority of them women. Conforming to prevailing cultural expectations, the association tried to find "married people with children" as their female staff members, to enable them "to understand more appreciably the problems of married people and of parents."[71] Male physicians comprised the medical advisory board, conducted research, and provided men's consultations, but female doctors actually performed examinations and supplied birth

control.[72] Women unquestionably managed the daily activities of the
Cleveland MHA. The situation represents a paradox: while exemplifying
some aspects of an acceptable gender norm (married women as nurturers),
the pioneer clinic challenged a fundamental tenet of that norm (women
as mothers) by assisting women in controlling fertility.

Despite legal, social, and medical proscriptions, the Cleveland Maternal Health Association opened in 1928 free from legal or medical challenges. Founders created the MHA as a private, low-profile voluntary
association, with neither hospital connection nor Academy of Medicine
backing but advised by a board of prominent local physicians. In its effort
to gain authority and avoid antagonizing its adversaries, the MHA stubbornly clung to its independence from national birth control organizations and local federations. Yet the Birth Control Federation of America
codified the founding strategies of the MHA and other pioneer clinics
into a model for new groups, as the cover for a BCCRB booklet illustrates
(see figure 17).

The MHA differed from the BCFA model, however, in its link to a
local philanthropy. The clinic's intimate connections with the Brush
Foundation and Western Reserve University consolidated financial and
institutional support to legitimize services. This close cooperation ensured
that the MHA would embody the prevalent eugenic justification for family limitation and follow a medical model. While providing a service generally unaccepted by the medical profession and of questionable legal status, the clinic successfully avoided controversy or public agitation. The
MHA courted support by quietly organizing along medical lines and
refraining from provocative tactics.

Based on such careful planning, the Cleveland Maternal Health Association garnered grateful clients, such as the woman who wrote, "I am very
pleased with your method and my husband and I thank you from the bot-
tom of our hearts for showing us the way." In the next chapter, more
MHA clients tell their stories.

# 4

## "Hubby and I think it's swell"

Maternal Health Association clients experienced birth control differently from the women involved in the clinic's creation and management. Continuing tensions about sexuality and birth control, both public and private, shaped personal experiences that, in turn, echoed the tensions. Staff, founders, funders, and board members held a three-fold vision of the MHA and its purpose: to demonstrate via statistics the scientific correctness of contraception; to improve the family, the community, and "the race"; and to provide women with relief from uncontrolled childbearing. Clients, on the other hand, came to the MHA for the third reason only—to space or limit their pregnancies. Some husbands encouraged their wives, others viewed birth control and the clinic with suspicion. This chapter explores the implementation of the MHA's purpose in its first decade by analyzing the diversity of experience.

Historians find it difficult to recreate the circumstances and reactions of people no longer alive to speak for themselves. We usually rely on annual reports, copies of lectures, personal papers, organizational histories, and local or national studies. These sources often reflect only privileged classes, however. The stories of others (ordinary people, who lectured only to their children, people who left no personal papers) often remain untold. In the fortunate case of the Maternal Health Association of Cleveland, a group of these voices communicates directly from the past through a collection of 231 letters kept by MHA staff and compiled in a scrapbook.

Before the telephone became ubiquitous, MHA clients wrote to the clinic to make or cancel appointments, to respond to staff queries, or to let the clinic know of changes in their family situations. Analyzing these communications does present some difficulties. Comprising only the letters that the clinic staff saved, the small sample does not accurately reflect client diversity in terms of class or personal circumstances. The letters represent only a tiny proportion of the over ten thousand women listed as new MHA clients between 1928 and 1938.[1] The clinic likely only preserved letters that portrayed the most extreme circumstances, positive or negative, and discarded much of the more mundane correspondence. The letters do not reveal the racial background of clients. Within these constraints, however, the messages disclose a variety of private encounters with birth control. Unaltered by the editing that characterizes Sanger's published collection of client letters, the MHA correspondence offers intimate insights into this reform and its personal consequences.[2] The preserved notes enrich the story of a social movement with the voices of clinic clients in addition to those of national and local leaders. The physical documentation of the letters themselves expands our knowledge base about the constituency of this early Midwestern birth control clinic.

## BACKGROUNDS AND BIASES

Examining the actual letters, one discovers that women came to the MHA from diverse backgrounds. Correspondents wrote to clinic staff on paper of all types, from monogrammed, deckle-edged, linen stationery, to lined notepaper, to pages from a child's school tablet, to paper fragments. They employed pencil, fountain pen, and occasionally a typewriter. Although the majority of women used plain stationery of some sort, more than 10 percent wrote on the backs of original MHA communications or other scraps. This particular choice of writing material demonstrates either extreme thrift or, more likely, strapped financial situations in the constraints of the Great Depression. One cannot generalize about social class based solely on the type of stationery that writers used, but the physical evidence suggests a broad spectrum of personal and familial situations among clients of the Cleveland Maternal Health Association.

Statistics from MHA annual reports confirm this heterogeneity with respect to economics. In her report of the first four thousand women served at the MHA, Dr. Ruth Robishaw stated that "sociologic data as to race, education, occupation of the husband, financial status, and housing conditions of the patients have been recorded to demonstrate that groups commonly considered socially and economically handicapped are found in the clinic's clientele in at least as large proportions as they are found in the general population of Cleveland."[3] In the MHA's first decade, most client families made less than twenty-five dollars a week (figure 18).

## Average weekly income of MHA Clients

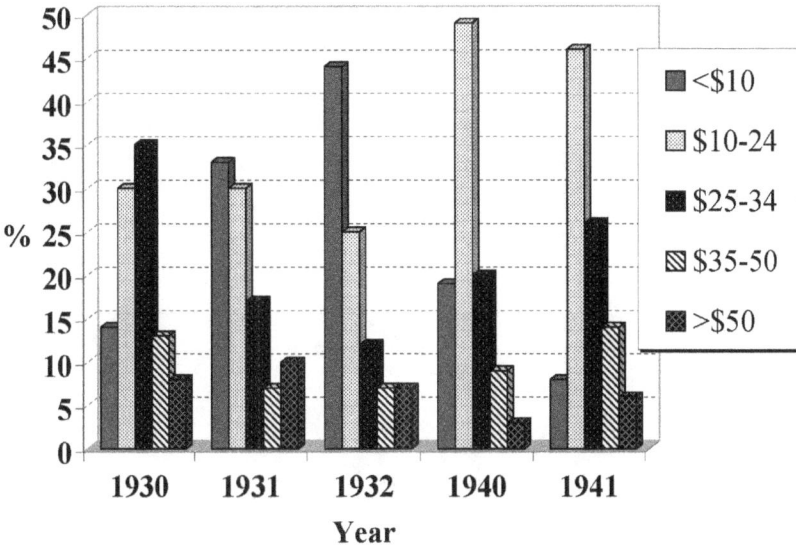

FIGURE 18. Average weekly income of MHA Clients.

Associated Charities of Cleveland estimated that this amount represented a minimum small-income budget for a family of five in 1930.[4] The *Encyclopaedia of Social Sciences* stated seven years later that as a national minimum to maintain a "standard of health and decency," a family of five needed about $38 a week. The *Encyclopaedia* estimated that 40 to 45 percent of Americans lived in poverty in the mid-1930s.[5]

The typical family size for MHA clients between 1928 and 1932 (the years for which numbers exist) was at least five people. The 1930 census indicates that the average Cleveland family numbered 4.01 persons. Almost 60 percent of MHA client families lay below the "health and decency" standard between 1928 and 1940. The people in more than half of these households subsisted on less than ten dollars a week, had irregular income, were supported by relatives, or were on relief. (See figures 18 and 19.) The majority of the MHA clientele during this time lived at levels far below poverty. Clearly the Cleveland MHA did not represent the middle-class phenomenon that other historians have depicted when describing the birth control movement. While never reaching more than a small percentage of the area's total residents, Cleveland's birth control clinic served a substantial portion of working-class and poor families.

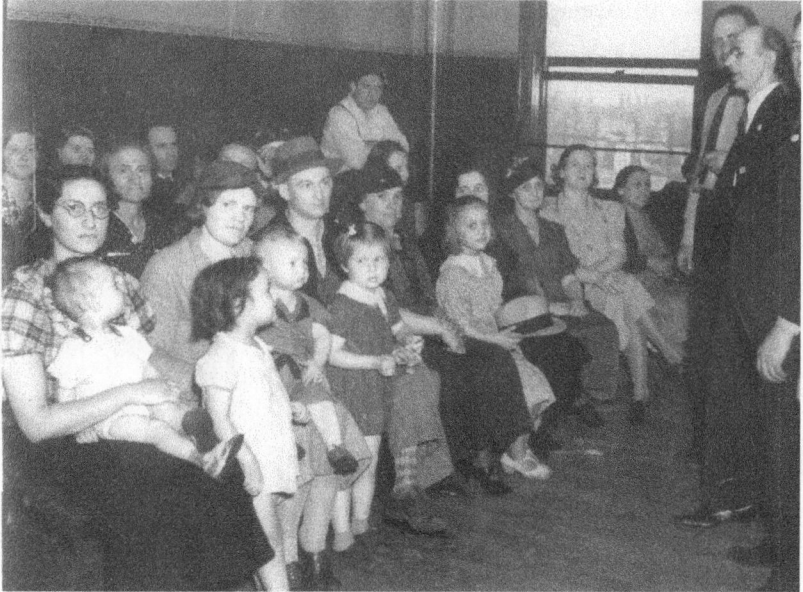

FIGURE 19. Clevelanders strike for relief. Sit-down strikers at Doan relief office, East 118th Street and Superior, 1938. *Cleveland Press* Collection, Cleveland State University. Fred Bottomer photo.

The MHA touted this fact in its early reports. By utilizing the clinic and successfully employing contraception, working-class and poor women disproved one class-based argument against birth control. Opponents who feared the deterioration of "human stock" maintained that while the elite increasingly limited the number of their progeny, less-privileged couples would not bother to use birth control even if given the opportunity. Some professionals argued that "people of this type" would not be able to employ contraception successfully if they chose to do so. In such a scenario, family limitation would lead to a proliferation of "the groups commonly considered as socially and economically handicapped." These people believed that contraception was "dysgenic," that is, pertaining to or causing degeneration, and would diminish the ranks of the middle and upper classes and threaten the social order. The MHA collected and published data about the race, occupations, housing conditions, and financial status of its clientele to refute this thesis. Even while contending that it made "no judgment as to inferior and superior groups," however, the organization exemplified race and class biases common to the nation in general and Cleveland in particular.[7]

Many Americans of African descent viewed Cleveland as hospitable during the early twentieth century. In 1916 Cleveland writer Charles Chesnutt described his hometown as "liberal and progressive," using as an example the fact that his daughter belonged to the College Club, along with white female college graduates.[8] Blacks in Cleveland did suffer less racist violence than in Southern cities. However, Cleveland citizens and institutions practiced outright discrimination and exhibited more subtle racism well into the twentieth century. During the first two decades of the century, city orphanages stopped accepting dependent black children. Cleveland Trust refused to hire a black woman as a teller, and Western Reserve University denied women of color admission to its nursing school. Black residents could not try on clothes in Higbees, a major department store, or watch a movie in a regular seat at the Loew's Ohio Theater or swim in the Brookside Park swimming pool. The Woodland Hills pool hired guards to protect its few black patrons from harassment, and Luna Park, an amusement park, lost lawsuits for discriminating against people of color.[9]

The confused nature of tolerance and racism in "liberal" Northern cities such as Cleveland continued through the 1930s and 1940s. The city's reputation did not accurately represent the reality of the policies and practices of its medical institutions, for instance. A *Saturday Evening Post* article titled "The Color Line in Medicine" praised conditions in Cleveland as exemplary in the 1920s compared to the rest of the country. The article noted that Cleveland City Hospital had first hired a black doctor in 1928 and opened its doors to black interns and nursing students three years later. St. Vincent Charity Hospital had three black nurses on its staff in 1926. People of color in Cleveland viewed the situation differently, however. The *Cleveland Gazette,* a popular newspaper in the black community, repeatedly disparaged City Hospital for waiting so long to offer professional training for black students. In 1939 Charles Garvin, M.D., who had practiced medicine in Cleveland since 1916, was one of only eleven of Cleveland's thirty-five African American physicians to hold a staff position at any hospital in the city. Garvin served on the staff of Lakeside Hospital beginning in 1919 and later taught in the School of Medicine of Western Reserve University. Most of the city's other physicians of color had no place to hospitalize their patients, however. Such discrimination prompted some black professionals to call for a separate hospital to benefit doctors and patients alike.[10]

Occasionally, opposition to African Americans in the city erupted in violence. In 1926 racists targeted Dr. Garvin and his family. They painted "KKK" on the side of their newly built home in upscale Wade Park and a few weeks later threw a homemade bomb that exploded inside the house.

A second bombing attempt was thwarted six months later. Although the Garvin family escaped physical injury, the incidents attracted national attention.[11] Discontinuities similar to those inherent in law and sexual policy, signaled by the local arrest and stiff prison sentence for Ben Reitman in 1916, also applied to race. Attitudes and actions in "liberal and progressive" Cleveland attest to and embody the complex dynamics of racial coexistence that affected both policy and daily life in early-twentieth-century America. The Cleveland MHA reflected this confused and generally oppressive climate.

The clinic began the statistical section of its 1930 report by comparing the ratio of its clients from "the colored group" to those of "the white race," and then labeling the African American women as "socially and economically handicapped and inferior." During the MHA's first three years, black women represented from 26 percent to 30 percent of the clinic's clients, more than double the proportion of blacks in the city's general population. This proportion declined in the next few years. By 1938 the ratio of black MHA clients relative to their numbers among Cleveland residents in general began to equalize: one in twelve of the women who attended the MHA were black, and the city claimed a ratio of one black resident in eleven. A 1939 study of 202 U.S. birth control facilities found that blacks comprised about 11.9 percent of the total clients and represented 9 percent of the total U.S. population.[12]

Birth control clinics across the country handled the race question differently. Many served black and white women separately. The Minnesota Birth Control League opened a branch for African American women in the Phillis Wheatley Settlement House in Minneapolis, and Sanger supporters ran a separate clinic for blacks in Harlem. Other facilities, like the one in Little Rock, Arkansas, did not serve women of color at all at first. On the other hand, some Southern states, such as North Carolina, initiated birth control as a state public health function in part to possibly limit the numbers of the poor, including white and black families.[13]

Maternal Health Association records do not account for the high percentage of black women who used the clinic in its early years or the decline in that percentage over the 1930s. However, the statistical reports of the clinic's third and fourth years offer some clues. These particular reports, more detailed than those of later years, note a jump in the proportion of middle-class women attending the MHA. Sociologist Charles Gehlke, author of the 1932 report, generalizes about class, based on the increasing percentage of MHA clients who lived in "spacious" quarters as opposed to "crowded" or "overcrowded" conditions. The clinic interpreted these adjectives as:

| Very spacious | 2 rooms more than the number of residents; |
| Spacious | 1 room per person more than the number of residents; or more than 1 and less than 2 rooms in excess; |
| Crowded | more than 1 and not more than 2 persons per room; |
| Overcrowded | more than 2 and not more than 3 persons per room; |
| Greatly overcrowded | more than 3 persons per room.[14] |

The number of those MHA families who enjoyed spacious residences jumped from 25 percent of the total client population in 1930 to 35 percent in 1932. During the same period, the number of MHA clients who reported crowded quarters fell from 54 percent in 1930 to 43 percent in 1932, and the ratio of those clients living in overcrowded conditions in Cleveland dropped from 10 percent to 8 percent.[15] These figures do not seem to fit the worsening economic conditions and warrant closer inspection.

As the 1930s progressed and the Great Depression spread its deleterious effects across class lines, couples on all economic levels began to rethink family size. More middle- and working-class mothers looked to acquire and use contraception. At the same time, the grave financial situation certainly limited access to medical care of any type for the area's poorest women. Even if the services cost little or nothing, getting to a clinic involved factors other than motivation. In reaction to the worsening economy in Cleveland and increasing employment discrimination against their male relatives, black women had turned to wage labor beginning in the 1920s. More married women, white and black, worked outside the home at some point during the thirties in order to make ends meet. Between 1930 and 1940 the number of married women in the American labor force grew by 50 percent compared to a 15 percent rise in their numbers in the population. Stretching the family budget to include transportation to the MHA and time off from work for a clinic visit must have been impossible for many poor women employed outside of the home.[16]

These elements certainly contributed to the MHA's diminishing proportion of black clients. The decrease could also indicate a dissatisfaction among black women with clinic attitudes or services. Historians have noted a general distrust among black women of medical institutions, especially those facilities run by whites. The location of the MHA in a building occupied by white doctors rather than in a settlement house or other more accessible neighborhood location did not especially attract black women. Perhaps women of color did not even know about the clinic, given the lack of publicity. News articles about the MHA focused on white, upper-class social events and did not appear in black newspapers. The poorest women, black and white, could not easily get to the MHA, especially as the Depression wore on and economic circumstances and living conditions deteriorated. Many black women desired to limit their families: in other locales, they helped establish contraceptive services.[17] Perhaps to avoid accusations of racism, MHA records and speeches are silent on the race question.

While race and class biases influenced the clinic's philosophy and services during the 1930s, the MHA helped some women of color to limit their offspring and improve their lives. A 1951 report looks back on the long-term participation of an African American family in the MHA. The 38-year-old mother, who had six living children after nineteen pregnancies, first came to the MHA in April of 1928, just after it opened. Not surprisingly, considering her situation, clinic staff described the woman as "too tired to care for her home properly," able to take "only a slight interest in her children." The MHA claimed that the woman's continued clinic attendance and consistent use of birth control over the years changed "the whole atmosphere of the home." This mother represented a determined client and bore no more children.[18]

In its early years the MHA served white and black women like this beleaguered mother, women who certainly could not afford engraved stationery or often food, carfare, or medical supplies. However, the clinic also assisted a few women of relative privilege. The names of at least seven MHA founders and board members appear in a clinic ledger (1928–1939) alongside the names of working-class clients. For example, although she had moved from Cleveland to Riverdale, New York, MHA founder Dorothy Brush used the services of the Cleveland MHA in 1931. Having married a second time, Brush bore her third and last child, a daughter, in 1930. Other board members also used the services of the MHA during the clinic's first decade.[19]

This fact disproves the assumption that birth control clinic founders obtained their own contraception from private physicians rather than from the clinics that they had created. While ignoring the preponderance of working-class and poor clients in early U.S. birth control clinics, researchers have at the same time portrayed clinic founders as remaining aloof from clinic operations. Scholars such as historian Linda Gordon and sociologists Robert and Helen Merrell Lynd note that early birth control advocates were removed by class and privilege from the women using their clinics. Gordon correctly contends that the increasing medicalization and professionalization of birth control in general in the 1930s distanced the movement from its radical working-class roots and clientele. The Lynds record a filtering down of birth control information from business- to working-class couples.[20] The information interchange ran both ways, however, and permeated all of the layers of social classes to some extent. In Cleveland, some women used the pioneer birth control clinic that they had founded or helped support for their own needs. No evidence exists to determine whether they acted purposefully to demonstrate solidarity with less fortunate MHA clients or whether they utilized the clinic out of convenience or because of a dearth of local physicians who would provide contraception in their practices. In any case obtaining their birth control at the new clinic rather than from a private physician proved their commitment to the venture.

Such profound commitment positively affected the character of service at the Cleveland MHA. According to staff descriptions of clinic clients and to clients' own correspondence, many women who came to the clinic sensed and welcomed the bond with founders, volunteers, and staff. As one client wrote:

> I want to thank you for the wonderful service which you have given to me and to my friends, and although we are mosttimes lax in expressing our thanks, I am deeply and sincerely grateful to the Maternal Health Clinic, and owe much of my present happiness to you. The friendliness of everyone connected with the clinic always makes a visit a pleasure, and I hope you may continue to make life more pleasant for a lot of worried wives and mothers.

Clinic executive secretary Gladys Gaylord, writing in 1939 about how a birth control clinic gains public acceptance, stressed the importance of hiring staff who were not only competent but interested in people. Gaylord explained, "Friendliness . . . must be evident throughout the service: in talking on the telephone, in meeting casual visitors as well as in routine procedure with patients or the Board." Social work student Goldie Davis, who researched and observed the MHA for over a year in the late 1930s, agreed with the client cited above about the clinic's particular practices. She noted "the keen interest [of] the personnel . . . in the lives and problems of their clinic families." One visitor reported that the MHA nurse had a "fine motherly personality."[21]

The physical surroundings of the Osborn building office reflected this commitment and concern. Like other pioneer clinics across the continent,

staffed by "sympathetic physicians, assisted by indefatigable and enthusiastic nurses" in a "wholesome and cheerful atmosphere," the MHA strove
for an informal environment, different from a hospital or dispensary. Staff
and volunteers decorated the place to soften the medical look. Board
member Julia McCune Flory had privacy screens made for the examining
room and painted them aqua with the popular lotus blossom design. (One
client, after studying the screens, asked, "Is that a picture of my insides?")
Observers described the homey appearance of the office and waiting
room, which featured a play area for children. Volunteers babysat for
mothers at the clinic and occasionally even shed tears with clients.[22] The
MHA endeavored to nurture as well as educate. Although the association
chose to work out of a building filled with other medical offices in order
to be considered reputable, it attempted to create a less institutional, more
welcoming space, to help women feel more comfortable.

## JUST THE FACTS

The Cleveland Maternal Health Association strove for a balance between
such an informal climate and the professionalism that was expected in the
medical and social service of the day. The clinic designed much of its
strategy and procedure along the Sanger and ABCL model.[23] The MHA
required an appointment for clinic service. A volunteer receptionist welcomed the prospective client to the Osborn building office. A nurse interviewed her and took a complete social history. She inquired about the
woman's religious convictions toward contraception, asked whether she
already had a private physician, and ascertained that she was married and
not already pregnant. The nurse also tried to discern if the woman came
voluntarily, perhaps to avoid any police "plants" such as those who troubled Sanger and others in the movement and to avoid charges of coercion.
According to the historical record, nursing staff and volunteers scrupulously avoided saying anything that could be construed as contraceptive
advice. To abide by existing laws, only the physicians discussed contraception with clients or prospective clients.[24]

The MHA pursued other cautious paths. Clinic staff advised Roman
Catholic women who did not know of their church's opposition to birth
control to go home and "talk it over" with their husbands. Staff counseled
women who had personal physicians to consult their own doctors first.
During the interview the nurse decided on the fee that the client would
pay for clinic services. Using a sliding scale, the MHA based its charges
on family income and responsibilities. A clinic visit cost from $.35 to
$10.00 in 1931. By 1938 the fees had risen to $1.15 to $15.00, with the

upper limit reflecting "the usual fee charged by the private physician." Although not always carried out in practice, according to Goldie Davis, the MHA desired "to refer those patients who are able to pay to a private physician and to concentrate its efforts upon the families who need this service but [for] whom the physician's price is prohibitive."[25]

In using such narrow qualifications for service, the MHA acquiesced to cultural constraints. By recommending that Roman Catholic couples agree on the use of mechanical contraception, the clinic presumably hoped to counter religious opposition. Likewise, clinic personnel did not want to rouse the ire of local physicians by infringing upon their private practices. By determining that a woman did not have a personal physician or that her physician had refused to provide contraception, the MHA helped circumvent such controversy.

This particular qualification implies that, in fact, some Cleveland physicians did dispense contraceptives during this era. An undated letter from an MHA client confirms this.

> Dear Miss Volk:
> . . . I am glad to report to you that I am in perfect condition and not expect-
> ing—an addition. I think I told you I sure had a family enough—
> Now regards why I have not called at your office—I have been so thin and
> since conditions improved a little with us my husband has had me go reg-
> ular to a doctor to try to build up—in weight. I have consulted the doctor
> regular and did get jelly from him. His advice and yours are alike. . . .

Because some area doctors provided birth control in their practices and would not welcome competition, the MHA took extreme care to win and maintain the good will of the medical community.

To avoid physician charges of propagandizing or allegations of eugenic coercion, the MHA declared that it did not actively seek out clients. An MHA report stated in 1931, "No effort is made to induce patients to attend the clinic." The original statement of purpose emphasized this philosophy: "to aid and support physicians in medical service and advice to married women." Annual reports repeated this assertion year after year. Acquiescing to social and moral compunctions as well the law, the MHA turned away unmarried women.[26] While the Ohio code did not specify that physicians could only give contraceptive advice to *married* women, the 1918 Crane decision had in fact made that exclusion. To abide by this legal interpretation, to diffuse any charges of contributing to sexual licentious-ness, and to stay within the bounds of "decency," most early American birth control clinics served only married women. In a list of twenty-five facilities operating in the 1920s, only Chicago's center accepted any adult, married or not, for contraceptive services. The married-women-only requirement held for most Planned Parenthood affiliates well into the 1960s.[27]

Ruth Backus, a former director of the pioneer clinic in Rochester, New York, regretfully remembered refusing to give birth control to two different women: a sexually active widow who already had nine children and an unmarried woman with two children by her common-law partner. Neither of these mothers planned to marry and thus did not qualify for assistance. Upon hearing that the latter woman had jumped from a bridge to her death, Backus said, "I wondered if I had given her a little push." Backus explained the reason behind these "heartbreaking" decisions: "The field was new, and public support was important to us. Also, we were constantly expecting challenges on legal grounds and so, we were very straitlaced."[28] The MHA faced similar concerns.

The Cleveland facility, logically, also refused to serve pregnant women until their babies arrived. One of the three women who came to the MHA on the day it opened, in fact, already was pregnant. "For her, the MHA had begun just too late," states one history. Publicly opposed to abortion, the clinic avoided situations that would compromise its reputation in this area. Most advocates in the early twentieth century argued for birth control as a way to prevent abortions. They did not publicly support abortion as a right or even an option.[29]

For the first year the MHA accepted women "for health reasons only," seeing only those women with health conditions that would make pregnancy or childbirth physically dangerous. In the first three months of the MHA's operation, it assisted only twenty-eight "active" clients (those who kept in touch after the first visit). The clinic accommodated these women in two-hour sessions twice a week. The limit of serving women "for health reasons only" severely circumscribed the potential service population. At its first annual meeting in June 1929, the association significantly broadened the qualifications to include patients whose economic and social situations warranted family limitation services. The MHA instituted these new requirements in January of the next year. Clinic leaders saw the policy change as a big step, opening its doors to more women while staying within legal, social, and moral conventions. The client population grew slowly but steadily. By October 1930 the MHA offered contraceptive services in four sessions each week, including Monday evenings and Saturday mornings. It served approximately five hundred women between 1928 and 1930, about the same number as the birth control center in Baltimore, Maryland, during the same period.[30]

The MHA began to welcome prenuptial clients in 1931. Area clergy had requested the service. Again treading a prudent path, staff requested proof of the upcoming weddings before serving the brides-to-be. Speaking before the 1939 American Congress of Obstetrics and Gynecology, Gladys Gaylord described this requirement: "Young people are accepted for premarital conferences only when they bring a guarantee of their plan to get married (marriage license, note from clergyman who is to marry them, or when [the couple is] brought [to the clinic] by parents)." The MHA welcomed the prospective husbands to these conferences and offered them the chance to speak privately with a male physician.[31]

By adhering to standards of propriety, early clinics downplayed birth control's association with promiscuity and set it apart from abortion. The restrictions also addressed arguments against the artificial control of a natural function, reproduction. Many physicians and other professionals who opposed birth control as unnatural asserted that contraception would free the "New Woman" from her traditional "duties" of marriage and motherhood. They argued that the widespread use of birth control threatened not only to sully or even eliminate women's sacred role as mother, but that it also threatened population quality by diminishing the ranks of the privileged classes. Some even warned that using contraception would lead to sterility.[32] Rather than directly confronting these arguments, the MHA remained quiet. Dr. T. Wingate Todd, director of the Brush Foundation and MHA board member, warned the MHA, "Neither records nor advice should be open to criticism." He further stated that the clinic should not recognize the desire of some to willfully avoid the responsibility of parenthood altogether, calling those individuals "undesirable patients."[33] The MHA carefully constructed its policies and routines within these parameters in order to achieve legitimacy and avoid conflict.

## LEARNING THE METHOD

After completing the interview and financial arrangements, the new MHA client headed for the examination room. Many of these women did not visit a physician regularly, if at all, and most had experienced at least four pregnancies with little prenatal or postpartum attention. The clinic physician took a detailed medical history, asking particularly about gynecological problems, history of pregnancies and abortions, and the results of contraceptive methods employed previously. Copies of blank MHA record forms from 1938 indicate that the physician also gathered information from each client about her sexual history. Fields on the form include "Frequency of coitus," "Do menses affect desire," "Attitude toward coitus," "Date last coitus," "Orgasm experienced (always, never, usually, sometimes, seldom)," and "Explanation for lack of orgasm" (see Maternal Health Association Patient Information Form, appendix). Answering these questions involved some level of openness about one's body and toward sexuality in general. Responses allegedly assisted the physician in deciding whether this particular client would be a good candidate for the diaphragm. Clearly, however, the questions sought many more details than necessary. Such intimate queries indicate the influence of Sigmund Freud's theories of personality as well as the burgeoning professional and popular interest during this era in determining the character of a "normal" couple's sex life. As part of the clinic's research agenda, the questions presaged the local and national Planned Parenthood's later emphasis on marital counseling.[34] The interview process embodied different strains within the MHA: treating clients objectively as subjects for study and treating them subjectively, as other women who desperately needed assistance.

After this thorough interview, the MHA doctor examined the woman, checking for conditions that needed medical attention or that might preclude prescribing a diaphragm. At the MHA and similar clinics across North America, women learned not only about birth control and disease but also more about their own bodies. Clinic physicians often discovered gynecological or other health problems that needed to be addressed. Since the MHA did not offer the resources for comprehensive health care, the physicians suggested that the woman visit another physician or dispensary for treatment of these maladies. Women often wrote to the clinic about following up on MHA physicians' recommendations. One client wrote in 1939, "The last time I was there, the doctor told me to go to a clinic about my womb because it was bad. So I am writing to you could you please write me a separate note or letter so I can take it to Lakeside Hospital . . . Friday morning." By 1944 Gladys Gaylord felt confident in claiming that the clinic was "a cancer prevention service," detecting preindications of cancer of the cervix in some women and referring them elsewhere for treatment.[35]

Given no contraindications, the clinic doctor then prescribed and counseled the client about a birth control method. The clinic most often suggested the rubber diaphragm, also called a pessary, coated with spermicidal jelly for extra protection. By offering this method almost exclusively, the MHA followed and perpetuated the medical model set by Margaret Sanger and others. To gain respectability, Sanger advocated the diaphragm over other commercial methods such as the condom. But increasing sales indicated the condom's growing popularity. It was cheap, easy to acquire and use, did not require medical supervision, and was more effective than other common methods even before the days of inspection and standardization.[36] Sanger saw the need to distance the "modern" birth control movement from the condom and other less-than-respectable for-bears, however, in part to attract the cooperation and support of physicians. The condom's association with prostitution and the prevention of venereal disease compromised its usefulness as a medical tool. Many doctors held it in contempt. The diaphragm, which Aletta Jacobs had proven safe and effective in Dutch clinics, seemed the perfect item. The need for medical control of birth control eventually did appeal to physicians, whom the commercial contraceptive marketplace of earlier days had cast aside.[37]

Fitting the diaphragm properly and placing it correctly represent the keys to the method's success. At the MHA a physician selected the appropriate diaphragm for the size and shape of the woman's cervix and demonstrated the device's proper insertion and removal. The client herself had to put in and take out the diaphragm in the physician's presence in order to ensure that she understood the procedure. One frank MHA correspondent thoroughly describes her use of the method and provides a clear idea of her interpretation, at least, of the instructions that she received:

> I have been useing the pessary in this way. I wash it in warm water before using and always stretch the pessary to see if there are any holes before we use it, then I put the jelly around the rim, and a teaspoonful inside the pessary, and after I insert the pessary I always feel to find the mouth of the womb through the pessary, then I douche about ten hours after useing, but I always lie down and douche half of the syrange of warm water then I remove the pessary and use the other half of the water. After using the pessary, I always wash it in warm soap water, and dry it and dust it with cornstarch.

This writer also graphically illustrates the diaphragm's major drawbacks, which often led couples to quit using it or even avoid it altogether. Not only was the device tedious to use and tricky to insert correctly, it required running water, hot as well as cold, and a private bathroom or other space. In the 1920s and 1930s many women in Cleveland and elsewhere lacked such luxuries.[38] Their life circumstances not only limited their access to the MHA clinic itself but also to the method that it commonly offered.

The personal nature of the interview, the exposure of private parts, and inserting a vaginal appliance in front of someone else certainly caused embarrassment and some discomfort for clinic patients.[39] These factors must have discouraged many potential users from even making a clinic appointment. Few clients' letters to the MHA speak of such feelings, however. One woman did write of confusion about the instructions she received: "I have not been able to use the supplies as yet as I can not make it work satisfactorily and am ashamed to come to you about it, so the best thing I could think of was to write and ask (if you'll forgive me) if I may come in and be shown again how to do so." Such letters offer some insight into the serious commitment with which many women approached their use of this method of birth control in spite of the awkwardness of clinic visits, the embarrassment of being questioned about personal matters, or the learning process involved.

Staff encouraged clients to purchase contraceptive jelly and other supplies at the MHA. The clinic scheduled follow-up visits at two weeks and again three months later, and an annual visit thereafter. At these appointments, a doctor checked for "pathological pelvic conditions" or other changes that might threaten the continued success of what was often called "the method." The MHA also advised women to contact the clinic after pregnancy, miscarriage, or childbirth to see if the conditions of the cervix, pelvic floor, or vagina had changed enough to warrant modifications in diaphragm size or type. Requiring return visits medicalized the process even further while enabling the clinic to track clients and their progress. The MHA maintained statistics for each woman as to the use or disuse of the method prescribed as well as the number of her pregnancies, accidental or planned.[40]

The clinic applied the businesslike rubric of scientific charity to intimate matters. Employing a specialized medical device, the diaphragm, attracted some physicians. MHA's procedures, from interview to follow-up visits to quantifying the results, modeled those of the first clinics such as Sanger's and became a model for the national movement. Clinic services differed significantly from those offered by the local pharmacist or mail-order company and helped distinguish clinical contraception from the marketplace variety.

While offering an innovative medical service, the MHA remained bound by convention and social expectations. The association cautiously screened clients, determined their marital status and religious orientation, and carefully noted personal details and family circumstances. Staff and volunteers worked to create a collaborative and nurturing environment but proceeded according to medical protocol. Finally, by focusing mainly on women and promoting the diaphragm as the preferred method of birth control, the MHA reinforced the cultural image of dutiful wife and mother as woman's proper role. Paradoxically, the woman-centered focus also drew other women to the cause as contraceptive users.

## TEACHING WOMEN TO BE HAPPY

While emphasizing "careful teaching and individual attention," MHA physicians and other staff reassured fearful clients with their matter-of-fact manner. Clients, in turn, generally impressed MHA staff with their "interest and effort." One person, probably Gladys Gaylord, observed that MHA clients "come willingly, anxious to be instructed, demanding no guarantee of infallibility, and ready to try something that shall serve them better than their wonted practices." Clinic observer Goldie Davis stated, "Seldom does a patient give any evidence of hesitancy. . . . The physicians feel that this is an indication that this service is, in the minds of these patients, regarded in the same light as any other phase of medical practice." Dr. Ruth Robishaw reasoned, "The determined search by the patient for something better than her past and fallible practices insures cooperation and gratitude." In one client's words, "This is the place where you teach women to be happy."[41]

Securing a reliable means of preventing pregnancy meant that these women did not have to confront decisions about abortion. Abortion represented the only way, albeit illegal, expensive, and dangerous, to end an unwanted pregnancy. Regulation of abortion lay with the states rather than the federal government.[42] Most states had criminalized abortion years before making contraception illegal. Ohio passed an anti-abortion statute in 1834, only thirteen years after the country's first law of that type passed in Connecticut.[43] The same late-nineteenth-century federal and state laws that proscribed information about family limitation also made it a crime to transport, sell, publish, print, or mail information on abortion, strengthening state anti-abortion provisions. Although providing contraception put physicians and patients in some locations at risk of legal action in the late 1920s and early 1930s, arrests and court battles occurred more often in cases of abortion. Fear of legal repercussions as well as medical consequences profoundly affected women's experience of abortion during this era and later. The secretive nature of procuring such a procedure deepened women's anxieties.[44]

Only a few of the letters in the MHA collection refer to abortion. One distraught pregnant mother wrote to nurse Rosina Volk, "I'm really desperate, if I would had the money I would not go through with it. don't think I'm such a sinner but it's terrible, the Dr. I went to wont do such a thing but told me where to go, but said it was a long chance as the thing had gone on to long, and of coarse I did not have the money for it was quit a sum, and no one would loan it to me for that . . . every-thing is against me." Studies confirm what this letter suggests—that women of all eras have utilized abortion as a method of birth control, at times with few moral compunctions, and that some physicians aided that practice. Still, trips to the abortionist triggered feelings of dread that women apparently did not associate with visits to birth control clinics.[45]

Clinics such as the MHA worked hard to counteract any apprehension that women felt. The friendly, chatty tone of the client letters testifies to the success of MHA's nurturing climate. Occasionally, clinic staff provided clothing to needy mothers, probably unofficially. One woman expressed her gratitude.

> The little romper's you gave me Saturday, they both pair fited them babies, so if it isn't any bother, if you would send me the other's you have there, and other little clothes by mail and I will pay postage. I am so glad these fited them even a little large. Mrs Johnson any time you have little clothes for my babies, do please send them out, I don't know how I will thank you. Hoping to hear from you soon. Thank you and bye bye.

A former clinic worker, after "retiring" from the MHA to full-time motherhood, wrote, "I congratulate you on having creat[ed] an organization with such an atmosphere. It has been a great pleasure to be associated with it." In a similar vein, a Cleveland widow and former MHA client sent a long, newsy letter, in which she told of feeling "so lost and alone I did not care to go on" after her husband's death. She then informed the clinic that she was engaged to an old flame and was happy again. The widow gratefully wrote:

> I am telling you all this because you have always been so kind to me I feel like you are a real Friend to me.
>
> I would like to come up for an examination just befor I am to be married and belong to your association again for I know I would not care for that worry of your children and my children and our children. I think three will [be] hard enough to raise and raise them well without any more added on Don't you? I hope this letter doesnt sound foolish to you and I do know you like to know your patients well and understand them in all ways. Thats what I like so well about you. . . .
>
> I remain your grateful Friend.

Such close attention to the physical and emotional needs of clients often characterized other female reform efforts of the era. Historian Molly

Ladd-Taylor notes that U.S. Children's Bureau staff sometimes sent gifts at their own expense to women who requested child care information. Ladd-Taylor recognizes that the bureau "functioned more like a distant relative than a government agency" at these times. The bureau's personal attention evoked a similarly intimate response from its clients.[46]

Not all MHA clients appreciated such a high level of concern. A few resentfully interpreted this personal approach as prying. One angry woman from a town outside of Cleveland vented her frustration in two typewritten pages. In the following excerpt, she referred to the intimate nature of the client interview.

> In the first place, I object to your third degree. You ask questions which you have no business knowing, no business asking. Probably you feel justified in knowing everything about a person you have on charity. But I question even that. If a person must be embarrassed answering personal questions, then anything you give in return is well paid for and could not be considered charity. . . .
>
> I came very unsuspectingly to you to buy a few tubes of antiseptic jelly. In [another city] I had religiously bought my jelly from the Clinic, even though at times it was rather inconvenient, because I knew of the very nice profit there was for you in it, and felt that it was one way of reciprocating. The nurse who interviewed me was extremely unpleasant, and she asked me why I didn't get my supplies at the drug store, a thing which I have since decided to do.

This correspondent resented the clinic's inquiry into her finances: "I could have gone to any doctor and had him perform a major operation without answering the questions you asked." She also objected to the nurse's insistence on a physical examination, claiming to have been recently examined elsewhere. Angry about waiting, as she described it, "wasting an hour of my time—which happens by the way to be just as precious as yours," the client felt exploited. She explained the lack of complaints by other MHA clients as resulting from female backwardness, saying, "Women will always humiliate themselves to gain an end."

Such objections, however articulately expressed, represent an anomaly in this clinic's collection of correspondence. The choice of letters saved by MHA staff may be partly responsible. There is no way to know how many women left the clinic dissatisfied other than from the MHA's own figures. Between March 1931 and March 1932, the Maternal Health Association reported that 166 women, or 15 percent, failed to complete their instruction in the technique, and 15 percent of all the patients who finished the "training" that year had discontinued the method. The existing criticisms from clients do indicate that some women perceived a condescending attitude on the part of MHA staff if not the clinic as a whole.[47]

Staff description and categorization of some clients in reports and other sources confirms that a judgmental outlook coexisted with womanly concern. For example, a 1931 report on unintended pregnancies among MHA clientele shifts from objective reporting to subjective interpretation, describing the new mothers as "lazy and ignorant," "apparently too shiftless to care," "careless," "questionable mentally," and "difficult" or "moderately difficult."[48] The MHA scrapbook containing its correspondence reveals something of the way the clinic viewed the women it served. Staff arranged the client letters under these headings:

> Failures
> Failures-Man Objects
> Failures-Religion
> Poor Background of Patients
> Planned Pregnancies
> Cooperative Spirit of Patients
> Good Reactions to Method
> Lack of Funds
> Requests for Help or Information.[49]

Labeling clients as "cooperative" and pregnancies as "failures" (of the woman or of the method, one wonders) indicates an appraisal of spirit if not character. Two categories in this list, Poor Background of Patients (rather than simply Background) and Lack of Funds, disclose an emphasis on—and judgment of—the poor. Other social service agencies, especially those serving the less privileged, often displayed such disdain. A 1935 speech on interviewing, filed with other MHA talks, reveals contradictory attitudes that some social workers held toward clients. On the one hand, the speaker explains, since clients often have psychological problems, it is critical that they identify with the social worker's (alleged) higher level of stability. On the other hand, the speaker claims that the social worker should not intervene in a client's life until asked to do so. Both nationally and locally, social workers and others who provided charitable service vacillated between condescending professional rhetoric and nurturing acts of concern for client welfare.[50] Efficiency sometimes conflicted with the demands of personal service.

Client letters describing contraceptive failures or a lack of understanding the contraceptive technique reveal the MHA's predilection to judge clients' behavior. Some of these letters appear above. A suburban woman wrote, "We have a nice baby girl, that makes 2 boys and 2 girls and that also makes enough. So I had better take care of myself. Please if I come back don't scold me. I am ashamed of myself." Another embarrassed client hid her pregnancy from a clinic worker.

> I'd like you to know that I realize what a fool I've been. Even the last time you were down I lied to you. I am pregnant again . . . I have felt so ashamed of being pregnant again, Ive even avoided my mother. But I had a long talk with the nurse at the Maternity Clinic and Ive promised her I'd return to your clinic as soon as I'm well, I don't even want to wait six weeks if I can help it. . . . Cause I really want to come, I can't possibly have any more children.

Filled with shame for her unintended pregnancy and unable even to confide in her mother, this woman shares her despair with an MHA nurse in order to have the chance to try and protect herself from yet another pregnancy. A cryptic note from another beleaguered mother expresses similar sentiments, "I have had a misscarriage so this explains the delay. Appreciate your interest and letter beyond words. I seem to be the world's champion fool, would like to return to the clinic if this is agreable." Women blamed themselves for contraceptive failures or for not using the diaphragm correctly. Their humiliation and the fear that they would be chastised, in part a reaction to medical authority, also implies a disciplining and perhaps disdainful posture on the part of clinic staff.[51]

Correspondence from women who needed care for other health problems manifests a lack of understanding on the part of the MHA physicians who had diagnosed these conditions. Many mothers found it difficult to obtain the extra medical attention that the clinic doctor suggested. The MHA advised one woman from a town south of Cleveland to seek help for her "protruding piles." Months later, the woman wrote to explain why she had not come to the clinic for her yearly checkup: she could not afford to see a physician for that problem. "I haven't the money to go to a doctor and there is no free clinic out here," she wrote. "Between embarrassment over the piles, lack of funds and no way to get in [to town] on clinic days I don't know what to do." Another client told of a potentially serious situation involving what looked to the MHA physician like precancerous lesions. This woman spelled out her reasons for not coming back to the birth control clinic as scheduled: "I have not been able to have the ulcers treated as [the doctor] said I should. I have tried most every way to find money to go for treatment but so far I have not found a way . . .

unless you have the money such treatment is impossible." The woman went on to say, "The Doctor was rather cross because I had not had this done before."

Both of these MHA clients worried about their particular physical conditions. Their financial inability to correct the health problems embarrassed them, however, and a fear of being judged made them reluctant to face the doctor who diagnosed the anomalies in the first place. Gaylord and other MHA staff who touted the MHA as a cancer prevention service ignored the financial challenges and other obstacles that kept many clients from attending to their personal health concerns outside of the birth control clinic.

Maternal Health Association clients felt disgrace at their ignorance or an unintended pregnancy, but no evidence suggests that they felt ashamed of actually using of birth control. Naturally, these mothers expressed some fear of the unknown and concern about the diaphragm's effectiveness. As one concerned woman explained, "Now if it is just safe allways everything will be fine but I still worry." None of the women represented in these letters displayed any shame or guilt about procuring or using birth control, however. In contrast to their attitudes about abortion, the women represented in these letters do not connect illegality or obscenity with their contraceptive actions or with the actions or services of the MHA.[52] Women acted out of the exigencies of their own lives and construed law and ethics based on intimate reality. In the area of reproductive policy in Cleveland and across the United States, a wide gulf separated law and the public moral code from personal experience.

A similar discontinuity prevailed in religious matters. About 17 percent of the MHA clients in 1929 were Catholic (as opposed to about 21 percent of Cleveland's general population at that time). Yet none of the letters in this group of over two hundred speak of a conflict with Catholic doctrine. Despite a 1930 papal encyclical condemning birth control, the two references in these letters to contraception as a sin do not refer to Catholicism. One represents a fundamentalist view but does not provide other details.[53] A Cleveland woman told the MHA: "I am writting to you to let you no why I am not down there this morning my Husban become a relious man since I was there and we lost one of our girls by a fire and We think it may be wrong for us to use the protation [protection] but I want to thank you for your help. and I will be sending your money soon." The second reference to faith matters appears in a record of a home visit by MHA staff. The following rather sarcastic description is included in the scrapbook of client letters, under Failure-Religion:

[The case worker or nurse quotes the mother:] "when you get convicted the Lord takes care of you so now I trust in the Lord." Oldest child 14, youngest 8 (4 children). one boy had infantile paralysis and girl born with club feet and dislocated hip, had bone trouble (increasing). . . . W[oman]'s church (Pentecostal) tells her it is a sin to prevent a germ from forming a child. W's sister has received (presumably from the Lord) her fifth baby. . . . Is convicted it is a sin to use method. . . . Record to be closed, religion.

Obviously MHA clients as a whole represented a motivated group, already convinced of the necessity if not the legitimacy of contraception despite legal or religious prohibitions. Some Roman Catholic parishioners and at least a few priests blatantly disregarded their church's teachings on contraception and the papal ruling—just as many people of all faiths disregarded the Comstock Law.

In 1939 Katherine Horner, R.N., a graduate student at Western Reserve University's School of Applied Social Sciences, closely studied ten MHA "cases." In one situation Horner found that a priest had tacitly sanctioned if not approved one Catholic couple's family limitation plans, perhaps moved by the wife's tubercular condition. Other Catholics in the same study experienced a difference of opinion among their religious leaders. For example, one woman explained that her own priest had tolerated the couple's use of contraception but that her husband's priest, an older man, took an opposing viewpoint. The older priest was, as the woman described it, "very much annoyed. He told him [her husband] we should have waited twenty-five years to marry if necessary rather than to use any such protection."[54] The prevalent cultural tensions around sexuality and the control of reproduction, between rhetoric and reality, reverberated within religious communities as well as the secular world. In the midst of this melee of conflicting messages, many couples sought guidance from clergy but then acted in their own best interest. Others simply ignored religious proscriptions and did what they felt was necessary to maintain their health and keep their families solvent.

In addition to women's commitment and matter-of-fact attitudes toward birth control, this collection of correspondence underscores other characteristic features of the MHA's clientele in the clinic's first decade. Often housebound and constrained by personal circumstances, many women faced considerable challenges in their quest for birth control. Yet some actively sought out and gratefully accepted the clinic's family limitation services when they could do so. The letter writers shouldered most of the heavy responsibility of managing homes and families. This coincides with historians' logical conclusions that the Great Depression added financial burdens and other tasks to women's usual familial duties.[55] Even if they worked outside of the home, the women made the child care arrangements, nursed ill family members, and scheduled visits to the MHA around their working hours and those of their husbands, paydays, or the availability of babysitters. A Cleveland woman preparing for a family move requested the MHA staff to "please pass this message along to the doctor, as I am so occupied during the day and in the evening. Even now my Son is hovering around grasping for the pen, and jerking the writing sheet, the reason for this unkempt page."

Mothers faced all types of difficulties in their attempts to limit family size, many of these associated with the problems and demands of daily life. One woman reported to the clinic that thieves had broken into her home and stolen "some strange things for a housebreaker. . . . Two blankets, a quilt, a large box of Kotex, and the first pessary I obtained was taken." Lucky for the client, already distraught from "foreclosure and sickness," she was "wearing the second one [diaphragm] at the time." Another client apologized for not returning to the MHA sooner and related a different kind of mishap: "One day when my family was under quarantine, I discovered that I had put my pessary, wrapped in a towel, in the washing machine. I used another method but it failed." Since women relied on their diaphragms for peace of mind and body, many endeavored to get accustomed to them outside of the bedroom.

One woman writes of perfecting her contraceptive technique but describes an unfortunate accident:

> Something terrible has happened, I misplaced that specery you see I had it in that same brown paper bag in the bathroom. I didn't put it away because I was putting it on twice a day—practicing how to put it on—and when I went to get it one morning I couldn't find it no where I looked and looked all over the house I caint find it. I think it was picked up and thrown out in paper basket and burned. So when I was to come down I didn't know what to do. I was to come in with it on, so I thought I better write first and you could mail me a card with an appointment on it for after the 24th because he gets paid the 22th. I am willing to pay a doctor for that one I was to bring down. I'm so terrible ashamed of myself of such carelessness I'm sorry. But what can I do. I caint find it. so send me a card with an appointment. please try to make it in the afternoon its so hard to get away in the morning with the little baby please. and I'll be down with the $2.15 For those things.
>
> Thank you.

Facing such daily struggles, mothers still found ways to obtain and use birth control.

If an MHA client could not get to the Osborn building for follow-up supplies, she often sent a brother, sister, husband, or friend. The reasons given for not returning to the clinic ran the gamut: "My husband has been ill"; "I have had poison oak"; "The children . . . have blood poisoning"; "I had a nervous breakdown"; "I don't have the carfare"; "I've been working two jobs"; "I work every Saturday"; "Mother broke her arm"; or "I have an ingrown toenail and cannot wear shoes." Some women felt too ashamed of their appearance to venture out to the MHA. One client summed up her particular obstacles: "I lacked carfare, lacked time, and lacked clothing."[56]

Despite the financial, travel, and other problems, however, these women welcomed and gratefully accepted the MHA's services. They actively sought the information they needed and made intricate arrangements to take care of themselves. Women's agency as clients sustained and pushed the birth control movement forward. Viewing contraception as a practical necessity, MHA clients and other women across America took control of their health and that of their families. One MHA client wrote from a sanatorium: "Within the next two months I expect to be discharged—apparently quite well. After that time I am sure to need the services of the Maternal Clinic. In fact I look forward to your help eagerly—my future holds no fear because of the method." These women acted out of a need for physical, psychological, and economic relief from the demands of large families.

Unlike MHA founders and staff, clients did not mention eugenic concerns or other broad philosophies as reasons for limiting their families. In fact, most women who wrote to the clinic did not go into elaborate explanations. The women would instead have agreed with these simple statements from others in similar situations: "I have had my hands full of trouble this summer" or "My husband wont let me rest at night" or "Things are not going so good right now." One woman who found herself pregnant, unexpectedly, fumed to the MHA nurse, "I am getting relief from S. S. and when I take the rent out, I haven't nothing left I hate to think of getting another baby, but I have to . . . hope it never happen again." Facing the harsh exigencies of life in the Great Depression, Cleveland women hopefully turned to the birth control facility for practical assistance. They wanted to improve the circumstances of their day-to-day existence. Maternal Health Association leaders, on the other hand, claimed that the motivations of clinic clients coincided closely with eugenics: "The Maternal Health Association is used by men and women who are thinking in terms

of the next generation and are trying to assure their children the best physical and mental heritage."[57] Such claims helped to promote and legitimize
the clinic's work but ignored the basic reality of many women's lives.

Mothers sought the services of the MHA in order to space their pregnancies. Most responded gratefully. One woman wrote in 1936, "I can
really say I have done the one thing she [the doctor] has been telling me.
My Baby will be 5 years old the 27th of this month. So for this I am
thankful." Even those who left the MHA expressed gratitude, as did this
woman from a town about thirty miles from Cleveland: "I am sorry to say
I will be unable to continue your methods. May I thank you a thousand
times for your kindness and personal interest in the past, also your much
needed help at the time it was needed so badly. I shall never forget you or
your associates." Two women expressed their thanks most succinctly. One
wrote, "I think there's nothing like it." Another exclaimed, "Hubby and I
think it's swell. Thanks to you."

## HUBBIES AND FATHERS

While the MHA directed most of its services to "worried wives and
mothers," it also attended to "hubbies" and fathers. In January 1931 the
clinic initiated a Men's Consultation Service. In order to educate men
about female anatomy, conception, and contraception, the MHA set
aside one night a week for husbands of clients to confer with male physicians. While staff welcomed any men to these consultations, clinic physicians specifically referred husbands of clients only "in selected and difficult cases." Maternal Health Association staff members also spoke about
the clinic's work to groups of clergy and lawyers, and at men's organizations. In 1938 they invited local businessmen, clergy, lawyers, and heads
of social agencies to luncheons in the Osborn building office. Despite
warnings in the advance publicity that "this was no sit-down affair with
hearty food," fifteen to thirty men at a time came to the MHA to learn
more about the clinic and birth control methods—and to enjoy a buffet
lunch of "thick meat sandwiches . . . , cheese, and doughnuts." The first
four events attracted a waiting list of over a hundred.[58] Although other
clinics across the country also tried to interest men in their work, these
men's luncheons may have been unique to Cleveland. In 1937 and 1938
the meals and the men's consultation service received national attention
in articles written by Gladys Gaylord in the *Birth Control Review* and by
Charles Higley, M.D., in the *Journal of Contraception*.[59] The MHA
offered woman-centered clinics and services but recognized the need to
involve and educate men.

Private North American birth control clinics promoted the feminization of contraception as well as its medicalization, beginning in the 1920s. The public over-the-counter trend headed in the opposite direction, emphasizing men's responsibility for contraception while continuing to court the attention of women, who most often purchased contraceptive devices. Condom sales increased after World War I, and the popularity of that method grew. Many men actively participated in the struggle to limit family size. Advocates and clinic leaders countered this trend in part to place the control of reproduction into the hands of women. Along with some physicians, they employed feminist arguments used in the nineteenth-century voluntary motherhood movement, depicting all men as unreliable and irresponsible in the area of sexual relations, especially sexual control.[60] While some husbands did in fact display such a disreputable character in the bedroom, other men joined their wives in the effort to control reproduction.

Spouses of clients occasionally contacted the MHA themselves to inquire about services or answer a query. One example is the letter cited in chapter 1, from the man who reported that his wife had not yet used the diaphragm because her brother did not believe in it.[61] After reading a book entitled *Facts and Frauds in Feminine Hygiene,* another man wrote from a Cleveland suburb to the American Birth Control League in New York City to inquire about the existence of a clinic in Cleveland. He reasoned, "We have one child and would like to limit our family to that for a while and at the same time take away the fear when we have marital relations." The ABCL forwarded his query to the Cleveland MHA. A Kentucky gentleman sent his request directly to the MHA: "I'm to be married in February and it is quite desirable that I have no children for two or three years. I am 23; my wife is 19. Please send or tell us the safest, sanest, and most practical method, etc. Thank you very much in advance." Occasionally men came to the men's consultations, called "night clinics," to find out about the MHA services before their wives began to utilize the clinic.[62] Obviously the MHA's nurturing extended to potential male supporters and spouses of clients: a few men felt comfortable enough (or curious enough) to come to lunch, utilize the consultation service, or correspond with the clinic.

The three letters cited in the paragraph above reveal ways in which the MHA related to its male constituents. The correspondence also attests to the powerful impact of public controversy and suspicion about contraception. The first correspondent makes clear that his family members and friends discussed the pros and cons of birth control itself, if not this particular couple's personal plans to limit their family size. The Kentucky man demonstrates familiarity with the common language about contraception in the 1930s and perhaps an acquaintance with popular literature on the topic. Two advice books of the period included the words "sane" and "safe" in their titles, describing the ideal marriage: *Sane Sex Life and Sane Sex Living* by H. W. Long (1919) and *Safe Counsel or Practical Eugenics* by B. G. Jefferis and J. L. Nichols (1925). Jefferis and Nichols actually employ the phrase "safe and sane" in their book to describe preferred methods of contraception (though, in order to abide by the Comstock Law, they do not provide any details).[63] The male letter-writers noted here demonstrate a familiarity with such language. Their communications disclose that concerns about birth control did not lie solely in woman's sphere.

The MHA increased its services for men between 1930 and 1940. The 1935–36 annual report stated, "Partly through the interest of the Men's Committee and partly because of the opinions expressed by social workers and others connected with industrial problems, greater emphasis is being placed on the man's attitude toward planned pregnancies and his responsibility for the mental and physical heritage of his children." Two years later the association's annual report included for the first time a section entitled "Projects for Men" and boasted "greater participation of *men* in clinic activities" as "an outstanding feature" of that year's work. The 1937–38 report says that 63 clergymen, male physicians, lawyers, and social workers attended the men's luncheons and that 245 patients used the men's consultation service. The report claims that more male physicians and social workers conferred about clinic services than in previous years, more men came in for supplies, and men took a more active part in fund-raising. The MHA began to give the husband of each new patient his own appointment card "so that he may use clinic service anytime." The association reported the addition of twenty-two men as members of the corporation in 1937–38 as proof of the clinic's attempts to broaden its masculine appeal.[64] An MHA lecturer pointed out in 1940, "The spacing of children is not a problem for women alone. It is usually the husbands who control the size of the family and unless we can carry the understanding of the men of our community, no program of this kind is going to be generally adopted."[65]

Birth control leaders Marie Stopes in England and Margaret Sanger in the United States received letters indicating that men shared their wives' interest in contraception. Men corresponded with Stopes and Sanger on a regular basis, though not as often as women. These men spoke in direct language, displaying no embarrassment or disdain. In addition to inquiring about contraception, they asked intimate questions about impotence, the propriety of certain sexual practices, penis size, and fertility. Some men wrote to express disapproval on moral grounds or to complain about failures of the diaphragm. Others showed respect for their partners and responsibility for their own role in preventing procreation.[66]

## "There is trouble brewing"

Unfortunately, such empathetic men represent the minority in the MHA collection of correspondence. Even for sensitive men, a distinct difference existed between them and their wives in the experience of birth control. While women surprised MHA staff with their willingness to discuss sexual matters, most men who came to the clinic represented the opposite extreme. In an early report of the MHA Men's Department, clinic physician John Hess explained, "Probably the greatest impediment in consultations with men is their natural or acquired backwardness in speaking frankly about sex relations. This reserve establishes a real barrier which it is difficult to overcome."[67] Perhaps it was easier for some men to express themselves on paper to relatively anonymous national leaders like Stopes or Sanger than to speak face-to-face about intimate matters with someone of their own gender in their own city.

Several women wrote to the MHA that they had decided not to use contraception at all because of their husbands. The clinic categorized such letters as Failure-Man Objects. As one potential MHA client explained, "I am not going to keep the appointment I have with you for Thursday. My husband wants me to drop it and in order to have peace in my home I must. Some day he may change his mind and I shall come to see you then." Another woman described a similar situation in her home: "I am sorry that I put you to so much trouble in trying to see me, but I have changed my mind as my Husband does Not think much of the idea. Will you please let me know if I should brings back [the things that] the doctor gave me. I have not used them at all." One woman bowed to her husband's wishes for additional family:

> I'm writing to tell you not to put me out of the clinic for I still want to be one of the members of it. for I took your method for 5½ years and it has helped me but my husband has a job and wants me to have one more baby so I am writing to tell you I am pregnant 4 mos and expect to have her the first week in May. Please answer me and tell me that I can still be one of your members when I get over this. Thank you.

Another woman explicitly blamed herself for contraceptive failure but implied that her marital relationship was the real problem:

I am ansering your letter sorry I didn't write sooner it isn't necessary for me
to come back as I have been pregnant for three months now
dont think it is your fault for it isent it is mine for being big enough D-F
for sleeping with such a man
so forget me sorry
and so long
better luck next time
maybe

Influenced by cultural as well as personal factors, some women relin-
quished sexual and reproductive control to the demands of their male
partners, and some men misused the power of that control.

In the MHA letters that mention unintended pregnancies, women
sometimes explicitly blamed their husbands, apparently with good reason.
One man burned his wife's diaphragm, according to her account, claiming that it was her duty to bear children. Another would not let his wife
use birth control because he feared that she would be promiscuous.
Nonetheless, he himself refused to use the condoms provided by the
MHA physician.[68] The most popular natural contraceptive methods,
abstinence and withdrawal, held obvious disadvantages for men. Despite
this situation, men often objected to other so-called mechanical methods
of contraception such as the diaphragm. "My husband is getting surly and
there is trouble brewing," wrote one woman requesting information from
the ABCL.[69] Unaffected by pregnancy and childbearing and much less
involved in child rearing than their wives, some husbands ignored the natural consequences of intercourse and displayed disregard for their offspring as well. One rural woman graphically depicted this attitude in a letter printed in the *Birth Control Review* in 1930: "I am a poor woman,
living in a very poor farming section. Children come by the dozen. If they
live, they live—if they die they die. There are men down here who don't
think any more about burying a baby than about burying a hog."[70]

Facing such callous attitudes, in some cases women lied to or tricked
their husbands in order to continue to space their pregnancies. There is
some evidence that MHA staff went along with this, condoning if not
encouraging the practice. The clinic tried to work with an uncooperative
spouse, offering opportunities for consultation and suggesting other
methods of contraception. If those initiatives did not succeed, however,
the staff talked with the woman about her husband's objections, "letting
her decide whether she will continue the protection without his knowledge." The diaphragm lent itself well to this type of subterfuge: the
woman controlled its use and could employ it without her partner's

knowledge. One woman said that, in response to her husband's complaint about his discomfort when she used the device, "I told him I don't use it no more and now it don't hurt him no more." In fact she lied and continued to use the diaphragm faithfully. She kept up the charade for at least nine years with plenty of motivation: she already had borne eleven children. As she approached menopause, this mother elaborated further on her lack of compliance at home. She explained matter-of-factly, "My husband says now, 'You don't need to go down there [the MHA] anymore, you won't have any more babies now.' But I'll come 'til you people tell me to stop."[71] Because of her success with the diaphragm as well as the gender bond, this client trusted the MHA more than her marital partner, at least in reproductive matters.

These surreptitious actions reflected the woman-centered nature of most U.S. clinical contraceptive methods of the period—and the woman-centered experience of pregnancy and childbirth. One mother expressed the burdens of that experience: "I worrie so much I almost go insane." Since the nineteenth century, advertisers often had touted means of family limitation on the basis of female control. Some ads encouraged duplicity, claiming, for example, that husbands "would hardly be likely to know that it [the contraceptive] was being used." The feminist roots of the birth control cause inspired some providers and proponents to tacitly or overtly approve and even advise secretive efforts by women to control their reproduction.[72] The wives and would-be mothers themselves, faced with harsh reality that differed greatly from moralistic rhetoric, chose the most practical course.

MHA clients viewed birth control as a necessity rather than a crime. Perhaps this was due in part to the legal practice of punishing contraceptive distributors rather than users (similar to that of punishing abortion providers rather than the women seeking abortions).[73] The reason also lay in the commonplace nature of childbirth and the prevention of conception in a woman's life. While cultural factors affected access to contraception, a woman's personal experience of birth control differed from legal and medical policy, from principles of eugenics or social science, from male experience, and from public pronouncements.

Although the particular segment of MHA clientele represented in this collection of correspondence does not depict the whole population, the written record does illuminate the nature of some women's experience with contraception. Almost all of these clients express tremendous gratitude for the services offered. Most describe the MHA as generally nurturing and caring. In their letters women remind us of the eternal binding nature of women's household responsibilities, responsibilities that often conflict with or mitigate the cultural expectations of women as happy mothers of better babies and fitter families. The correspondence clearly demonstrates the determination with which some women took charge of their reproductive lives because of and in spite of extremely trying situations. These communications also reveal differing and changing male and female experiences of sexuality, contraception, childbirth, and child rearing.

MHA founders correctly perceived women's need and desire for contraception but misinterpreted their motives. Separated from their clients by privilege, advocates and leaders underestimated the strong motivation of living in desperate straits. Struggling to keep home and family solvent on a daily basis, clients gratefully welcomed clinic services for very different reasons than the lofty ideals posited by the MHA. Using whatever means necessary, some women even deceived their husbands in order to control childbearing. Many Cleveland-area mothers made elaborate arrangements to obtain and continue to use birth control. Their dedication surprised and impressed clinic leaders, who in turn supported clients' efforts. Women's eager acceptance of clinical birth control, unfettered by concerns about legality or morality, contributed greatly to the success of this clinic and others across North America.

Gender affected the way clients and their spouses experienced birth control. So also did gender issues shape the ways in which clients and leaders sustained the Cleveland Maternal Health Association, the subject of the next chapter. To ensure the clinic's future, MHA leaders employed whatever means seemed the most practical at the moment, from sponsoring classy public events to participating in surreptitious civil disobedience.

# 5

## *Friends of the Movement*

Cleveland MHA leaders maintained and nurtured the pioneer birth control clinic in a variety of very different ways, from transporting diaphragms in their luggage to organizing ice skating galas. Rather than adhere to a fixed plan of outreach over the clinic's first decade, these women chose paths that seemed practical and productive. The MHA interacted with the city as a discreet collaboration between and among individuals and organizations. Women of community stature and with experience in social organizing established the Cleveland Maternal Health Association. Founders and leaders employed networks to garner clinic clients and ensure stability. Strong connections resulting from social status and experience in the voluntary sector supported nontraditional acts as well as more common fund-raising activities.

Clients in turn sustained the low-profile MHA with referrals through their own channels. Clients and founders alike informally manipulated webs of relationship to their advantage. The effort evolved from women's daily lives, alliances, and actions in other reform causes.

### FAMILY TIES, GENDER BONDS

Family networks among local MHA trustees, introduced in chapter 2, played a critical role in the clinic's founding. They also supplied credibility and helped ensure longevity for the new venture. During the Maternal Health Association's first decade, family ties existed among many of its trustees. By recruiting their mothers, sisters, daughters, in-laws, and spouses as board members, clinic leaders followed the pattern set by founders Dorothy Brush and Hortense Shepard. Relatives often shared views on social issues and supported each other's causes. In Susan Ostrander's study of the voluntary activities of Cleveland's wealthy women, participants mention their duty to society, their obligation to give back some of what they possessed, and the importance of carrying on the family tradition. As in other cities, upper-class Cleveland families passed on to their progeny a sense of responsibility to improve the welfare of the less fortunate. Ostrander also notes the significance of class for her group of volunteers. Supporting certain causes helped to create and preserve class consensus among upper-class families. Just as the interlocking relationship with the Brush Foundation and the Brush family helped to inaugurate and sustain the MHA, other kinship ties provided a close-knit base for the clinic.[1]

Among the MHA's fifty-seven original board members, at least sixteen, or 28 percent, were related to at least one other board member (excluding their spouses). Many of these people had two or more relatives on the board. The constellations included mothers and their daughters or daughters-in-law, sisters and sisters-in-law, aunts and nieces. The Brush family connections have already been explored (see chapter 2). In another example of the various kinship bonds at work in this organization, Roberta Holden Bole served on the first MHA board with her sister, Delia Holden White, and niece, Delia White Vail (who was married to state legislator Herman L. Vail). White and Vail, in turn, were the sister-in-law and niece (respectively) of another charter board member, Ella White Ford.[2]

Within a few years of its founding, the MHA board of trustees included even more relatives. The White family, whose wealth derived in part from the White Sewing Machine Company (later White Motor Company) dramatically expanded its involvement in the association, with eight additional relatives serving as trustees in 1934. Another family, the Eells clan, had begun to participate on the MHA board by 1929, represented by Maud Stager Eells and her daughter-in-law, Adele Chisholm Eells. By 1934 Maud's daughter and son-in-law, Maud Eells Corning and Warren Corning, had joined the MHA ranks.[3]

Memoirs and biographies such as *Cleveland's Golden Years* and *A Long Way Forward: The Biography of Francis Payne Bolton* make clear the import of blood ties to the local business and social relationships of the community. Looking at the larger picture, scholar Francie Ostrower explores the relationship between philanthropy and elites. Among other things, she says, donors develop strong personal commitments to certain causes and organizations. Family connections with a particular charity often lie at the base of those commitments. Ostrower explains, "Involvement with particular organizations becomes part of the donors' own identity." As one Cleveland volunteer told Susan Ostrander, "I did the things my grandmother and my mother did, and so it was a tradition, and it was good." The extensive familial involvement in the Cleveland Maternal Health Association and its successor, Planned Parenthood of Greater Cleveland, arose out of this phenomenon, which Peter Hall calls the "culture of trusteeship."[4] The connections among relatives and across generations stabilized the association and became part of its corporate identity. In building a strong foundation, the MHA also crossed gender lines.

Created at a time when the character of women's organizations was changing across the country, from its founding onward the Maternal Health Association included men as well as women on the board and as corporation members. Of the fifty-seven original MHA board members, eighteen, or almost one-third, were men. The wives of all but five of these men also served as MHA trustees. With such a constituency, the Maternal Health Association embodied a step in the evolution of women's associations in the United States. All-female groups of the nineteenth century had at times depended on men for public leadership and authority, and women in the mixed-gender organizations of the mid-twentieth century often gave up the reins of leadership to men or were pushed into subordinate positions.[5] In board composition and governance, the MHA of the 1920s and 1930s lay in the middle of this spectrum. Examining the original MHA board in terms of gender and class provides insight into the choices of founders and early leaders. These choices affected the organization's direction.

Records indicate that female professionals and volunteers handled the day-to-day operation of the MHA, as stated earlier. Nurses and female social workers interviewed clients, directed the clinic, and conducted home visits. Women physicians performed examinations and dispensed birth control, while male physicians conducted the consultations for men. Women volunteers kept records, helped with correspondence and reports, took charge of the lending library, decorated and furnished the suite, cared for the children of clinic patients in the office nursery, and made telephone calls. Maternal Health Association leaders, employees, and volunteers organized, managed, and staffed fund-raising events. Between 1928 and 1933 women held all MHA offices except assistant treasurer and second vice president; for many years afterward men did not hold any association offices.[6] Looking at the occupations of male MHA charter board members helps to develop a clearer picture of the group's social foundations.

Thirteen men served with their wives on the first MHA board. This group included three lawyers, three physicians, five businessmen, an architect, and an engineer. By including these men and others as members, the MHA associated itself with local hospitals such as Lakeside; the city's health department; and the School of Medicine of Western Reserve University. Other connections linked the organization with prestigious law firms including Thompson, Hine and Flory; local industries such as Great Lakes Engineering; banks such as Union Trust; and civic groups such as the Cleveland Chamber of Commerce.[7] The broad range of affiliation among MHA trustees and their spouses sustained the clinic with support in a variety of professional venues. In securing its first board, the MHA tapped into the city's sources of power. The group used such a tactic, common to the founding of voluntary organizations, not only to gain influence but also to downplay its connections with a questionable social movement.

In 1935 the MHA restructured its administration. Until that point the clinic had simply added each of its new supporters to the existing board of trustees. By 1934 the board had become quite cumbersome, at 235 people. The association established a new category of supporters by 1936, dubbed "members of the corporation." The 1935–36 MHA annual report lists five officers and eighteen people on the board of trustees, a much more manageable group in terms of size. The report designates the rest of the over two hundred people involved as members of the corporation. Between 1936 and 1942 the board remained small, around twenty-five, and the members of the corporation continued to increase in number, to 395 by 1942.[8]

The MHA built its first board on the familial and social connections of the founders and their husbands. After the restructuring, MHA women strategically kept the power of policy making as well as daily management of the clinic in female hands. Between 1936 and 1960 the smaller MHA board of trustees consisted solely of women. Their spouses and male relatives and friends served as members of the corporation rather than trustees. From 1934 until 1966 men did not hold any MHA office outside of the all-male Medical Advisory Board.[9] With that notable exception, women led the MHA throughout the clinic's first decades. They purposefully claimed and maintained the control of the board of trustees and its leadership positions. Maternal Health Association annual reports, historical accounts, talks, and correspondence do not specifically proclaim its identity as a woman's group. However, the documents do focus almost exclusively on the achievements of the female founders and leaders and the characteristics of the clinic's female clientele. An MHA officer concluded in 1960 that the MHA "has always been a women's organization." The women of the Cleveland Maternal Health Association focused on a reform critical to other women. They considered their voluntary health association a women's effort and acted accordingly.[10]

No evidence links MHA leaders with organized feminism. They did not identify themselves as feminists nor did their contemporaries. But within their own cultural constraints, they fit into a feminist framework. One historian defines feminism as "a critique of male supremacy, formed and offered in the light of a will to change it, which in turn assumes a conviction that it is changeable."[11] The MHA acted as a feminist catalyst. It stretched legal, medical, and social policy to benefit women yet remained firmly planted within the strictures of reverence for motherhood, preservation and enhancement of the white race, the constraints of social class, and the authority of physicians. Rather than pursuing political or legal action for contraception in the public arena, women in Cleveland and across North America acted individually and collectively in voluntary health associations out of common aspirations for control of private, reproductive rights. Although bound by popular cultural ideologies, these women implicitly, rather than explicitly, criticized male supremacy.

While leading the organization themselves, MHA founders and board members strategically sought a mixed-gender support base. As with the male charter board members mentioned above, they purposefully incorporated their husbands and other men into corporation membership if not leadership. Although each of these women could claim a certain social status, most of them did not hold professional positions themselves. Their marital relationships linked them to important financial, social service, and cultural institutions in the city and state. The very presence of distinguished community leaders such as their husbands within the MHA membership added weight and import to the association's actions and facilitated its search for support. It also aided the organization's quest for legitimacy.[12] Further pursuing this goal, the MHA turned to the city's religious community.

## COURAGEOUS CLERGY AND CONTROVERSY

One anonymous historical account reflects that the MHA sought "the advice and sponsorship . . . of the more courageous and liberal ministers of the city" in addition to social and public health agencies. The courageous clergy on the first MHA board all served upper-class or upper-middle-class congregations. The men included T. S. McWilliams, professor of religious education at Western Reserve University and former pastor of Calvary Presbyterian Church in Cleveland; Joel Hayden, pastor of Fairmount Presbyterian Church in Cleveland Heights; Ferdinand Q. Blanchard of Cleveland's Euclid Avenue Congregational Church; and Abba Hillel Silver, rabbi of Temple-Tifereth Israel, then the largest Jewish

Reform congregation in the country, located at Cleveland's University Circle. The Rev. Philip Smead Bird became a board member during the MHA's second year. He served as pastor of the Church of the Covenant (Presbyterian) near University Circle. Many Protestant pastors and some Jewish leaders across the country had expressed support for birth control. Debates on the topic raged at national meetings of religious organizations during the 1930s. Securing the backing of prominent clergy helped the MHA to create a basis on which to counter opposition from Roman Catholics and fundamentalists.[13]

In an intriguing twist, however, these clergy, all of whom were married, served on the first MHA board without their wives. In fact, in the whole group of clinic trustees, only one other man, Charles B. Sawyer, participated without his wife in the early years. (A close friend and business partner of Charles F. Brush Sr., Sawyer headed the Brush Beryllium Company.) The Rev. Dilworth Lupton of the First Unitarian Church of Cleveland was the sole clergyperson in the MHA's first two years who belonged to the board with his wife, Mary Helen Bell Lupton. The Rev. Bird, on the other hand, served the MHA without his spouse for eight years.[14]

It is unclear whether the MHA selected clergy as trustees, and not their wives, or whether the pastors chose to serve alone for the first couple of years. In either case the fact that clergy participated on the clinic's early board by themselves indicates the illicit nature of contraception. Due to the shady reputation of family limitation, the MHA recruited prominent religious leaders to add moral authority and an air of propriety to the cause. Social connections and family ties certainly provided a strong base on which the MHA could build and from which it could recruit other support. But the clinic also required a firm moral foundation to counteract possible charges of acting against faith precepts or the laws of nature. The critical need for a secure grounding within the city's Protestant and Jewish faith communities overrode the issue of class in this case.[15] These "courageous" pastors, wary of the potential social ramifications for their families, could well have been protecting the reputations of their wives by participating in the new venture by themselves at first.

The clergy spouses did not stay out of the endeavor for long, however. The 1931 MHA annual report lists Susan Nigpen McWilliams, Ethel West Blanchard, and Hazel Petty Hayden among its trustees. Virginia Horkheimer Silver became a member of the corporation during a 1937 MHA membership drive. Margaret Kincaid Bird joined the next year. Either the pastors had tested the clinic's legitimacy by this time and found it secure enough for their spouses, or their wives had insisted on being included. Probably both of these factors, together with the MHA's increasing stability and active search for new members, influenced the spouses to sign on and the clinic to welcome them.[16] Recruiting key area clergy who committed themselves to supporting the clinic's work began a long history of MHA involvement with local churches and synagogues. Meanwhile, religious conflict over birth control came to a head in the United States and in Catholic countries around the world.

On December 31, 1930, Pope Pius XI issued *Casti Connubii,* an encyclical that condemned every means of contraception including sterilization, for any reason. It was the first papal encyclical in fifty years. Only a few months before, in August of 1930, the Lambeth conference of Anglicans in Great Britain had turned from a similar position of opposition and adopted a resolution approving methods of family limitation as long as they were used morally and "in the light of Christian principles." The Catholic edict responded in part to the Lambeth report as evidence of a growing popular acceptance of contraception. Reactions to the Anglican and Catholic statements filled the national and local press.[17]

The furor spurred some Cleveland religious leaders to join others across the nation in speaking out on these intimate matters. Episcopal bishop Warren Lincoln Rogers sympathized with the Pope's statement and bemoaned that "conditions, even in America, are such as to make such a document necessary." Maternal Health Association board members Silver and Lupton disagreed. Silver stated that the Jewish tradition was not so "uncompromising" as that of the Roman Catholics. He told the *Plain Dealer,* "Judaism recognizes that there are situations where considerations of health and economic stress make the begetting of offspring dangerous and undesirable, and when birth control through contraception is the best solution for general marital well-being." Lupton employed stronger language, calling the Pope's declaration "unreasonable and unscientific." He posited, "Were his [the Pope's] decree carried out to the letter, society itself would be menaced." Other local pastors who commented favorably included Blanchard.[18] The 1931 news articles offering the comments of these religious leaders did not mention their involvement with the Maternal Health Association, but their public advocacy of the cause helped to strengthen the clinic's position nonetheless.

In Cleveland and other urban areas during this time, the birth control controversy found its way into pulpits on Saturday or Sunday mornings. In a sermon on marriage and the home at First Unitarian Church, the Rev. Lupton called for legalizing birth control in order to create smaller and better families. At the Euclid Avenue Temple (Anshe Chesed), Rabbi Barnett Brickner advocated for a state law legalizing the dissemination of birth control information by anyone, to anyone. In July 1930 visiting pastor and religious editor William H. Leach preached at the Lakewood Congregational Church. Having just returned from a trip to Great Britain, Leach said that English clergy had trouble comprehending "the particular prudery of America" in matters of contraception. He claimed that some English churches had actually established birth control clinics. While religious bodies in Cleveland did not go that far, their leaders continued to speak boldly and publicly about the subject. Blanchard countered Catholic arguments in a speech before the MHA annual meeting in 1931, calling birth control "a new step in man's attempt to regulate the ways of life in accordance with his highest intelligence."[19] The Cleveland Maternal Health Association used other strategies to promote such "regulation."

## NEXT-DOOR NEIGHBORS

In addition to inviting their marital partners, other relatives, and clergy to support and participate in the MHA, organizers also recruited neighbors, for many of the same reasons. All of the clinic's original board members with the exception of two Lakewood residents lived on the city's east side. The suburban east-side residential pattern among MHA's original trustees indicates once again their race—white—and socio-economic status—middle class, upper middle class, and upper class. In 1931, 66 percent of Cleveland-area residents in general who were named in the city's elite *Blue Book* lived in the eastern suburbs of Bratenahl, Cleveland Heights, East Cleveland, and Shaker Heights. During the 1920s and 1930s descendants of elite Euclid Avenue families often migrated to these new and growing areas as the former Millionaires' Row evolved from a posh residential neighborhood into a commercial district.[20] Steeped in traditions of obligation to the community and bolstered by family ties, many MHA board members also enjoyed geographical proximity.

Neighboring families would have been likely to be at ease with each other. Bound by similar experience and background, they held some attitudes, values, and commitments in common. Working together for social reform helped these citizens promote and sustain community standards and stability. Maternal Health Association leaders lived near each other in several east-side neighborhoods. For instance, in 1928 nine MHA trustee families (twelve trustees) lived within a two- to three-mile radius in the southeastern corner of Cleveland Heights. Only a few miles from University Circle, the new suburb had been designated a city in 1921 and attracted young white families.[21] Many of these folks could walk to each others' homes. They attended neighborhood luncheons, parties, and other social gatherings together. Five of these nine Cleveland Heights families had links to Millionaire's Row.[22]

Another cluster of seven MHA leaders enjoyed views of Lake Erie about six miles east of downtown Cleveland, in Bratenahl. Within the Cleveland city limits but incorporated as a separate village in 1903, Bratenahl had evolved from farmland into a tiny but wealthy community characterized by lakefront mansions. This contingent grew between 1930 and 1940 as more Holden and White relatives joined the MHA.[23] Four other MHA members lived in what was then a rural area near Mayfield and Richmond Roads. Of these last two groups, only two couples were not former Euclid Avenue residents or directly related to the same.[24] The small geographical area represented by each pocket of MHA trustees must have facilitated committee meetings, education and planning sessions, and the assignment and completion of volunteer tasks. Perhaps a few of these folks would not have been involved in the birth control venture at all were it not for their proximity to one or more of their heavily committed neighbors. Such networking is not limited to the privileged. Writing about the Ladies' Auxiliaries of labor unions in the 1930s, Sheila Rowbotham notes that the mobilization of working-class women was often based on their connections to families and neighbors rather than ideas about their own rights to equality or even their own welfare needs.[25] As one Cleveland woman explained motivations for voluntarism in another context, "People do things for people as well as causes."[26] MHA leaders acted out of both of these motivations.

## PROTECTED CARGO AND COMELY SKATERS

With a solid base in family, community, and neighborhood networks, the MHA directly but quietly challenged cultural mores around contraception. State and federal laws severely restricted the interstate commerce of devices for the prevention of conception. These regulations hampered the procurement of supplies for the MHA during its early years. The clinic ordered its stock wholesale from New York City companies but feared the risks of shipping diaphragms and spermicidal jelly to Cleveland. Buoyed by deep commitment, fierce determination, a sense of adventure, and some naivete, these birth control advocates confronted the problem directly but discreetly. Cleveland women utilized the business connections of their spouses and other family members and friends to undermine transportation restrictions and advance their cause.

Accompanying their husbands on business trips to New York City, MHA board members and volunteers—"any friend of the movement"—

carried empty suitcases onto the passenger trains. In New York suppliers filled the luggage with diaphragms and tubes of contraceptive jelly that the Clevelanders then took back to Ohio for clients of the MHA. Clinic supporters later remembered that they "never went to New York without calling Miss Volk to find out if supplies were needed and often came home with cartons piled high in their Pullman berths." Occasionally the contraband even boasted police protection. Such was the case when Frances Goff, widow of Cleveland Trust president Frederick Goff, traveled to New York. According to MHA historical accounts, the bank's police escort guarded MHA "valuables" in transit, along with Cleveland Trust's financial securities. A local business also facilitated the subterfuge. Morris Black, married to MHA trustee Lenore Black, presided over the fancy Lindner's department store in Cleveland. At his wife's request, Black and store buyers transported "packages" containing contraceptive items from New York into Ohio, along with the store's own merchandise. With physicians authorizing the purchases and private individuals rather than "public carriers" conveying the goods, these upstanding citizens convinced themselves that they had solved the supply problem "within the law."[27]

These actions directly contradicted the legal opinion that MHA founder Jerry Fisher had constructed in 1922 for the clinic's protection. The last sentence of the opinion states, "Not even a physician can legally use the mails, or common carriers in interstate commerce, for the conveyance of contraceptive information" (see figure 7, chapter 2). Passenger trains certainly qualified as common carriers. Yet some MHA leaders firmly remained convinced that carrying suitcases full of diaphragms and contraceptive jelly across state lines was legal. Their acts and beliefs embodied and reflected a deep confusion within legal policy involving the control of reproduction and in the popular interpretation of that policy. Despite the Comstock Law and its successors, Americans did not hold a united view on the regulation of sexuality or obscenity.

Statements by MHA founder Hortense Shepard convey the muddled state of the popular mindset during this era toward laws regulating contraception. In 1929, at the organizational meeting for the Middle Western States Birth Control Conference, Shepard explained the way that the MHA procured its supplies. She proudly—if naively—proclaimed:

> The Cleveland group is the only clinic that is operating without breaking any Federal and State law. We are doing that because we want to give the illustration that it could be done. We have someone who brings all our supplies back and forth on the train. People go individually. It may be ridiculous just

to prove that we can do that, but we are very interested in having something done about the Federal Law. If we preferred to pay higher prices for supplies, we could buy them, right in Cleveland, we would not be breaking the law.

Shepard seemed to have difficulty in understanding that a law could actually be wrong. At the same time, she did not see herself or her colleagues in voluntarism as criminals. She even contradicted herself within this brief summary of the MHA's activities. Shepard said on the one hand that the clinic is not "breaking any Federal or State law" but later stated that if the MHA chose to buy its supplies in Cleveland, *then* it would not be committing a crime. At that same meeting, Mr. Park, whom federal officials had previously arrested and fined under the Comstock Law, challenged Shepard's conclusions. He protested, "You now have to take a bootlegged article or you have to take a train and go down to New York and bring back a suitcase of them just in order to get them to the people." Shepard retorted, coming back to her first point. "I beg your pardon, we are not breaking the law." Park disagreed, pointing out that transporting diaphragms from one state to the next was illegal, that "the people moving them" clearly risked arrest.[28] No record exists of Shepard's answer or of an immediate change in the MHA's *modus operandi*. At some unspecified later point, according to MHA documents, the Western Reserve University School of Pharmacy developed a formula for contraceptive jelly, and a local business began to manufacture diaphragms and other necessities. By 1938 the MHA purchased its stock through "Cleveland agents of various supply houses."[29]

Restrictive public policies toward sexuality and contraception encouraged creative thinking among other advocates as well. Margaret Sanger engaged in smuggling supplies for the Clinical Research Bureau in the early 1920s, with the invaluable assistance of admirer and industrialist J. Noah Slee, who later married Sanger. His company brought diaphragms in Three-in-One Oil cartons from Germany and shipped them through Montreal, Canada, into the States.[30] With or without knowledge of Sanger's subterfuge, friends of the movement smuggled diaphragms and jelly into Cleveland for an indeterminate length of time. It is unclear whether the process continued for weeks, months, or years. What is clear is that, at some point, founders of the pioneer birth control clinic in Cleveland supported their fledgling endeavor with civil disobedience, although they would not have described it as such. Advocates did recognize the crucial nature of their actions on some level, however. They kept the tales of the clandestine train trips alive and always described the New York ventures in clinic histories.

Before the MHA even opened, its leaders structured existing laws for their benefit. They avoided medical opposition by interpreting the state law in the form of a legal opinion. They approached the difficulty of stocking the clinic in a less traditional manner, however, focusing on practicality rather than technicalities. Their covert actions again took advantage of ambiguities within the statutes governing the transport of "obscene" materials and challenged the very foundation of those statutes. Maternal Health Association leaders and advocates ventured into gray areas of the law out of a firm belief in the legitimacy of contraception. They acted to broaden women's access to birth control, manipulating a strong and broad web of support and ignoring the law when necessary.

Familial and social networks also undergirded more conventional activities, such as fund-raising events for the Cleveland Maternal Health Association. In the early 1930s, along with the rest of the city and country, the association suffered from financial troubles. MHA caseloads rose while its income fell. The clinic cut staff salaries by 50 percent in 1932. During these years, spending twenty-five cents for a lampshade for the office waiting room involved great debate. Nurses reportedly had to "get along with a string" rather than the towel rack they had requested "for at least the next month." By early 1934, according to one account, the clinic needed five thousand dollars to continue its work.[31]

Maternal Health Association leaders decided to sponsor a large benefit to raise the money. The women turned to sports instead of society's usual cabarets, dances, or teas. Several MHA families enjoyed ice skating with their friends at the Elysium Ice Carnival, located downtown at the corner of East 107th Street and Euclid Avenue. The Clevelanders heard of the wonderful performances of the Toronto Skating Club in Ontario, Canada. Early in 1934 Adele Chisholm Eells, her sister, Helen Chisholm Halle, Margaret Allen Ireland, and Gladys Gaylord traveled to Canada and invited the Toronto club to perform in Cleveland. The Canadian skaters, amateurs rather than professionals, represented "the cream of Toronto society." Maternal Health Association leaders counted on the wide appeal of sports in Cleveland and the unusual nature of the event to transcend tight economic circumstances and draw a crowd. The women also factored in Cleveland's stellar reputation for philanthropy in the face of adversity—and the power of their own social and charitable connections.[32]

Industrialist and philanthropist Howard Eells Jr., Adele's husband, loaned office space in the Hanna building downtown and the use of his telephones to the event's organizers. The committee included Roberta Bole, Geraldine Walker Brown, Gladys McNairy White, and those who had made the trip to Canada. The women telephoned friends and acquaintances to sell as many tickets as possible. One account claims that, if the idea of an ice show "drew yawns" during the phone conversations, the callers "mercilessly sold civic responsibility and shamelessly called in their reciprocal markers" from others whose causes they had supported in the past. A historical account of a clinic organized in 1932 in Morristown, New Jersey, explains the pressure on friends to attend fund-raising gatherings there: "They didn't dare not come. It was a social event."[33] Likewise, MHA women manipulated any and all alliances to further the clinic's work.

On March 18, 1934, according to news headlines, seventy-two Canadian ice skaters put on the "Spectacular Ice Ballet" in Cleveland on behalf of the Maternal Health Association. The clinic enlisted the help of other community groups for the show. The local Hruby Brothers Orchestra provided the music, and Junior League members, debutantes, and representatives of social service organizations assisted MHA board members as hostesses. The *Cleveland Press* called the upcoming event "undoubtedly the most notable society undertaking for March." While the crowd did not fill the Elysium's twenty-five hundred seats as hoped, the gala inspired rave newspaper reviews and cleared enough money to make it worth repeating.[34]

Maternal Health Association bookkeeper Minnie Brow recalled the problems in selling skating show tickets for that first event in 1934: "Another woman and I sat in the lobby of the Hotel Statler all day without selling a single ticket," she remembered. The situation changed after the 1934 show, Brow said. "After we had shown Cleveland what a skating carnival was, everyone wanted to come."[35] The next year the show played to a sold-out audience and garnered $7,500 for the MHA. The fund-raiser had succeeded socially and financially. Planning for the 1936 benefit hit a snag, however. The Toronto Skating Club at first refused to return to Cleveland. The group feared that one more performance held at a public arena, outside of the venue of a skating club, would jeopardize its amateur status. Faced with this dilemma, Adele Eells asked her husband to add yet another a local association to his already long list of community activities. He agreed and became president of the new Cleveland ice skating club. Organized by MHA supporters and their friends, the Cleveland Figure Skating Club's first twenty-five members included seven MHA leaders.[36] The MHA had extended its connections into the world of sports as well as philanthropy, reform, and health care.

Having resolved the issue of amateur versus professional status, the Cleveland Figure Skating Club hired the Canadian group to again perform in Cleveland for the benefit of the MHA, calling the show an ice carnival this time. Two sold-out performances in March 1936 featured one hundred members of the Toronto Skating Club with the addition of twenty-four Cleveland skaters, some of them MHA leaders. All delighted the crowds. Dubbed "the most important financial event since the books of the Association were audited," the 1936 show netted ten thousand dollars in profit. The next year, the MHA and the Cleveland Skating Club split the revenue from the ice carnival, and the clinic cleared almost five thousand dollars The MHA measured the carnival's success not only in financial gain, however, but also "in terms of beauty, skill, and international friendships."[37] These women knew how to entertain! They successfully used their extensive experience of attending or staging similar social events to further their chosen cause.

The Cleveland Skating Club claims to be the first private figure skating organization in the United States to build its own indoor rink. The direct evolution of this club out of the MHA's fund-raising efforts demonstrates once more how well clinic leaders knew their cohorts. In addition to health care and reform, the women understood local sports and entertainment, men's interests as well as women's. They built on Cleveland's affinity for athletic events and expanded the city's interest in ice skating while raising money for birth control. Maternal Health Association leaders again demonstrated their knack of tapping into a previously untouched area of avid interest at an opportune moment. Their actions helped sustain the birth control clinic and spawned a long-standing sport and social club.[38]

Local newspapers noted the skating shows as important social functions. Before the productions and afterward, the papers ran many pictures of organizers and skaters on the society pages and in the Sunday supplements (see figures 20 and 21). An enthusiastic *Plain Dealer* reviewer in 1936 emphasized the appearance and talent of the performers: "It's conceded by practically everyone that comely young women are good to look upon. Grace on a dance floor is admirable, but when you have beauty on skates you have the summit of perfection. And when they are set off by young gentlemen with well-turned limbs, who can skate like the devil while handling themselves like angels, then you have an elegant show indeed."[39] The real news seemed to lie in the show's beauty and social significance rather than its charitable objective. Press coverage avoided mentioning the services offered by the MHA or its very reason for being. While the skating carnivals fulfilled their monetary functions and influenced the future of sports in Cleveland, they contributed little to public understanding about the purpose of the Maternal Health Association. Brief ads directed people who wanted to purchase tickets to borrowed

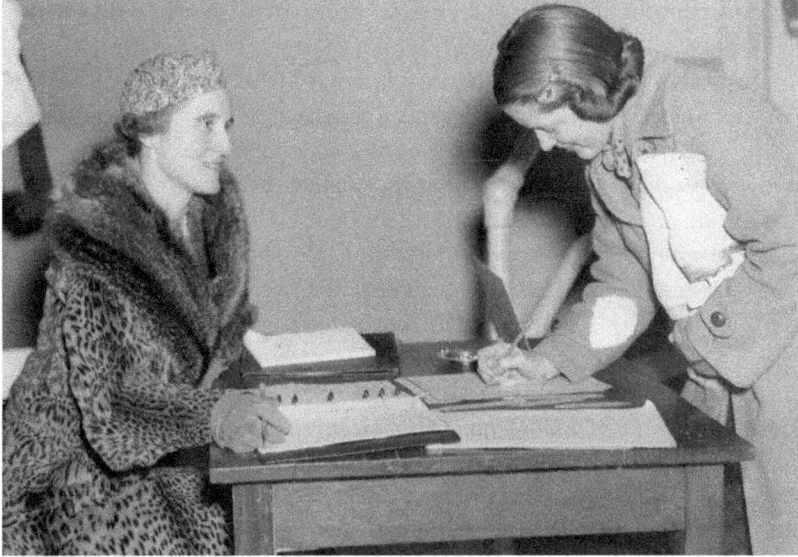

FIGURE 20. Selling skating gala tickets. MHA board member Adele Chisholm Eells (left), Dorothy Osbourne, 1930s. *Cleveland Press* Collection, Cleveland State University. Louis Van Oyen photo.

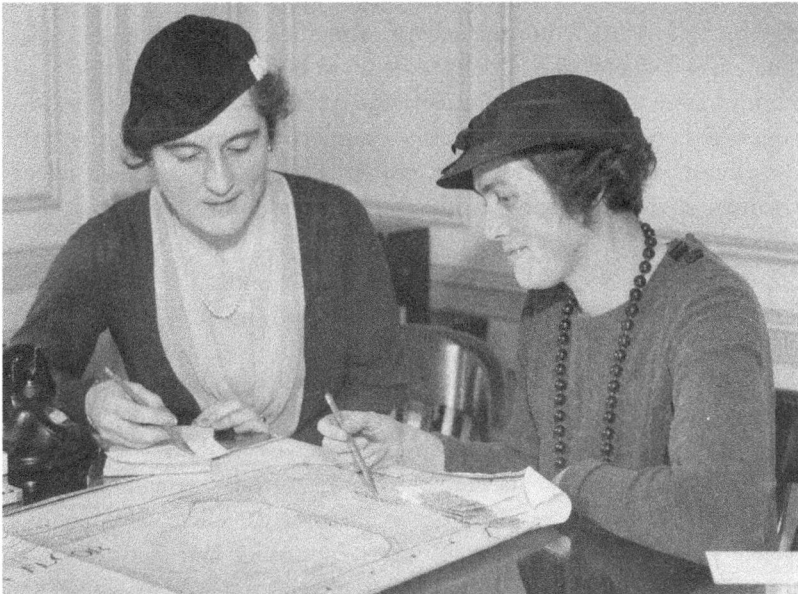

FIGURE 21. Planning the seating for a skating gala. Adele Chisholm Eells (left) and Geraldine Walker Brown study the floor plan of the Elysium skating rink in preparation for the 1934 MHA fund-raiser. *Cleveland Press* Collection, Cleveland State University.

headquarters in the Hanna building rather than to the MHA's own Osborn building offices. The ads did not even mention the clinic.[40]

Reporters who did include the Maternal Health Association and its function in their articles wrote in veiled language, as in previous press coverage. One piece of news about a skating gala, for example, obliquely paraphrased the MHA's statement of purpose as "co-operating through physicians in helping mothers in the health of their infant children." This could easily have described a prenatal or children's dispensary rather than a birth control clinic. Several articles described the events as fund-raisers and spoke of the MHA's need for money but did not address the ways in which the clinic would use the funds.[41]

Later reports of other MHA activities continued this pattern. Describing a 1939 MHA luncheon meeting presented for nurses and social workers, newspaper reports did not mention birth control at all. Other articles spoke of "the unique work" of the clinic or the "association's work."[42] Given its fear of adverse publicity, the MHA probably encouraged this practice. By making a new health care service available to women and families, the MHA advocated social change. But the organization did so quietly and without confrontation, conforming to acceptable standards of behavior. The successful skating shows and later benefits provided opportunities to educate Cleveland citizens about specific services that the MHA offered or the subject of reproductive control in general. The clinic did not take advantage of those opportunities, however, but trod its usual careful path. Publicly the MHA sidestepped the volatile issue that lay at the heart of its mission and instead emphasized the social contributions of individuals and events. Due to this lack of general advertisement about clinic services, the MHA resorted to indirect means to attract clients.

## "ALL MY FRIENDS"

The strong and diverse connections among MHA founders, trustees, volunteers, and the reform community sustained the new clinic. But examining only those elite networks omits a key part of the story. Maternal Health Association clients employed similar strategies and developed links of their own to recruit other women for the clinic. Their actions enabled the association's survival. Correspondence and statistics prove that women depended on and utilized their personal webs of association to obtain birth control at the MHA and elsewhere. Contented clients spread the word about the new service more effectively than any news articles of the era. Pleased with the assistance that they received at the clinic, women shared the news about the service with their neighbors, family, and friends. Searching for reliable methods of family limitation, clients and their relatives supported one another with child care, information, and transportation to and from Cleveland. They delivered messages and contraceptive supplies to each other. Networking out of concern for the health of friends and families rather than for the MHA's future, they nonetheless contributed to the clinic's longevity. Given the clinic's limited publicity and the restricted nature of the contraceptive work in public agencies during these early years, the client-to-client network sustained the MHA. It played as critical a role in the association's continued existence as the links fostered by founders, trustees, and staff.[43]

An unidentified MHA staff member speculated that the knowledge that "friends have been treated successfully" inspired clinic clients and helped them to "maintain confidence." Cleveland mothers spoke of directing other women to the MHA out of appreciation: "I am very grateful and would like to send all my friends in. Several have come." Sometimes women referred pregnant acquaintances to the MHA for postpartum assistance in limiting their families. After expressing her own satisfaction with the diaphragm in a letter to the MHA nurse, one new client wrote about a pregnant friend with whom she had discussed the clinic. The client explained that her friend "has not yet had her baby so it will be at a later date that I will bring her in." Kathleen Horner's case study described another woman who, while she "didn't 'broadcast' her [own] clinic attendance," recommended the MHA to neighbors when "she felt there was a need."[44]

Other clients helped people who had already heard about the MHA to overcome their initial reluctance and take advantage of the service. A woman from a town south of Cleveland told this story of persuading another out-of-town friend: "[She] is very much interested. She is the mother of four children and her Doctor suggested the Clinic to her but she . . . didn't do anything more about it until I talked to her and offered my assistance." This MHA client planned to accompany her friend to the clinic, since the mother of four was "not acquainted with Cleveland." When writing to the MHA to schedule or change visits, clients often made or canceled appointments for other women as well. An inquiry to the MHA during its first decade often contained two or more such contacts. For example, one woman wrote, "Quite unexpectedly a friend offered to drive me in to Cleveland this week so that I could come earlier in the day instead of the evening as before." The client then asked the MHA to cancel an appointment that she had made for another friend who would be unable to "come in town for a few weeks yet." This woman had one friend who offered transportation to the clinic while she herself assisted another woman in obtaining birth control.

The supportive network crossed gender boundaries and enabled women to access MHA services. Women often depended on husbands or brothers for transportation to the clinic or for child care during MHA visits. They sent their menfolk as well as female friends and family to the clinic office with messages or to pick up supplies. One Cleveland woman wrote to the MHA in 1937, "Please give my brother a tube of jelly. It's very difficult for me to come down, because the girl who used to watch my baby is married I hope it is all right for my brother to stop for it." As was the case with the woman whose brother opposed her use of birth control (see chapter 1), this is another instance where a man knew something of his sister's private life. Clearly the urgent need to continue this successful method of contraception overcame issues of modesty in some instances. Another woman who lived a good distance south of town had her husband bring a note to Cleveland and mail it to the MHA from there, "to save the extra penny postage," she explained. Some men as well as women made special arrangements to facilitate child spacing in their own families or even those of their relatives.[45]

Given the low public profile of the MHA, the wide-ranging nature of client networks provided an essential bond between clinic and client. Personal contacts among clients promoted clinic services and assisted out-of-towners in keeping up with their appointments and supplies. One client wrote from London, Ontario, Canada, "I just mailed $5. to my sister last Saturday for to get me supplies so she likely will be coming in soon as I ask her to put it in with the Xmas parcel. I would certainly would appreciate it very much if you could let her have a P-#85 [identifying number of the diaphragm] as the one I have is very thin and has a crack in it. It isn't very safe." This Canadian resident explained why she wanted to remain an MHA client, although there was a birth control clinic in Hamilton, Ontario, by this time.[46] She claimed, "It really is more convenient for me to go to your clinic. I usually alway go home once or twice every summer." The MHA and its supportive staff inspired deep loyalty among its clients.

Friends, family, and acquaintances drove women from all over Ohio to the Cleveland MHA office. Women inquired or responded from Portsmouth, in the southern portion of the state, to Toledo, in the northwest corner, and from many towns in between. A mother living about fifty miles south of Cleveland does not explicitly describe how she discovered the MHA but mentions friends who would bring her to the clinic when they came to the city. This writer outlines the problems presented by living so far from this health service—and the desperation of a family living on the fiscal edge:

> Your letter came this morning stateing that Cleveland may be far too expensive a trip for me. I am sure it would be as we are . . . not working and I am so worried that another baby will come is there any way that you can get help from a birth control center when you are not able to pay? We have two children living and had (4) four miscarriages I dont want to bring children into the wourld and cant support them.
>
> . . . please let me know what you can do about it I will go to Akron if you will send me the name of Physicians there or . . . I could ride to Cleveland with some friends of mine when thay come over I did not know that you had to visit a Doctor more than once I didn't know any thing about it I was told to use Jelly but I did not beleve Jelly alone would do any good. Oh there must be some way to help me.
>
> Please answere soon

MHA clients maintained contact with the clinic from states as distant as Connecticut, Missouri, and Nebraska, and even from foreign countries. The wife of a navy man wrote:

> My indefinite stay in France makes it rather difficult to keep in touch however I would appreciate the opportunity of making a visit to the clinic upon my return to the USA. The advice I received at the clinic had given me and my husband great comfort and satisfaction, and I wish to express my appreciation to you for the benefits which your association dispenses.

Sometimes strangers rather than relatives or friends told other women about the MHA. Clinic nurse Edna Rusch recalled the experience of a mother approaching menopause. The woman had endured two pregnancy scares, Rusch said, "before she overcame her embarrassment sufficiently to ask the advice of a clerk in the 'Women's Department' of a large drug store." Fortunately, the wise clerk referred the desperate mother to the Maternal Health Association.[47] Women's great need and desire for a reliable method of preventing or spacing pregnancies led them to confront such embarrassing situations head-on. Social attitudes toward contraception and sexuality must have deterred many women from seeking help in the public way that this particular mother employed. However, very different private views, especially among peers, encouraged women to question the people closest to them. Women asked or told their family and friends about birth control services and then often relied on a web of personal contacts to gain and maintain access to MHA services.

In its first decade, client-to-client referrals increased dramatically each year that the clinic was open. The proportion jumped from 2.2 percent in 1928–29 to 14.9 percent in 1932. Dr. Ruth Robishaw had predicted the effect of such networking in 1931: "The [Maternal Health] clinic attendance will receive another great impetus when patients learn to know they may fearlessly refer friends and neighbors as possible candidates for admission to the clinic."[48] Statistics indicate that by 1935 clients, friends, and "interested individuals" referred more women to the MHA than social agencies (which were the largest source before this date—see figure 22). Client networking supported the MHA as well as other birth control facilities across the country.

A 1930 description of the Los Angeles Mothers' Clinic indicated that personal contact provided the best advertisement for contraception on the West Coast as in the Midwest. Likewise, a 1932 study of the Newark, New Jersey, birth control clinic reported that almost 40 percent of its first two thousand clients were referred by another client or friend. In small towns as well as cities across North America, mothers passed messages through letters, personal visits, or from one person to another—and then another. The informal system often covered great distances. For example, pregnant women in rural Montana who lived far apart from each other still contacted neighbors and family members to locate midwives or abortionists and to find out about contraceptive methods.[49]

These one-on-one referrals crossed generations as well as gender lines and geographical space. In Iowa in 1937, the mother of twenty children had three babies among her many progeny. How did she finally get to the Maternal and Birth Control League of Sioux City? Her husband's grandmother directed her there. Similar connections supported birth control clinics elsewhere across the country. Some scholars assert that working-class black women disseminated birth control information among their peers even more effectively than white women. In addition to uncovering sources of family limitation, women of all backgrounds used similar methods—contacting family members, friends, acquaintances, or generally "asking around"—to locate abortionists while abortion was illegal.[50] The MHA depended on such quiet, one-to-one proselytizing among its clients while also working closely with other organizations.

## REFORM LINKS AND THE COOPERATIVE SPIRIT

Maternal Health Association outreach depended on contacts beyond those of family, friends, neighbors, or client networks. Staff and volunteers obtained clinic referrals through their other reform work and that of friends and acquaintances. One history states that three close advisers to the MHA founding committee, Marion Howell, Elizabeth Folckemer, and Hanna Buchanan, sent or actually brought the first patients to the MHA. These same administrators had helped the MHA select its first nursing staff. Cleveland hospitals and other health and social service agencies also directed clients to the MHA, sometimes in an unofficial capacity. Some local government relief authorities ignored prohibitions and guided women to the clinic on the condition that the referring individual or organization remain anonymous.[51] This active interchange among service organizations—Cleveland cooperation—bound the city's reform community. That collaboration helped inaugurate and maintain the city's pioneer birth control clinic.

In order to enhance well-being of clients and meet their complex needs, many female health care and social service professionals stressed interagency cooperation rather than assigning a separate expert to each function. Emphasizing such interprofessional connections ran counter to the specialization trend in medicine, a trend generally associated with male physicians.[52] One student of sociology explored the extent of such "cooperative use of resources" at the MHA and declared, "The Maternal Health program is not an isolated effort but part of a coordinated program of social and health agencies to build family solidarity and to help create homes where children may learn to make a desirable social adjustment."[53]

For MHA staff and founders, working with the clinic emerged from their own involvement in the reform community. Most board members already served as founders, officers, or on the boards of other organizations geared to improving the lives of women and children or the underprivileged in general. In fact, these people often worked together in the same organizations, providing an example of the power of interlocking boards. These organizational interconnections, introduced in chapter 2, warrant further exploration.

Maternal Health Association founders and trustees played critical roles in a plethora of Cleveland's service groups. Mabel Wason assisted in creating the Cleveland Day Nursery and Free Kindergarten Association in 1894 and presided over the Day Nursery, the first group established in Cleveland to specifically address the needs of young children. Katherine Bingham (later Katherine B. Fisher) came to Cleveland to serve as the

## Maternal Health Clinic, 1931, Cleveland, Ohio:
### Sources of Clinic Cases.

| REFERRAL SOURCES | NUMBER OF REFERRALS | | |
| --- | --- | --- | --- |
| | 1928–29 | 1929–30 | 1930–31 |
| **Health Agencies** | | | |
| Babies Dispensary | 24 | 40 | 43 |
| Board of Health | 0 | 0 | 3 |
| City Hospital, O.P.D. (out-patient dept.) | 0 | 0 | 11 |
| City Hospital Sanatorium | 0 | 0 | 9 |
| Cleveland Clinic Hospital | 1 | 0 | 2 |
| Cleveland Heights Hospital | 0 | 0 | 1 |
| County nurse | 0 | 0 | 2 |
| East Cleveland Clinic | 3 | 3 | 0 |
| Lake County Public Health League | 0 | 0 | 1 |
| Lakeside Hospital | 0 | 0 | 3 |
| Lakewood Hospital Clinic | 6 | 5 | 10 |
| Out of town nurse | 0 | 0 | 4 |
| St. Luke's O.P.D. | 4 | 1 | 28 |
| University Nursing District | 46 | 43 | 58 |
| Visiting Nurse Assn. | 11 | 27 | 10 |
| Western Reserve Maternity Dispensary | 2 | 0 | 12 |
| Woman's Hospital | 0 | 0 | 1 |
| Other Clinics | 37 | 32 | 12 |
| **Total Health Agencies** | **134** | **151** | **210** |
| **Social Agencies** | | | |
| American Red Cross | 6 | 5 | 7 |
| Associated Charities | 12 | 31 | 95 |
| Friendly Inn | 1 | 0 | 0 |
| Humane Society | 1 | 2 | 0 |
| Jewish Social Service Bureau | 7 | 15 | 22 |
| Juvenile Court | 0 | 3 | 1 |
| Lorain Social Worker | 0 | 0 | 1 |
| Mothers Pension | 1 | 0 | 0 |
| **Total Social Agencies** | **28** | **56** | **126** |
| **Other Agencies** | | | |
| American Birth Control League | 12 | 6 | 11 |
| Association for the Blind | 0 | 1 | 1 |
| Child Guidance Clinic | 0 | 0 | 5 |
| Cleveland Board of Education | 0 | 1 | 7 |
| Clinical Research Bureau | 1 | 0 | 3 |
| Fresh Air Camp | 2 | 0 | 0 |
| Philadelphia Birth Control League | 0 | 0 | 1 |
| Social Hygiene Association | 1 | 0 | 0 |
| Women's Protective Big Sisters | 0 | 1 | 1 |
| Y.M.C.A. | 0 | 0 | 1 |
| Y.W.C.A. | 1 | 0 | 0 |
| **Total Other Agencies** | **17** | **9** | **30** |

FIGURE 22. Maternal Health Clinic, 1931, Cleveland, Ohio: sources of clinic cases.

| Maternal Health Clinic, 1931, Cleveland, Ohio: Sources of Clinic Cases (cont'd). | | | |
|---|---|---|---|
| REFERRAL SOURCES | NUMBER OF REFERRALS | | |
| | 1928–29 | 1929–30 | 1930–31 |
| **Individuals** | | | |
| City Nurse | 1 | 0 | 0 |
| Company Nurse | 0 | 1 | 1 |
| Friend | 0 | 0 | 15 |
| Interested Individuals | 11 | 22 | 15 |
| Minister or Pastor's Assistant | 1 | 2 | 11 |
| Newspapers | 9 | 2 | 4 |
| Osteopath | 1 | 0 | 0 |
| Patients | 5 | 14 | 60 |
| Private Nurse | 0 | 1 | 3 |
| Private Physicians | 15 | 18 | 37 |
| Self | 3 | 9 | 23 |
| Source Unknown | 0 | 0 | 1 |
| **Total Individuals** | **46** | **69** | **170** |
| **TOTAL REFERRALS** | **225** | **285** | **536** |

Letter from G. Gaylord to Mary MacAulay, May 1, 1931, MS-LC, reel 7.

FIGURE 22. (cont'd.) Maternal Health Clinic, 1931, Cleveland, Ohio: sources of clinic cases.

nursery's executive secretary in 1914; in 1931 Helene Narten was vice president. Frances Goff, Margaret Ireland, Gertrude Judson, and Julia Flory also served as Day Nursery trustees. Edna Perkins, Frances Goff, Elizabeth Baker, Helen Bassett, Roberta Bole, and Lenore Black helped charter the Cleveland Women's City Club in 1916. All of these women served as MHA board members during the 1930s.

Associated Charities, organized in 1900, benefited from the energies of the same women. With almost eighty years of service to Associated Charities between them, Wason and Black led boards and committees of that organization and its successors, such as the Family Service Association. May Oliver served on the Associated Charities board for twenty-one years. At least seven other MHA board members also volunteered for the group. Maternal Health Association trustees had been involved, directly or indirectly, in creating and supporting Western Reserve University's School of Applied Social Sciences. The school opened to train social workers in 1916.[54] Many of the same people managed these and other social service groups in the city. Interlocking boards assured cooperation among the organizations and provided a rich resource for fledgling efforts such as the Maternal Health Association.[55] MHA leaders created, governed, officiated over, and served diverse organized reform causes.[56] Linked by class, family, and geography, these people had a long history of working together in a variety of configurations to improve the welfare of Cleveland's needy citizens—especially the poor, women, and children.

Although not all of the MHA founding trustees had previously engaged primarily in health care reform, their activities in woman suffrage, education, and family service provided contacts, leadership experience, and a basis for action. Many former suffragists joined the national and international movements for birth control, among them Katherine Houghton Hepburn in Connecticut and Katherine Dexter McCormick in New York.[57] Figure 23 lists the local service agencies and other organizations in which three or more MHA supporters participated between 1928 and 1940. As noted in chapter 3, links to Western Reserve University topped the list, with at least forty-nine MHA trustees or corporation members, both women and men, having some connection to the university and its various schools. At least thirty women from the MHA belonged to the Women's City Club between 1928 and 1940. Thirteen men and women of the MHA served on the board of the University Public Health Nursing District. At least nine participated in each of these other agencies or special events: American Red Cross, local chapter; Brush Foundation; Chamber of Commerce; Junior League; League of Women Voters; and the National Conference of Charity and Corrections annual meeting in Cleveland in 1912.[58]

Even social clubs acted as resources for the MHA. The Junior League of Cleveland provides one example. Organized in 1912 to promote voluntarism, develop women's potential, and improve the community, the league held high standards and required social service experience for admission to its ranks. Junior League membership opened doors of voluntary action and offered leadership opportunities to middle-class, upper-middle-class, and upper-class white women in the 1920s and 1930s. The organization trained and supplied volunteers for many Cleveland organizations. At the MHA, Junior League members performed daily duties such as baby-sitting and acting as receptionist, and assisted at special events. In fact, Junior League voluntary work at a prenatal clinic elsewhere in town first inspired founders Dorothy Brush and Hortense Shepard to create the MHA.[59]

The wide variety of social and reform links among MHA leaders greatly aided the clinic in securing interagency cooperation for the cause of birth control. For example, the Jewish Social Service Bureau considered

**Local activities of MHA founding trustees**
Local organizations in which three or more MHA founding board members served

Academy of Medicine
American Red Cross
Anti Tuberculosis League
Associated Charities (and succeeding organizations)

Brush Foundation

Chamber of Commerce
Citizens League
City Club
City Hospital
Cleveland Health Council
Cleveland Playhouse
Cleveland School of Art
College Club
Community Chest
Consumers' League
Council of Sociology

Day Nursery and Free Kindergarten Assn.

First Unitarian Church
Flora Stone Mather College
Frances Payne Bolton School of Nursing

Hiram House
Humane Society

Junior League of Cleveland

Lakeside Hospital
League of Women Voters (and earlier suffrage groups)

Maternity Hospital

National Conference of Charities and Corrections, 1912 meeting in Cleveland

Phillis Wheatley Assn.

Rainbow Hospital for Crippled and Convalescent Children

St. Luke's Hospital

University Hospitals
University Public Health Nursing District
Urban League

Visiting Nurse Assn.

Welfare Federation
Western Reserve University
Women's City Club
Women's Council for the Prevention of Future Wars
Women's General Hospital

YWCA

FIGURE 23. Local activities of MHA founding trustees.[60]

"family regulation" integral to its relief work. The bureau's case work supervisor told social work student Goldie Davis in 1938 that "if family regulation were not already founded on a firm basis in Cleveland, our Agency would be obliged to establish this service as a department of our own organization."[61] Davis surveyed the MHA's relationship to other services in the city, gathering her information primarily from interviews with leaders of local relief and reform groups. She found that the MHA based its work on a strong network of give and take among these organizations, involving mutual cases. The system even included sharing the personal details of individual family situations among agencies.

Davis asserted, "The Maternal Health Association reports back to the referring agency on all cases that fail to keep the first appointment. On all who have been accepted [for clinic service], a report is sent to the referring agency stating that the patient has been in, whether or not she was given contraceptive instruction, and what method was advised; or, if she was not so instructed, the reasons why instruction was not given, and the

conditions found upon pelvic examination." During this era, professionals believed that revealing facts about the personal lives of their clients to
other agencies was integral to the efficient coordination of social service.
One example lies in the relationship between the Visiting Nurse Association (VNA) and the MHA, as outlined by Davis.[62]

The local VNA did not officially dispense birth control advice and had
"no established policy governing the matter of referral," according to
Davis. Some VNA nurses acted as agents for the MHA, however, by individually directing some women who sought contraceptive advice to the
birth control clinic. They gave referral cards to pregnant clients and
advised them to consult the MHA after the babies were born. But the
VNA did not stop there. This public health association also apparently
passed on the names of possible MHA prospects. Goldie Davis found
that the VNA reported to the MHA the names of those VNA clients who
gave birth. The birth control clinic then followed up with home visits and
contraceptive advice to the new mothers. One VNA stipulation for service
coincided with an MHA qualification: a woman should consult her family physician, if she had one, before coming to the VNA. Davis reported
that the VNA acted as carefully as did the MHA with regard to religion
and contraception, "maintaining the same policy," though Davis did not
provide details.[63]

Cooperation between the birth control clinic and the nursing service
worked both ways. Clinic nurse Edna Rusch told a gathering of Ohio
nurses in 1940 that the MHA referred some pregnant clients to the VNA,
especially women who requested prenatal advice and information, and
sent along any background on the patients to give the VNA "a better
understanding" of each situation. Rusch also detailed other instances in
which the MHA used the resources of medical specialists, the Child
Guidance Clinic, and other local child welfare and social work agencies to
assist clinic clients. In all of these examples, the MHA took a proactive
social service role. The clinic explained each family's circumstances (as
interpreted by clinic staff) to the cooperating organizations.[64]

Sharing such intimate details about individuals and families among
social agencies indicates the relative invisibility of clinic patients and the
clients of other organizations as individuals and their lack of autonomy in
the larger system. Twenty-first-century standards of confidentiality did
not generally apply. The social and medical establishment of the 1930s
viewed its clientele, especially poor or working-class people or those of a
different ethnic or racial background, through a moralistic lens. The system did not separate patients or clients from the medical and social problems endemic during the Depression, such as tuberculosis, malnutrition,

poverty, illiteracy, or unemployment. In spite of claims that "modern" social work employed a scientific, psychological approach rather than a moralistic one, many professionals still viewed their clients as embodying social ills.[65] They often treated them as subjects for study rather than as people who needed assistance.

According to this way of thinking, the economic level and class of many of the women who came to the MHA warranted what would later be viewed as intrusiveness into the private lives of clients. In 1932 Cleveland hospitals began reporting instances and the circumstances of maternal deaths to a common body, the Cleveland Hospital Obstetric Society, despite ethical questions. As one local historian noted, "It was generally felt that charity cases could be reported but that private patients could only be included with the consent of the attending physician." Distinctions between public and private blurred under the authority of providing healing or assistance.[66]

Occasionally, such treatment drew criticism. One observer of relief procedures in Cleveland described the new methods used in interviewing the people who applied for assistance from welfare agencies. She complained that "a bunch of embryo psychiatrists and amateur psychologists . . . feel that they are eminently fitted to 'reconstruct' these families less fortunate than themselves."[67] By participating in such institutional give and take of personal details about its patients, the MHA assumed contemporary medical and social service standards. The clinic acted to benefit women, but it acted within a system that took advantage of the vulnerability of its clients and intruded into their private lives. The Cleveland Maternal Health Association used its broad web of links to access the existing configuration of local agencies rather than to challenge prevailing policies. The clinic needed support from this segment of the Cleveland community to raise professional awareness about clinic services and to continue its own quiet work.

## RESULTS AND OPPOSITION

Broad and wide-ranging client, trustee, and reform networks and the cooperative use of resources could not accomplish everything, however. By shunning publicity, advertising, and public advocacy, the MHA limited the number of women it could serve. Knowledge of the MHA's very existence eluded many interested people, such as the woman above, who "didn't know any thing about it." Another example is the man who in 1936 wrote to the ABCL in New York City asking if there was a birth control clinic near his Cleveland home (see letter in chapter 4). By 1936 the MHA of Cleveland had served an average of about eight hundred clients a year for eight years. Yet this man, who was someone actively seeking family limitation information, had no awareness of the services offered in his own city. News of the MHA's work had not reached him. One couple who chanced to hear of the MHA complained in 1939 about the clinic's lack of advertising. Some medical professionals remained ignorant of the clinic's existence. A 1937 report indicated that many Cleveland physicians—especially specialists other than gynecologists— did not know about the MHA.[68]

Amenability, dedication, and intensive networking did not always ensure interagency cooperation, either. Social and moral stigmas attached to contraception affected not only clinic outreach but also its community acceptance. Many organizations in town officially distanced themselves from the services of the MHA. Bound by policy not to "superimpose upon clients a particular point of view," the local unit of the federal Emergency Management Relief Administration advised those women who requested contraceptive information in the 1930s to consult a dispensary or medical professional. The Cleveland Division of Health gave similar advice and did not refer patients to the MHA. Researcher Goldie Davis found that even Associated Charities, whose board and volunteer force closely intertwined with those of the MHA, officially directed women to the birth control clinic only when the clients exhibited health problems in addition to wanting information about child spacing. As for the policy of Associated Charities with respect to religious beliefs, Davis explained, "If a client whose church does not oppose family regulation asks for advice, the workers of the Agency [Associated Charities] tell her where the [Maternal Health] Clinic is located, but the client makes her own appointment. It is the policy of the Agency through an agreement with some religious bodies not to discuss the Maternal Health Clinic with their membership." Such policies deferred to the strong hold of the Roman Catholic Church in Cleveland during this era. Associated Charities worked closely with the Catholic Charities organization in Cleveland and with individual Catholic churches among its many contacts. These deliberate attempts by organizations to disassociate from the MHA, especially in religious matters, embody the volatile nature of birth control information in the 1930s and the prevalent negative attitudes toward its dissemination.[69]

The Academy of Medicine of Cleveland, the local professional association of physicians, did not recognize the pioneer health care venture in their city during these years. The Academy neither endorsed nor opposed the work of the MHA, according to Davis, but left the matter to individual physicians. A few doctors did tell their patients about the MHA or directed women to the clinic from hospital out-patient departments.[70] Social workers also remained wary about supporting birth control, especially collectively. In 1934 Henry Busch of the Cleveland MHA spoke about contraception at the Social Workers Club in Akron, Ohio. According to a news article, the Akron club president carefully pointed out that, although the group had invited and hosted the speaker, it was not "sponsoring the movement."[71] Many health and social service groups and professionals opposed, ignored, or deliberately steered their work away from contraception during the 1920s and throughout the 1930s.

In such a hostile climate, MHA leaders spurned publicity and confrontation. One board member described a strategy that the clinic used, based on experience from "old suffrage days": "We absolutely refused to debate [birth control] because it pulled in an audience for the opposing side. However, we made a speech when we had the chance."[72] The Clevelanders quietly nurtured and utilized their connections to acquire funding and gain respectability for birth control and the MHA. The activists circumvented the law when necessary but used tried-and-true fund-raising methods.

A few women and men of Cleveland took risks for the cause of birth control, expanding the boundaries of philanthropy, social responsibility, and voluntarism. Clients, on the other hand, utilized the MHA in order to *minimize* risk—the risk of unintended pregnancy. One MHA client wrote, "I think fear is at the base of all this" (referring to trouble with the particular birth control method). Fear certainly lay at the base of this reform. Fear of being labeled radical or immoral and of provoking opposition motivated leaders to work quietly. Private couples and public officials feared the results of uncontrolled childbearing for individual women, families, and the race. Female founders, board members, volunteers, and physicians closely identified with the biological reality behind women's fears and thus empathized with clients. They acted out of feminist concern, attempting to empower clients to control their reproduction. At the same time, they utilized eugenic rhetoric, which had a lasting negative impact. The clinic followed conventional patterns of service delivery at the expense of client privacy.

Maternal Health Association leaders and clients alike based their actions on a firm foundation of interconnections. Formalizing loosely structured kin, social, and acquaintance networks often sustains voluntary associations and social movements. In the birth control cause, with its questionable reputation, personal and social links played even more

crucial roles. Local connections solidified support, ensured the cooperation of many other organizations, attracted clinic clients, and lent an air
of propriety. Based in strong voluntary action networks and ties of family
and friendship, MHA advocates collaborated for the common good.
Women's enthusiastic promotion of contraception to other women as
clients sustained early clinics such as the MHA across North America and
propelled the continental birth control movement from the local level.
The final chapter explores how the Cleveland Maternal Health Association expanded from this local focus and shaped the wider movement.

# 6

## A New Point of View

In the best tradition of early-twentieth-century social science, the Maternal Health Association of Cleveland embraced science as well as service. The organization assisted women on a personal level and, at the same time, worked publicly to make birth control acceptable to both the medical and the scientific communities. With other facilities across the country, the Cleveland MHA touted and tested the viability of clinical contraception. The close relationship between the MHA and the local Brush Foundation, introduced in chapter 3, broadened the focus of the clinic's work to include research into methods of birth control and related areas. Paradoxically, this relationship negatively affected local MHA service while it extended the influence of the pioneer birth control clinic far beyond the Cleveland area.

### BRANCHING OUT

During its first decade the MHA expanded to other sites in Cleveland despite limited funds and staff and concerns for adverse publicity. The need and demand for family limitation information grew as the Depression worsened. The community's positive response to clinical birth control built the MHA's confidence, and the clinic's strong support base facilitated local outreach. In 1936 and 1940 the MHA established its first clinic branches. A facility located on Cleveland's West Side, across the Cuyahoga River from center city, opened on April 1, 1936. The MHA stated in its annual report that year, "The opening of the West Side Branch . . . marks the beginning of a decentralized service which should give greater opportunity for the development of the marital-adjustment and pre-marital service, while making the regular clinic service accessible to greater numbers of people. . . . Plans for decentralization will . . . take into consideration the industrial sections of the community." After eight years, the MHA was taking its services into residential neighborhoods. Even with only limited hours, the West Side branch served increasingly higher numbers of women in its first five years. The first year, 126 new clients used its services along with 137 women who were transferred from the Osborn building clinic. The MHA described the group as a whole as having a "particularly low income." By 1940 this clinic served patients on Tuesday afternoons and evenings, and Friday mornings and afternoons. By 1941 the number of active clients at the West Side branch had climbed to 1744.[1]

Keeping the West Side branch, in 1939 the MHA moved its main downtown offices and clinic about a hundred blocks farther east to University Circle, close to Western Reserve University and University Hospitals. In the next year, the association opened two additional East Side branches. One was located on Woodhill Road, at the edge of the poverty-stricken Central Avenue area, near East 93rd Street. That facility was short-lived, but the other new clinic, at the East 35th Street Dispensary, served area women for years.[2] Coincidentally, this dispensary was the very place where volunteer work with young mothers had first convinced Dorothy Brush and Hortense Shepard to open a birth control clinic in Cleveland (see chapter 2). The dispensary's clientele had changed since the 1920s, however, from immigrants to migrants.

An MHA annual report observes that the East 35th Street clinic was "convenient to patients in the congested Central Avenue Area of Cleveland," an area that had housed black families since the Civil War. Many blacks who came to Cleveland during the Great Migration between 1870 and 1915 settled on the East Side, west of East 40th Street near Central Avenue. Overcrowding, disease, crime, and other problems plagued residents of the Central district, which by 1930 extended to East 55th Street. Between 1940 and 1971, when the Cleveland Division of Health took over the East 35th Street MHA branch, that clinic served people of color almost exclusively.[3] Maintaining a clinic to control births in an all-black neighborhood diversified the MHA clientele and made this health service more accessible for some of the city's poorest women. At the same time, establishing the new branch fueled eugenic and racist controversies. African Americans across the nation cited similar efforts as targeting the country's black citizenry for extinction.[4]

Unlike some institutions created by whites for people of color, the MHA did involve local citizens in clinic governance. By 1951 (the first year for which this information exists) black women did serve on the Committee of Management of the East 35th Street clinic. The management committees for each branch worked with the general MHA board of trustees, and the chairpersons of the committees served on the MHA board. The main MHA clinic provided physicians, nurses, and clerical workers, and office and medical supplies for the auxiliary facilities. Responsibilities for the committees of management of each satellite included stimulating community interest, acquiring volunteers, and securing funding. Services offered by the branch clinics changed according to need and funds available. For a time the East Side and West Side clinics provided only contraception, while the main clinic offered marriage counseling and infertility clinics in addition to the basic services. Only the main clinic participated in the training of medical personnel, at least for the first few years.[5]

When the MHA opened in 1928, its first physicians, Ruth Robishaw, Leona Glover, and Sarah Marcus, learned the technique of fitting diaphragms at Margaret Sanger's clinic in New York City. Medical school curriculum generally did not address issues of women's day-to-day reproductive health, including contraception. Early in its first decade, the MHA itself took on this responsibility and became an educational center. Senior women medical students from the Western Reserve University School of Medicine first came to the clinic as observers in 1933. Other doctors, nurses, and medical and nursing students soon began to visit the MHA to observe and actually participate in clinic sessions and to learn about clinic programs. Researcher Goldie Davis briefly described this training in 1938, saying that clinic doctors felt it "advisable for a visiting physician to spend at least three days observing and practicing if he [sic] anticipates opening a clinic elsewhere." The MHA also educated public health nurses, who came on a voluntary basis rather than as a formal part of their training. Students in the public health nursing course at Western Reserve University could choose to spend a day of observation at the MHA during their field experience. By 1948, according to one MHA historical account, Western Reserve University required its medical school students to attend a series of lectures on birth control given by an MHA staff person. Local doctors and students learned contraceptive methods at the MHA into the 1960s as did personnel from clinics across the country.[6] The MHA not only served women who might not be able to afford to obtain birth control from a private physician but it also educated the physicians (and future physicians) themselves. In doing so the clinic encouraged the acceptance of birth control by physicians as a legitimate medical matter.[7]

Hospitals and clinics in the United States had long served as training grounds for young clinicians. By operating as a teaching clinic, the MHA set and followed a common pattern among early birth control providers as well. Sanger's Birth Control Clinical Research Bureau trained nurses and doctors as did clinics in Rochester, Minneapolis, Denver, and elsewhere. Advocates saw this specialized education as one of the main functions of pioneer birth control clinics.[8] Clients must have held a different view, however, although their reactions are missing from the historical record. Being examined and fitted for a diaphragm involved its own embarrassment. Having those intimate procedures witnessed by a group of students or other visitors intruded on women's privacy and compromised their rights. It also certainly made the women uncomfortable. According to all accounts, the MHA did not recognize or address their clients' needs in this regard. Subjecting its clientele to the humiliation of being the objects of observation, the clinic acted according to the mores of major medical facilities of the time.[9] In matters of science, it sacrificed individual well-being for the public good of winning respectability, approval, and medical acceptance for birth control.

To this end the Cleveland MHA served as a resource for physicians and new clinics from other locations. In 1930 Gladys Gaylord reported that "New York" had asked to refer to the MHA "all inquiries regarding the organization and procedure for starting new clinics." The American Birth Control League, located in New York City, probably made that request; it received queries for assistance from across the nation.[10] In 1931 the MHA recorded visits from Dr. and Mrs. Stuart Mudd from Philadelphia; a physician from a birth control clinic in Pittsburgh, Pennsylvania; and "two workers" from Hamilton, Ontario, Canada, who studied the Cleveland facility's "methods of organization." The three-year-old clinic in Cleveland also received written inquiries for information from Missouri and Iowa that year. The new birth control center in Rochester, New York, sent its first director, social worker Ruth H. Backus, to the Cleveland MHA in 1933 to learn how to manage a clinic. Backus later recalled, "I found the highest professional standards prevailing" at the MHA, "one of the best services in the U.S."[11] The Cleveland birth control clinic spread its service patterns and philosophy to other areas of the state and country and into Canada, encouraging observation by visiting medical students, nurses, social workers, and physicians. Players in the national movement sought assistance from the pioneer facility in Cleveland.

In addition to establishing clinics in the 1930s and acting as a professional resource, the MHA took its message to the general public. Gaylord and others from the MHA lectured around Cleveland on birth control and family life. They spoke to area librarians, parent-teacher associations, nurses, social workers, clubs such as the American Association of University Women, and settlement houses. Topics included "Men and Maternal Health," "Contraception: The Woman's Point of View," and "The Eugenic Value of a Maternal Health Center." These lectures addressed a general "lack of understanding of the place of family regulation in the social problems" of the era, according to MHA sources.[12] Clinic leaders hoped to educate Clevelanders about contraception as a suitable social concern and as a possible solution to Depression-era problems. While the speeches helped to interpret the clinic and its work to professionals and other Cleveland citizens, the MHA also aimed to affect a larger population. Acting as a center for research in cooperation with a local philanthropic organization, the association stressed its place within the national movement to legitimize contraception. The resulting philosophy of service embodied the clinic's interdependent and at times conflicting goals: to improve family and child health; to nurture and educate women; to prove the viability and respectability of contraception; and to improve population quality.

## BENEFICENT RESEARCH

Brush Foundation monies not only helped establish, support, and maintain the Cleveland Maternal Health Association, as explained in chapter 3, but they also modified the association's agenda. Because of these intimate ties, the MHA committed itself to research and extensive outreach as a demonstration center for the philanthropic foundation.[13] The Cleveland MHA carefully monitored its own work and provided data to the developing cache of knowledge about sexuality, reproduction, and contraception. In doing so it played a key role in the wider movement. A brief history of clinical birth control in the *Birth Control Review* in December of 1932 (published nationally by the American Birth Control League) listed the Cleveland MHA, which was then four years old, as making "important contributions" to the "consistent study" of clinic statistics.[14] The MHA carefully recorded clients' attendance and tracked their pregnancies.

This focus was not unusual in the birth control field: Margaret Sanger named her clinic the Birth Control Clinical Research Bureau. The BCCRB and most other early clinics in the United States purposely kept detailed records and published sociological reports to demonstrate the safety, usefulness, practicality, and—most importantly—scientific authority of their efforts. At the same time, by emphasizing the importance of statistical studies, these clinics participated in a larger effort to justify the study of sexuality as integral to the analysis of social reform.

Across the United States, researchers such as Katherine Bement Davis, Marie Kopp, and Robert L. Dickinson hoped not only to remove the stigmas from sexuality in general but also to offer scientific solutions to what they understood as social problems (divorce, family disintegration, and gender identity). Some social scientists and physicians viewed companionate or ideal marriage, informed by sex education and enabled by contraception, as the pinnacle of human experience. Since little published data existed on "sex adjustment," fertility, or contraception, national organizations such as the Bureau of Social Hygiene, the National Research Council's Committee for Research in the Problems of Sex, and Dickinson's Committee on Maternal Health sponsored investigations in order to create a base of knowledge.[15] Brush Foundation support of Cleveland's pioneer birth control clinic guaranteed the MHA's participation in this pattern.

In 1931 Cleveland's Brush Foundation began to study the menstrual cycle in an attempt to perfect the safe period method of contraception (now known as the rhythm method). Physicians T. Wingate Todd and Theodore Zuck, the originator and director of the study, designed the project in part to identify a reliable and acceptable contraceptive option for Catholic women and others who were forbidden by religious doctrine to use artificial birth control. The Brush Foundation had stated at its founding that its purposes included "the furtherance of scientific research in the field of eugenics and in regulation of the increase of population," with the self-serving goal of producing more "well-born" children (see chapter 3).[16] The foundation took this purpose seriously.

Investigators hoped to confirm that women generally ovulated on or near the fourteenth day of their menstrual cycles, and that impregnation was impossible—or at least improbable—at other times during the month. The research project involved a long-term commitment from each client who, in following the study's protocol, took the distinct risk of becoming pregnant. Participants first kept detailed records to attempt to ascertain individual ovulation patterns, determined in the early years of the study by observable signs such as cramping and later by recording fluctuations in body temperature. As instructed, clients used the diaphragm when they had intercourse anytime during the twelfth through the sixteenth day of a menstrual cycle. During the next cycle the women were to avoid any contraception *except* on the fourteenth day, when they were to use the diaphragm. The diaphragm was to be used at all times throughout the third cycle *except* on the fourteenth day. Subjects were to record the dates of every instance of sexual intercourse (which Zuck called "coital exposures"). They were instructed not to employ any other means of birth control for the duration of the study.[17]

Abiding by a plan for cooperation between the MHA and the Brush Foundation, the clinic provided subjects for the Brush research project. The agreement stated: "That the Cleveland Maternal Health Clinic and any other Maternal Health Clinics which it may establish will endeavor to cooperate in [any] contraceptive or eugenic research which the Brush Foundation may undertake." The MHA promoted the "Research Department" to its clients as a "preconceptional service" that would help parents determine the optimal time for conceiving and bearing their "well-born" children.[18]

Zuck summarized the research results in 1938 in an article in the *American Journal of Obstetrics and Gynecology*. The article concluded, among other findings, that "basal body temperature is a guide to the period of fertility" in women.[19] The published results indicate that the investigation uncovered other facts as well. Zuck noted in his summary, for example, the short viability of both the sperm and ovum and described signs of pregnancy that often take place before the first missed menstrual period. With regard to the results that he sought, Zuck reported: "In 35 cases . . . conception occurred from the tenth to the twentieth days of the menstrual cycle regardless of cycle length."[20] The foundation and clinic participated together in the study until 1940. Zuck's study did not represent a research landmark but did contribute to the gathering body of knowledge about gynecology and reproduction.[21]

The Brush-MHA ovulation project was unique among North American birth control research trials in that it informed prospective subjects of the risks and did not target poor clients.[22] The study required participants to keep accurate and detailed records and to be financially and emotionally able to handle another pregnancy in case the precautions failed. Exhibiting considerable class bias, the MHA at first recruited "suitable" research subjects solely from the middle class and upper-middle class. In 1930 Todd asked the MHA to "extend their present service so that the number of patients from the privileged classes may be augmented in order that we may be reasonably sure of securing . . . enough cooperative patients willing and able to work with the Foundation."[23] This presented a problem early in the project. MHA executive secretary Gladys Gaylord described the situation: "Those who would normally use this service [i.e., wealthier women, whom the MHA thought to be the most reliable record keepers] left town for summer vacations. . . . It was therefore felt advisable in the beginning to include *regular* patients in this session." ("Regular" most likely referred to the general MHA patient population.) In the end only 26 out of the 119 total number of women first recruited for the study were rated as "cooperative patients—those interested and able to work with Dr. Zuck on various research problems." The final results tracked nearly two hundred couples.[24]

Other birth control clinics conducted research projects during the thirties and forties as did concerned eugenicists such as Clarence Gamble. A 1930s source briefly mentions that a doctor in Denver, who was associated with the Maternal Health Committee there, was experimenting with spermatotoxins, that is, preparations to disable sperm. The 1944 draft of a clinic handbook for Planned Parenthood of Columbus, Ohio, states, "Planned Parenthood centers are laboratories for social and scientific research in the field of conception control."[25] The autonomous status of many early clinics facilitated their initiation of and participation in such studies. Working as voluntary associations, free from institutional restrictions, the facilities pursued their chosen paths. One observer declared, "Every family situation offers unlimited opportunity for such research."[26] Initiating studies such as the Brush Foundation ovulation project took advantage of women's great need and desire to control reproduction. However, the research subjects themselves sometimes welcomed the chance to contribute to the growing body of knowledge about women's health.

Participants in the Cleveland study demonstrated high motivation and aided the success of the investigation. Unlike the subjects of many other medical research efforts elsewhere, these women willingly and knowingly participated in the project.[27] One research client, a social worker herself, found keeping track of the details of her intimate life tedious at times and a little unnerving, especially when the MHA selected her meticulous records (including the number and dates of "coital exposures") for publication as an anonymous example. "Imagine," she reflected years later, "the details of my sex life spread out for all to see!" However, the possibility that her efforts eventually might help others inspired this woman to continue. One study participant expressed her satisfaction with the "temperature control method" of birth control and said, "it makes me very happy to think that perhaps I, in a very small way, am contributing toward a better understanding of the fertility and sterility in women." Another research client reported to the MHA for an examination each week for ten weeks. Apparently, as Gaylord claimed, "Many people are willing to go to great personal inconvenience in order to assist in a Research program."[28] Maternal Health Association clients demonstrated their own commitment, not only to their personal well-being and that of their friends and family but also to the larger cause of birth control. Their dedicated support of studies at the MHA and elsewhere, as represented in their continued participation, helped move the research agenda along.

The ovulation project eventually added a new service to the MHA program. Although initially directed toward preventing conception, the study evolved to include a focus on fertility problems. Like other contemporaneous clinics in the 1930s and 1940s, the MHA began to assist couples who were attempting to conceive as well as those trying to limit their families. A dearth of medical knowledge about the intricacies of conception as well as its prevention offered little or no hope for "barren" couples of the early twentieth century. Pioneering researchers in gynecology such as John Rock, M.D., of Massachusetts addressed fertility issues in addition to studying ovulation and contraception.[29]

Zuck's Cleveland project strengthened support for adding a concern with infertility to the MHA's philosophy and services. The association recognized that medical professionals ignored women's problems with conceiving children as well as controlling conception, leaving another gap in health services. The MHA stepped up to fill that gap. By 1940 the clinic's program statement included among its ten goals "to assist parents in planning a pregnancy where sterility, health, or economic factors have proven an obstacle." The Cleveland MHA officially began an infertility clinic in 1946.[30] As its founding purpose had proclaimed, the MHA provided services and conducted research that stressed the importance of a heritage of good health to the family unit rather than the health of mothers in particular.

By addressing the inability of some couples to conceive, the MHA not only identified a new service group, but it also countered opponents of birth control. Approaching infertility as a medical issue demonstrated the association's concern that families continue to reproduce but at a slower rate, to ensure well-born children. Infertility research fit well into a eugenic agenda. Many viewed childlessness, whether voluntary or involuntary, as a social problem that contributed to diminishing population quality. Experts often equated voluntary childlessness with selfishness and predicted a "national decline" if women, especially educated white women, continued to shirk their childbearing duties.[31] The MHA always aimed its work at helping women to better fulfill the high calling of motherhood rather than avoid it. As T. Wingate Todd stated in 1930, "The Maternal Health Movement more and more clearly stands out as the supreme effort of Motherhood to safeguard her offspring." Fitter families included fewer children and healthier children. Childless women or couples did not fit the ideal.[32]

Birth control promoters across North America, not only in Cleveland, emphasized better maternal health as a means of producing better babies—white or black. Historian Susan Smith finds that the black community emphasized children's health in its rhetoric and voluntary work during the early to mid-twentieth century. Smith notes, "Black women, in particular, argued that the survival and uplift of the race depended on healthy children." Black physicians like Cleveland's Charles Garvin also promoted increased attention to public health, especially to improve the well-being of black children. Garvin encouraged other doctors of color "to discover and disseminate knowledge that will prepare our race to go forward in the battle for survival, physically fit." Using the same arguments as white eugenicists, he further urged attention to "the preservation and betterment of our racial stock."[33]

The popular press, meanwhile, also encouraged high standards for the rearing of children of any ethnicity. African American neighborhood newspapers like the *Cleveland Gazette* ran articles that romanticized motherhood and called for attention to children's dress, for example. In 1930 one such piece extolled the virtues of fashionable nightclothes for children: "Most amusing and most winsome do little tots look in these fantastic garments, and the vogue is gaining in popularity. . . . It behooves every mother who is interested in togging her little folks in the latest to turn her attention to the pajama theme."[34] In a time of increasing financial woes among area residents, black and white, such an image promoted an unrealistic and unattainable goal.

Some birth control advocates and other leaders employed eugenic arguments and practices as a tool of racial oppression rather than racial uplift, targeting various groups in different geographic areas. Historian Johanna Schoen notes that in Ontario, Canada, birth control leaders hoped to reduce the French-Canadian population, while in the state of Rhode Island, immigrants represented the least desirable group. Eugenic ideology assigned a population's inferior status according to levels of poverty and economic dependency. In the Deep South during the thirties, many birth control advocates focused their efforts on poor whites as well as blacks, considering both groups as threats to the status quo. Proponents conflated social class and race. Assumptions about inferiority based on class and race continue to circumscribe reproductive rights more than a century later. As one scholar contends, "Reproductive politics in America invariably involves racial politics."[35]

In the 1930s in Cleveland, MHA rhetoric focused on class. Case studies used in MHA annual reports to illustrate the acute need for contraceptive services typically depict a family with many children living in extreme poverty. The examples usually pay no attention to the race of the people involved. The 1931 MHA annual report, for example, focuses on four cases. The descriptions highlight overcrowding, such as a family of

# Nobody Wanted Jimmy
## But He Was Born Anyhow

His mother was sick with worry before he was born. His father was an unskilled laborer, out of work for 17 months. The family is on relief, without enough food for the other five children. Which one of us under these circumstances would look forward to the birth of Jimmy?

The community didn't want him. Cleveland is already spending $312,000 a month for relief.

Jimmy didn't want to be born; life meant only misery to him.

### But Anyhow
He was born November 21, 1931

| | |
|---|---:|
| His mother was given pre-natal care by a public health nurse | $11.00 |
| He was born in a hospital | 35.00 |
| The social service department furnished baby clothes | 2.50 |
| The City gave him a quart of milk a day for 4 months | 8.40 |
| He was supervised by a doctor and nurse during his brief life | 40.00 |
| The home was so cold he contracted pneumonia; hospital care, 7 days was | 14.00 |
| He died March 30, 1932, and was buried "free" by the community | 28.00 |
| So his short and painful life cost us all | $138.90 |

### Now Honestly
Was it fair to Jimmy to be born at this time with no chance for a happy childhood?

Was it fair to the children when the family is on relief at $5.00 a week, for food only, with no money at all for rent or clothing?

Was it fair to the community, that is already supporting 21,000 families?

Physicians at the Maternal Health Clinic instructed 2,072 women in contraceptive methods during the past 4 years. These mothers, half of them with unemployed husbands, desperately feared the birth of another child.

### The Clinic Believes
That a child's first right is to be wanted.

That hunger and fear cannot create a wholesome home for a baby.

That during this crisis the birth of those babies whose coming is now cause for dread should be postponed until a better time. The community cannot keep in health and decency the children that are here.

That the knowledge of how to "space births" now open to those who can afford it should be made available to the very poor.

The work of the Maternal Health Clinic has doubled each year.

The past year 1,026 women were given contraceptive information by our physicians.

This next year we want to care for 2,100.

The cost of instructing a mother in contraception is $5.00.

We refused 25 women in June because of lack of funds.

### If You Believe
that it is essential for us to help those people who seek us, please send a contribution immediately.

Make checks payable to Maternal Health Ass'n., 609 Osborn Building.

MRS. H. P. EELLS, JR.,
*Treasurer.*

FIGURE 24. Nobody wanted Jimmy, 1931. PPGC, box 3, Western Reserve Historical Society.

ten living in four rooms over a store, or note dire financial straits, such as sixteen children and two adults existing on a daughter's income of fifteen dollars a week, supplemented only by the father's occasional work. The report concentrates on the issues of financial status and family well-being rather than race.[36] Likewise, an early MHA fund-raising letter offered a class-based (and eugenic) argument for supporting the association (see figure 24).

The 1932 MHA annual report offers further evidence of the use of class-based rhetoric to promote the ethic of family stability. Designed to emphasize the excessive burdens that some women carried, burdens that the MHA could help to relieve, the report charts statistics on thirteen separate clinic cases but does not include race. The data include the mother's age, how many years she had been married, the number of her pregnancies, and the number of children born alive. The information supported MHA arguments that large families hindered upward mobility and strained the health of mothers. (It is conceivable that all of the women in this group were white.)

The clinic was in no way free from the burgeoning racial prejudice in Cleveland and the country during the 1920s and 1930s, however. Sarah Marcus, a native of Sommerville, South Carolina, and an MHA staff physician during this era, revealed her own prejudices against "colored girls" in a 1974 interview. The MHA did not hire its first black staff person until 1953. During the MHA's first decade, though, it directed eugenic rhetoric and philosophy of service toward specific classes rather than a specific race.[37] As a model for other facilities, the Cleveland MHA promoted this class-based rhetoric and philosophy, and its inherent racism, across the state and beyond.

## SPREADING THE WISDOM

Maternal Health Association leaders kept in touch with their peers across North America through existing familial and social networks as well as new contacts. Many clinic founders across the continent had an acquaintance with Margaret Sanger: for example, Mary Chambers Hawkins in Hamilton, Ontario, Canada; Dorothy Brush in Cleveland; and Ruth Vincent Cunningham in Denver, Colorado.[38] These crucial bonds placed the pioneer efforts within the national and international movements and pulled the far-flung clinics together in a loosely strung web. The connections facilitated the sharing of ideologies and patterns of service. Being among the first fifty freestanding birth control clinics in North America, the Cleveland MHA eagerly embraced the opportunity to act as a demonstration center and used its link to the Brush Foundation to that end.

In addition to focusing clinic work on eugenics, research, and infertility, the foundation extended the MHA's influence beyond Cleveland and Ohio. In 1929 the Brush Foundation provided five thousand dollars to the MHA to pay the salary of an executive secretary. Social worker Gladys Gaylord held this position, funded by the foundation, for nearly twenty years. She performed managerial duties, spoke in Cleveland and around the country about birth control and the MHA, organized and led a statewide birth control group, and assisted with the formation of clinics in other areas. Hiring an expert for these tasks helped the MHA secure professional authority and promote itself as a reputable service organization. Hiring a woman to fill the position kept the leadership power in female hands. Gaylord promoted clinical birth control on the Sanger model and disseminated the design of the Cleveland MHA and the policies of the Brush Foundation throughout Ohio and outside of the continental United States.[39]

By 1937 the Brush Foundation mandated that the MHA "release practically the whole time of Miss Gladys Gaylord to education and extension work, particularly outside of Cuyahoga County."[40] The MHA seems to have supported this decision. The outreach work took the local association to a new level of state and regional leadership. The efforts outside of Cleveland fulfilled one of the clinic's stated purposes, to act as a demonstration center for other facilities, and pushed forward the Brush Foundation's agenda. With the financial support of the foundation, the MHA moved beyond service and research to education and advocacy.

Birth control clinics directly modeled after Cleveland's began in cities across Ohio, as far north as Ontario, Canada, and as far south as Puerto Rico. People from Columbus, Ohio, contacted the MHA in 1930 to discuss beginning a clinic there. That year, Gaylord reported "no immediate action in Toledo, Painesville, or Akron," Ohio, regarding the opening of centers for contraception, but optimistically noted that Youngstown residents were considering forming a clinic. Members of the Young Woman's Mission in Springfield, Ohio, visited the Cleveland MHA two years before opening the Mother's Health Clinic in that southwestern Ohio town. These women, already engaged in assisting the "sick poor," patterned their birth control effort after the Cleveland and Columbus facilities. Philanthropist and eugenicist Clarence Gamble, of the Procter and Gamble Company, helped to initiate and support the Ohio clinics in Springfield, Columbus, Toledo, and his hometown of Cincinnati. One history of the Cleveland Maternal Health Association claimed in 1948 that Gladys Gaylord was the "primary organizer" of eleven out of the twelve Ohio birth control clinics then in existence.[41]

Gaylord assisted other groups around the United States and in Canada. While in Minneapolis for the National Conference of Social Work in 1931, she witnessed the formation of the Birth Control League of Minnesota and advised that organization about opening a clinic in Minneapolis. The Hamilton Birth Control Society (BCS) in Ontario, Canada, opened in 1932, two years after its founders first visited the Cleveland MHA. The Hamilton BCS sent its first nurse and a physician to Cleveland for training.[42] Without the Brush Foundation's subsidy of

Gaylord's salary and expenses, her extensive outreach would not have been possible. Other staff members also took the MHA's message and model to the state and national levels. The Rev. Ferdinand Blanchard gave a talk at the National Conference of Social Work in 1937, for instance, and Ruth Robishaw spoke before the Ohio State Nurses' Association in 1939. Both speakers focused on the eugenic benefits of contraception, especially for children and families. Blanchard noted that birth control clinics had a "widening field of opportunity . . . to spread the wisdom" of family limitation.[43] The MHA took this task to heart and spread the wisdom throughout Ohio and across the U.S.-Canadian border.

As the first birth control clinic in Ohio, the MHA served a wide geographic area. A 1934 report issued by the American Birth Control League (ABCL) listed two other clinics in the state, one in Cincinnati and one in Columbus. Three more Ohio clinics formed over the decade, in Dayton (1935), Springfield (1935), and Youngstown (1937).[44] In the early thirties, before these other clinics took hold, the ABCL directed requests from Midwesterners and nearby Canadians for birth control services or information to Cleveland. Maternal Health Association clients also referred their out-of-town relatives and friends to the Cleveland facility (see chapter 5). Clinic physician Sarah Marcus remembered that a car full of women once drove the 120 miles from Toledo to be fitted for diaphragms at the Cleveland MHA.[45] Apparently distance did not deter some women from their pursuit of reproductive control.

The Cleveland MHA and Gladys Gaylord coordinated the state clinical birth control effort. When the Maternal Health Association of Ohio formed in 1933, Cleveland's MHA served as its first headquarters. The state organization circulated information among Ohio's birth control clinics, held joint meetings, and helped establish more facilities. Gaylord acted as "field secretary" for the MHA of Ohio during the 1930s and early 1940s. Some officers of the Cleveland association also served as officers in the state MHA group. This cooperative effort continued until at least 1949. The Cleveland MHA also organized a statewide Association of Maternal Health Nurses, which met twice a year, once in conjunction with the Ohio State Nurses Association.[46]

The Brush Foundation funded Gaylord's activities around the state, activities that the foundation and the MHA considered "education and extension work."[47] Having support for such efforts allowed the clinic to broaden its impact beyond northeastern Ohio. The education and extension work combined MHA's Midwestern influences and Brush Foundation ideology with the methods and ideals of the national birth control movement. New clinics throughout Ohio and elsewhere connected to the national effort through the MHA. The Cleveland clinic's outreach efforts did not stop at the state line, however.

Gaylord carried MHA practices and Brush Foundation philosophy even farther afield. Dorothy Bourne, social worker and founder of the University of Puerto Rico's School of Social Work in the 1930s, invited Gaylord to Puerto Rico in 1934 to help plan the island's clinical birth control strategy. Bourne was married to James Bourne, the director of the U.S.-funded Puerto Rico Emergency Relief Administration (PRERA). Appalled by Puerto Rico's desperately crowded and unsanitary living conditions, the Bournes wanted to address these issues through population control, to be funded by the PRERA. As a U.S. territory, the island was subject to the Comstock Law. Predominately Roman Catholic, Puerto Rico also faced religious proscriptions against contraception. In spite of these obstacles, Bourne and the PRERA took on the task of investigating the possibilities of setting up a birth control clinic in Puerto Rico. The MHA granted Gaylord release time. She spent four months on the island during her first visit in 1934 and two months the next year. With the aid of the PRERA, Gaylord and gynecologists working in the area opened a trial birth control clinic in Puerto Rico in 1935. By the end of that year, services extended island-wide.[48]

No direct evidence connects Brush Foundation monies with this overseas effort.[49] However, rhetoric and research strongly suggest strongly that Gaylord brought the influence of both the foundation and the MHA to Puerto Rico. The first Puerto Rican clinic was designated a demonstration center, for instance. Leaders there called for the formation of a Race Betterment Association "to improve racial stocks," and clinic physicians investigated the rhythm method.[50] The Brush Foundation's emphasis on utilizing the MHA as a model and conduit for research directly influenced the direction of Puerto Rico's movement for family limitation. As an agent of the foundation and the Cleveland MHA, Gladys Gaylord used her contacts and professional expertise to implement this outreach.

Controversy soon developed in the mainland United States around the federal support of contraceptive services in Puerto Rico as well as around religious issues. Roman Catholic groups in Washington condemned the effort. As a result of this opposition, all PRERA-sponsored clinical birth control activity in the territory ceased in September 1936, which was, not coincidentally, a United States presidential election year.[51] The movement on the island continued, however, sponsored in part by private individuals such as Clarence Gamble. In 1936 twenty-three clinics opened in Puerto Rico under the auspices of the Maternal and Child Health Association there. By 1959 the small island boasted an extensive

| Date | Clinic Hours per Week | New Clients |
|------|----------------------|-------------|
| 1928–29 | 4 | 385 (225)+ |
| 1929–30 | 5.5 | 285 |
| 1930–31 | 10 | 536 |
| 1931–32 | 17 | 1026 |
| 1932–33 | – | 1043 |
| 1933–34 | 22 | 1045 |
| 1934–35 | 26 | 1057 |
| 1935–36 | 27 | 971 |
| 1936–37 | 29 | 986 |
| 1937–38* | 31 | 1216 |

+ Figure given for 1928–29 in second annual report.
* Figures include the West Side branch.
– Missing data

Men's consultations are included in the hours but not in numbers of clients.

FIGURE 25. MHA hours and numbers of clients: data from MHA annual reports.[52]

system of birth control clinics; researchers studied the effects of the birth control pill using the clients of these clinics. The Cleveland MHA's involvement overseas, short-lived though it was, helped create the structural and ideological base for later contraceptive clinics as well as for international research on women's health and population control.[53]

In retrospect, such heavy emphasis on outreach beyond Cuyahoga County and outside of the continental United States limited the number of Cleveland women served by the MHA. Certainly a comprehensive visiting nurse or physician program would have reached many more women than the MHA average of about eight hundred to nine hundred new clients per year between 1928 and 1939. Although some contemporaneous facilities served smaller numbers of women than did Cleveland, clinics in Los Angeles (est. 1925) and New York (est. 1923) reached about 3,800 and 4,300 women, respectively, by 1929. They did this by maintaining clinic sites in a variety of locations for up to twenty-two hours a week.[54]

Cleveland's MHA also held clinics for twenty-two hours a week after 1933 (figure 25), but that time included men's consultations and other services such as the Brush research clinic. Evidence indicates that the MHA chose to focus on international instead of local outreach. The association had earlier proposed "to continue its work along conservative and scientific lines, cooperating with recognized social and health agencies wherever possible, limiting its functions to those activities in keeping with the highest standards of medical practice."[55] The active pursuit of more birth control clinic clients in Cleveland might have jeopardized the MHA's relationships with other social service organizations. While the clinic maintained this position to stay within the law, win medical approval, and keep peace within the local reform community, its conservative approach limited the numbers of women it could assist.

Comparable time and effort spent on publicizing the clinic locally, hiring more physicians, sending nurses into the community, or adding clinic hours might have dramatically broadened access to and increased the use of the MHA's clinics in Cleveland. While the MHA took steps in this direction with its branch sites, those clinics did not approach full-time status for decades. The time and money spent on extensive outreach in the state, on the continent, and overseas stretched the MHA's influence beyond Cleveland. The extension efforts contributed to the national and international movement but negatively affected the clinic's local course.

The MHA executive secretary would not have agreed. Gaylord stated in 1930 that only "slow, sane progress" with strong medical backing helped clinics "lay a foundation that will hold." She claimed that "clinics [that] started less carefully in other cities" had failed. Gaylord stressed the necessity of foundation support for the MHA's efforts outside of Cleveland: "We cannot render service to other communities without the financial and moral backing of the Brush Foundation." An anonymous note taker clarified the foundation's stance on outreach eight years later: "Never has the Foundation been interested in a birth control clinic as such. But they have been interested in educating the public to a new point of view." This new point of view recognized the social import of contraception and viewed it as a matter for scientific study. In 1939, in a speech to the Birth Control Society of Hamilton, Ontario, Gaylord weighed the short-and long-term benefits of "working quietly." She insisted that convincing a community to support an innovative demonstration service required continual education and interpretation. An unidentified MHA leader, probably Gaylord, gave another reason for acting as a model facility. In a speech in Jackson, Michigan, in 1936, she stated that a "demonstration service . . . is often a necessary means of changing . . . medical opinions."[56]

The pioneer birth control clinic in Cleveland, Ohio, shared the larger movement's visions of birth control as an agent for social change and a means for women to help other women. Other clinics and their advocates implemented those visions through voluntary activity, collecting and publishing statistics, and quietly networking. The MHA moved beyond service and data keeping and added scientific research to its program. The clinic's connection to the Brush Foundation, its founding as a demonstra-

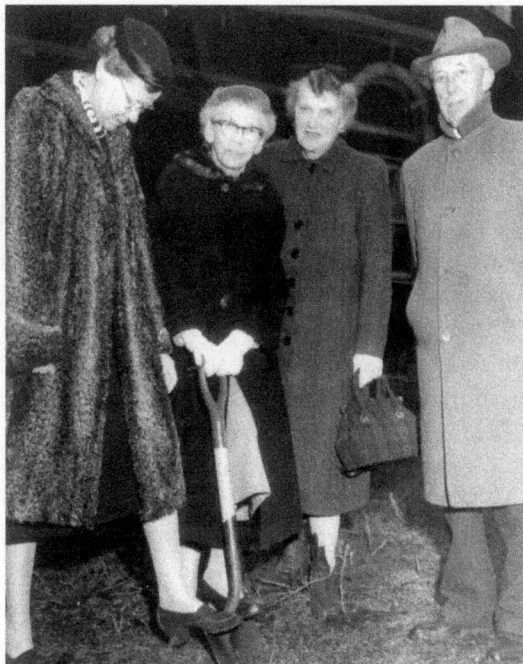

FIGURE 26. Katherine Bingham Fisher, Roslyn Campbell Weir (honorary MHA president), Dorothy Rogers Williams (president), and the Rev. Dr. Ferdinand Q. Blanchard, pastor emeritus, Euclid Congregational Church, break ground for a new MHA building on Cornell Road, March 22, 1956. All except Williams helped to found the MHA.
© Nixon, Cleveland Public Library Photograph Collection.

tion center, and its focus on research all demonstrated its commitment to social betterment in the best tradition of the Progressive Era. Though characterized by compassionate nurturing and personal service, the MHA always held true to its heritage of professional reform.

The close cooperation between the MHA and the Brush Foundation attached a scientific focus to the clinic and extended its influence beyond Cleveland. At the same time, the link to the foundation limited the number of local women served by the MHA and planted the clinic firmly within the prevalent eugenic justification for family limitation. Through its bond with the foundation, the MHA emphasized its role as a model, a demonstration center for contraception. Together the voluntary association and the philanthropy applied the aims of twentieth-century scientific charity to the birth control movement throughout Ohio and outside of the continental United States. The close relationship of the MHA with private philanthropy rather than medical institutions or public health organizations embodied the ambiguities inherent in sexuality and birth control.

# Conclusion

In the 1920s a few Cleveland women perceived a need that the city's health care community refused to address, the need for reliable birth control. They believed that medical and social service professionals denied women, especially poor and working-class women, critical health care information. Like other reform-minded citizens of their era, they created a voluntary health organization to solve the problem. Unlike other reforms, however, birth control stood on the edge of respectability and at the boundaries of the law. Acting for the good of individual women and society as a whole, as well as in the interest of their race and social class, these women took female voluntarism in new directions. They entered the illicit domain of sexuality and reproduction.

This case study illuminates the critical nature of several interlocking factors. Voluntary action, gender, networking, the power and limits of the law, and a conflicted cultural unease around sexual matters and policy—these elements all shaped the MHA's history and future, as well as the history and future of the larger struggle for reproductive rights.

Social tensions and legal prohibitions directly influenced women to establish birth control clinics such as the MHA as private organizations. Inspired by Mary Ware Dennett, Margaret Sanger, and other national leaders, these women took advantage of a legal system that proscribed such activity as obscene but only sporadically enforced those proscriptions. Like the successful commercial vendors whom they scorned, birth control leaders of the 1920s and 1930s found a market that physicians had ignored. American citizens wanted and needed reliable ways to limit their families. Some even went to great lengths, traveling long distances and making intricate arrangements to acquire the means to do so.

To establish their birth control clinic, MHA founders also went to great lengths. These upper-class women, whom some disparage as self-centered or flighty socialites, supplemented traditional voluntary tactics with direct involvement. Due to contraception's shaky legal standing, they at once utilized and bypassed existing laws. By publishing a legal interpretation and including lawyers on the MHA board, founders recognized and used the power of the legal system for their own ends. However, by bending the law through civil disobedience, founders and supporters enabled the clinic to actually provide contraception in its early days. Refusing to accept the legal definition of contraception as obscene, MHA leaders and clients disclose in their beliefs and by their actions the limits of the power of the law and policy in private matters.

When hospitals and other institutions in Cleveland and other cities dismissed the controversial idea of sponsoring clinics for contraception, women created freestanding clinics and ran them as volunteers. Women secured funding and recruited women physicians, nurses, and social workers as staff. Operating out of the voluntary sector offered the autonomy to provide new services such as contraception and eventually infertility assistance. Unaffiliated with any national group for years, the MHA took advantage of that independence to act in an unorthodox manner at times, smuggling diaphragms from New York, for example. "The power of the unofficial sphere is that you can make decisions that would be impossible in the official one," says historian Catherine Allgor, speaking of the influence of women's private actions on nineteenth-century politics.[1] The MHA demonstrates and embodies that critical element of women's voluntarism and philanthropy.

Serving women's reproductive needs from the voluntary sector rather than in a medical or governmental institution limited the influence of early birth control clinics, however. In studying the patronage of artistic pursuits, Ralph Locke finds that voluntary reform often "colludes in the very problems it claims to be fighting," by not forcing government or other institutions to attend to the issues.[2] Although birth control pioneers acted alongside, and at times outside of, the perimeters of institutionalized medicine and social service, they structured their new clinics firmly under medical authority and adhered to accepted service standards. Guided by the carefully selected Medical Advisory Board of prominent male physicians, the MHA organized under their purview to avoid confrontation and safeguard its future. By focusing exclusively on the diaphragm, a method that required medical supervision, the MHA and other clinics distanced their efforts from the illicit trade in contraceptive goods and sexual favors. The choice placed birth control firmly in the hands of doctors and encouraged a reluctant medical profession to take charge. Working toward the end of improving women's health by expanding family limitation options, the MHA and other early birth control providers in fact circumscribed those very options by focusing almost solely on the diaphragm. The fact that the condom steadily remained more popular among American couples indicates that the diaphragm held limited or no appeal for many women.[3]

The MHA's involvement in Brush Foundation research programs led to and reflected a detached philosophy of scientific philanthropy rather than a more involved social work or public health philosophy of birth control. However, in the actual provision of services, the clinic took a personal, warm approach, though tinged with condescension and rooted in the racist and class-based biases of the era. In clinic design, for example, founders added a nurturing component, softening the harsh medical atmosphere with art and furnishings from their own homes. They combined the prevailing private practice model of one-to-one, expert physician/passive patient consultation with a social welfare model of outreach, education, and empowerment. Rather than setting a fixed fee for service as did private physicians, they accepted payment on a sliding scale. By popularizing "modern" barrier methods of birth control, especially the diaphragm, birth control clinics helped to raise the level of women's knowledge about their bodies and attended to related health problems. The dual service agenda embodies the conflict within much of philanthropy: a conflict between the racist, class-based ideal of scientific charity and the person-to-person actuality of helping individuals.

The story of the MHA uncovers layers of other complexities within this reform movement. Motivated in part by a shared biology, MHA clients and founders acted to change their lives and the lives of other women, using personal rather than party politics. They challenged and modified policies—for example, expanding the basis for offering birth control from strictly health concerns to include psychological and economic needs. After 1918 national and local birth control rhetoric emphasized the eugenic improvement of progeny and the race rather than the value to women of spacing their pregnancies. Yet clearly a major reason for local clinics' success lay in women's desperate need and gratitude for affordable, accessible, reliable birth control information and services, as revealed in their correspondence. Mothers cited practical considerations—financial stability, health, family concerns, peace of mind—rather than eugenic reasons for limiting their families. Their motivations help explicate how private citizens interpret and utilize the ideology of experts to their own ends. Clients' silence about the illegality of birth control both reflects the lack of enforcement against users of contraception and indicates the deep discontinuity between policy and practice, between law on the books and law in action. Like MHA founders and leaders, clients rejected the notion of contraception as immoral or obscene. Within the strictures of increasing emphasis on expertise and authority, usually defined as male, these women created a female dominion.[4]

The Maternal Health Association was a women's organization in its early years, run by women for women. Within the context of maintaining the patriarchal family system and class and racial hierarchy, MHA supporters acted as feminists in the broadest sense. The choice of the diaphragm by the MHA and most 1930s clinics both furthered and restricted the feminist goal of increasing woman's control of reproduction, however. The female-centered method emphasized and maintained woman's cultural role as the mother of the race while setting the control of reproduction in her hands. Relegating the condom to second place in the hierarchy of birth control methods despite its popularity only reinforced its distasteful public reputation and promoted the common view of men as irresponsible in reproductive matters. The almost solely female-centered direction of research and development in the areas of contraception and fertility into the twenty-first century manifests one long-term policy result of this decision.

Social status and extensive philanthropic connections enabled MHA leaders to accomplish what they did, but the fear of losing that status or corrupting those connections limited their accomplishments. Courting the support of the Brush Foundation strengthened the MHA's ties to modern philanthropy. The clinic stressed its purpose as a demonstration center. This role mandated participating in research and using businesslike, efficient methods, at times compromising the women who came to the clinic. Such conservative strategies maintained the status quo and limited the number of clinic clients. Concurrently, though, this approach established a firm base for peaceful coexistence with other social agencies. Cleveland's clinic escaped the protest and prosecution that other facilities experienced.

"We look to the time when every child shall come into this world through the gate of deliberate planning and not through the portal of chance," declared MHA physician Ruth Robishaw.[5] While this goal has yet to be reached, the MHA and its peers did effect change. By initiating birth control clinics as voluntary associations outside of, yet connected to, the medical establishment, American women identified a need, provided a service, and helped persuade physicians, social workers, and the general public to accept contraception. An MHA spokesperson explained in 1944, "As is usual in any new development, it is lay people through private agencies who first demonstrate the need for new types of service, therefore, it is not surprising to find that clinics and services dealing with the spacing of children have been started throughout the United States. . . . [by laypeople]."[6] Laywomen helped bring the common private practice of birth control before the public eye. Without much publicity or drama, women in early clinics—supporters, founders, leaders, and clients—quietly kept the subject alive and pushed the movement forward. Although such efforts reached a small proportion of women, they effectively vitalized the birth control movement at the local level.[7]

Evidence from the MHA and similar facilities calls for a characterization of the 1920s and 1930s as an era of the legitimization of birth control rather than simply professionalization. "Legitimize" in this case refers not to making birth control legal by law but rather to transforming it from disreputable to acceptable in the public eye. Most pioneer birth control clinics avoided legal confrontations and employed a variety of means to that end. While these clinics tried to stay out of the limelight, however, their very creation and existence drew attention to contraception in communities across the country. Birth control clinics raised local awareness among physicians, clergy, social workers, and health professionals, as well as private citizens, as the story of the MHA reveals. Wide-ranging networks spread this awareness of women's demand for safe and effective family limitation to other regions, states, and outside the United States.

Local facilities like the MHA sustained the birth control movement during the 1930s. Clinics across the continent easily attracted clients from a variety of social classes with little advertisement, indicating the extent of women networking on each other's behalf as well as the extreme nature of the need. The clinics demonstrated that some women wanted a birth control method that differed from the commercial variety. Women and men, laypeople and professionals, donated money, volunteered time and talent, served on boards, and advised, managed, staffed, and patronized the clinics. Grounded in local efforts and shaped by local influences as well as national ideologies, such leaders as Dorothy Brush and Gladys Gaylord acted beyond Cleveland and the MHA.

Brush, Gaylord, and other Clevelanders lectured publicly, published articles, served on state, regional, and national committees, advised other clinics, trained staff, organized state groups, and attended regional and national conferences. Through such outreach and their connections with other clinics, these activists added MHA tactics and Brush Foundation philosophies to the larger movement.[8] Other birth control clinics that organized in the 1930s likewise contributed to and helped shape the broader effort. Focusing on the separate but connected stories of local efforts expands and modifies other historians' depiction of the national birth control effort as lethargic and depressed during the 1930s.[9]

Women organizers, funders, physicians, social workers, nurses, volunteers, and clients acted in birth control clinics as agents for change, both purposefully and by chance, to legitimize contraception. Their roles equaled and often surpassed that of male physicians, managers, and funders. This evidence from the Cleveland MHA and other facilities modifies another historical argument, that the professionalization of birth control in the 1930s led to male managers (professionals) and female workers (amateurs). The biggest discrepancy between this claim and the documentation lies in the assignment of the category "amateur" to clinic organizers and staff. On the national level, female professionals actively pursued the goals of female visionaries such as Margaret Sanger and Mary Ware Dennett as well as male leaders such as Clarence Gamble and Robert Dickinson.

The argument ignores the women physicians, nurses, and social workers who staffed most clinics in North America. Some of these local professionals such as Gladys Gaylord actively worked within the national arena. Applying the term "amateur" to former suffrage activists such as Edna Brush Perkins or social service organizers such as Lenore Schwab Black negates the skills and experience that women gained through voluntary activity. As for directing and consulting, in the Cleveland example, women led the board of the MHA through the 1960s and often that of the Brush Foundation as well.[10] The stories of local clinics, standing separate from but within the context of the national movement, highlight voluntarism, networking, and gender in addition to the role of professionals as critical factors in the history of birth control in this time period.

The Rev. Ferdinand Blanchard claimed in 1937 that the previous decade had witnessed a "changed outlook upon the use of contraceptives." He explained, "Once a subject unfit for decent conversation, it is today an accepted element in social organization. Once outlawed not less by public opinions than by legal statute, it now occupies a respectable place in the study of wisely organizing our life. Once the indecent fantasy of irresponsible fanatics it has become a well considered principle for dealing with our modern but age old problems of disease, crime and poverty."[11] While Blanchard overstated the case, the thirties did see a profound change in attitudes and policy towards birth control. The histories of local clinics suggest that private action and professionalization each played critical roles in moving contraception from outside the bounds of polite society, closer to the mainstream.

Birth control clinics of the 1920s and 1930s embodied ambiguities and discontinuities between women's rights and the duty of motherhood; between individual benefits and the eugenic good of the race; between physician authority and patient agency; and between civil disobedience and the letter of the law. Within these overlapping cultural confusions, clinics like the MHA modified and shaped reproductive policy. Clinic founders and leaders helped to reframe birth control as respectable rather than immoral by taking it on as a reform cause. Their voluntarism recognized and promoted contraception as a serious matter worthy of the energy, time, and money of prominent citizens. Clinical contraception did not eliminate the commercial birth control market but rather added another dimension, that of medical authority, to reproductive control. Clinics paradoxically increased birth control's acceptability while limiting accessibility by requiring marriage licenses and medical supervision. By offering birth control to women of all classes and races in woman-centered, voluntary health organizations like the MHA, middle-class and upper-middle-class women helped set an ongoing pattern for such services. The national birth control movement incorporated tactics common to female voluntarism, tactics perfected in local clinics like the MHA.

Looking backward, the twenty-first-century feminist historian wishes that early-twentieth-century birth control activists and clients had agitated for self-determination and a broader spectrum of service rather than for medical authority and control. The eugenic philosophy of clinic founders and funders directly affected attitudes toward family planning among people of color. The philosophy reverberates worldwide in the present day.[12] The actions of leaders such as Sanger and the women of the MHA bound the effort to control fertility within tight conservative parameters. Those limits affected the many individual women who could not access centers for birth control or who did not qualify for their clinic services. The conservative parameters circumscribed the movement and greatly lessened its impact. Despite the continued existence of the MHA and many other clinics founded during the thirties, they reached and continue to reach only a handful of the women and men who seek and need family planning counsel.

The story of women and voluntary action as revealed in the records of the Cleveland Maternal Health Association discloses the power and the limits of women's individual and collective agency driven by vigorous networks across boundaries of gender and generation. Rather than a progressive tale of accomplishments, then, this study of local activity within a national social movement analyzes a distinct moment in the history of the complex efforts of women to get out—and to help others out—from under "the shadow of maternity."[13]

In 1962 a Planned Parenthood Federation of American report titled "How to Improve Communications About Birth Control" suggested three ways for such organizations to legitimize their cause: identify with authority symbols in the community; utilize existing networks; and avoid challenging the power structure.[14] The strategies used by MHA leaders to gain respectability for birth control had found their way into organizational policy long before 1962. The MHA clinic, begun as an autonomous experiment, a demonstration center, had become a North American model.

In the realm of sexuality, discontinuity and tension between policy and practice, rhetoric and reality continue in the twenty-first century. Heated debates around abortion and other sexual issues, such as AIDS, teen sexual activity and pregnancy, homosexuality, and, yes, birth control, often ignore or minimize actual practices. In March 1992 the hallowed halls of the Harvard Divinity School exhibited artwork created with condoms. The display was designed to improve the public image of the age-old contraceptive. However, according to the Associated Press, the "Sacred Condoms" exhibit was not highly publicized and opened only "90 minutes a day for two weeks, mostly while the university [was] on vacation."[15] Late-twentieth- and early-twenty-first-century attempts to regulate indecency in music and over the Internet, in the name of protecting children, smack of Comstockery. Comstock-like fear of the private and public expression of sexuality exists in a society that at the same time encourages and profits by exploiting sexuality in fiction, advertising, film, and television, and on the Internet.

American society remains bound by sexual taboos and stigmas in some areas while openly manipulating sexuality in others. Since the 1980s the United States government has cut funds for family planning and abortion programs. The cuts and court decisions reveal a dramatic reversal in the state's attitude toward reproductive rights. The instability and fragility of public policy toward reproduction indicate that the volatility of the issues endures and still negatively affects women's lives, individually and collectively, in the control of reproduction; in invasive, imperfect, expensive yet highly touted fertility technologies; in an increasing emphasis on fulfillment through motherhood; in a renewed eugenic drive for the perfect baby; in experiments in genetic engineering and cloning.

The struggle over freedom to choose a method of family limitation versus social, political, legal, or medical control of reproduction began before Anthony Comstock in the early nineteenth century, was circumscribed by twentieth-century domestic and international population control experiments, and continues. A 1940 statement by MHA nurse Edna Rusch applies over half a century later: "Even greater than our concern for the health and happiness of this present generation of adults is our concern for the next generation, which after all constitutes a tangible expression of our hope for the future."[16]

I lament that my younger sister, my sons, my nephews, my nieces, and my younger friends face moralistic sexual policies set in place before my grandmother's lifetime, policies that hamper personal experiences of sexuality and circumscribe reproductive choices. Paying attention to the voices and agency of individual women and men and the power of local organizations, historians must continue to unearth the complexities of birth control policy in order to comprehend and confront current dilemmas. Perhaps we can even illuminate past peregrinations and pitfalls that may, again, lie ahead.

# Epilogue

In 2003 the Cleveland Maternal Health Association, or rather its direct descendant, Planned Parenthood of Greater Cleveland (PPGC), celebrated seventy-five years of continuous service. Over time PPGC expanded its range of health services, added and relocated clinics, and moved and improved its administrative offices. The organization embraced new technology in the areas of information retrieval, communication, and record keeping as well as contraception, and lobbied aggressively rather than quietly for women's reproductive rights. Yet the social and political climate of 2003 resembled the association's early years: a negative, almost punitive attitude towards family planning prevailed among government policy makers in the United States and abroad. PPGC employed a large paid staff but continued to rely on its staunch supporters—board members, donors, volunteers, and grateful clients—in marketing, fund-raising, and service. Below are a few highlights of the years between 1940 and 2003.

The MHA joined the reorganized national birth control organization Planned Parenthood Federation of America in 1942, but maintained its own identity in many ways, for example, keeping the Maternal Health Association name until 1966. The agency employed a couple of male directors, but women continued to comprise the majority of staff members and directors over the years. The association diversified its leadership, however, hiring its first staff person of color, Alice Malone, a registered nurse, in the 1950s and continuing to increase the representation of people of color as officers, staff, and board members through the century.

For nearly forty years PPGC provided contraception and related services in Cleveland as the sole public organization to do so, yet it experienced few significant challenges and stayed out of the city's courtrooms. In 1953 Margaret Sanger returned to Cleveland to speak at the MHA's

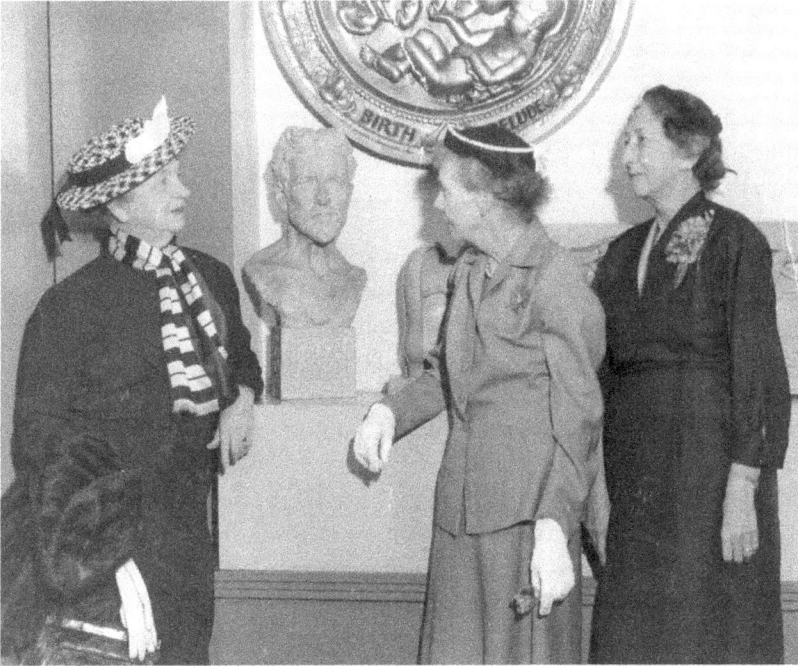

FIGURE 27. MHA celebrates twenty-five years. On the way to the MHA's anniversary celebration, (from left) Margaret Sanger, Roslyn Campbell Weir, and Dorothy Brush stop at the Cleveland Health Museum and admire a bust of Robert L. Dickinson, 1953. Sophia Smith Collection, Smith College. © Health Museum of Cleveland.

twenty-fifth anniversary celebration; she was introduced by her friend and associate, MHA founder Dorothy Brush (see figure 27). The organization constructed a new building on Cornell Road in the University Circle area of Cleveland in 1957, a building that was among the first American structures to be built solely to provide family planning. PPGC began a mobile clinic in 1965. Hospitals in Cleveland did not officially offer family planning until the 1960s; the city health department provided family planning advice in its health centers only beginning in the 1970s. In the same decade PPGC relaxed its age and marital restrictions and addressed the city's high rate of teenage pregnancy and single mothers by educating and serving young people. Cleveland's needs in the area of reproductive health continued to increase. While 5 percent was a standard growth rate for other Planned Parenthood groups of the era, PPGC experienced a 14 percent growth in demand for services, reaching 10,800 clients in 1987 as compared to 5,000 in 1982. During its sixtieth anniversary in 1988, Planned Parenthood undertook a $2.3 million campaign to increase the number of clinics, endow future work, and make services more accessible for low-income people.

Planned Parenthood of Greater Cleveland assumed an advocacy role in the face of an often hostile political and legislative environment beginning in the 1980s. The Cleveland Planned Parenthood Action Fund organized in the 1990s to manage political lobbying and issue advocacy on behalf of PPGC. In 1993 the American Jewish Committee honored PPGC with its Isaiah Award for Human Relations. Planned Parenthood of Greater Cleveland participated in national Planned Parenthood projects such as Global Partners and collaborated with city schools and community groups in training, programming, and advocacy.

After careful in-house planning, negotiation, lawsuits, and countersuits, in January of 1997 Planned Parenthood of Greater Cleveland began to offer abortion services for the first time in its history, joining two other Planned Parenthood locations in Ohio in providing these services. Women responded gratefully and positively; donations actually increased.

The physical location of the organization changed a few times between its sixtieth and seventy-fifth anniversary years. PPGC closed the deteriorating Cornell Road building in 1982 and moved its headquarters to the Bulkley building in downtown Cleveland, while opening clinics in Bedford, East Cleveland, and Lakewood. Seven years later PPGC moved its administrative offices farther east on Euclid Avenue to a building in the Midtown Corridor, where it opened a large resource center for interested professionals and the public. In 2003 PPGC again relocated its administration, to the Adam Joseph Lewis Cleveland Environmental Center on Lorain Road, only a few miles west of the organization's first home.

In 2003 the agency served more than sixteen thousand clients at five clinics as the largest single provider of reproductive health care in Cuyahoga County, maintaining a consistently high rate of patient retention. In the twenty-first century, PPGC championed the reproductive health and rights of women, provided health services and educational programs for all ages, and offered all approved options for child spacing. As in its early years, however, PPGC reached only a tiny portion of the women and men who needed and wanted low-cost family planning in the Cleveland area. Still, as other agencies cut back reproductive health care, PPGC asserted upon its seventy-fifth anniversary, "No other organization exists primarily to serve—and to fight to serve—Cleveland-area women, and to preserve their right to make and carry out decisions about their fertility." That long and affirming history inspired one client to state, "I've been going to Planned Parenthood for years. Why would I go anywhere else?"[1]

# *Appendix*

## Maternal Health Association Patient Information Form

### Maternal Health Clinic     Case No ..........

Date first clinic visit .......................................... Branch No .........
Name ........................... X Reference ........ Birth Date ............
Address ................................................ Tel. No ...............
.............................................................................
                                    Private         Private
Housing— Single ... Rooming ... Ten ... Bath Common ... Toilet Common ...
Persons ....Rooms ......
                F ....................       Yard

              M .....              M .....        M.................
Nationality      W ................ Citizen W ... Religion W.................
         M ....................                M.................
Education W .................................    Mentality W.................

Husband's Name .............. Health ......... Habits ....... Birth Date .........
Trade or Profession .................. Income ...... Unemployment dates .........
Present Occupation .................. Income ......... Other income ............
................................... Extra Financial Responsibility..............
.................................. House rented, owned, encumbered ..........
               M ................
Date Previous Marriage W ....................... Attitude M .................
Referred by ......................... Pt.'s Reason ...............................

---

***Source:*** Goldie Davis, "Appendix II," in "The Maternal Health Association of Cleveland, Ohio," master's thesis, 1938, xxi–xxiii.

## Maternal Health Association Patient Information Form (cont'd.)

### Clearing House Report

Age of First Menses ........... Present Character ............ Last Period ........
Marriage Date ................ Age of First Pregnancy ...... Nursing Mother ....
Living Children ....... Children Dead ..... Still Births ..... Miscarriages ........
Number of Pregnancies, date and result of each:

| | | |
|---|---|---|
| 1) | 6) | 11) |
| 2) | 7) | 12) |
| 3) | 8) | 13) |
| 4) | 9) | 14) |
| 5) | 10) | 15) |

Miscarriages, Therapeutic............. Accidental ............. Induced ..........
Character of Labors .............................................................
Remarks.........................................................................

### Sex History

**Contraceptives Used:**

W .... How long .... Result ....     Sup ....... How long ..... Result ......
C................................     LAJ ...................................
P ...............................     Others...............................
D................................

Frequency of coitus .......... Dysparaeunia ...... Do menses affect desire ........
             M.............
Attitude toward coitus  W ............................ Date last coitus ..........
Orgasm experienced (always, never, usually, sometimes, seldom) ...................
Explanation for lack of orgasm ......................................................

# Maternal Health Association Patient Information Form (cont'd.)

## Physical Examination

General ........................................................................

Pelvic .........................................................................

Doctor's reason for giving contraceptive advice ....................................

Reason no contraceptive advice given ............................................

Method Recommended ........................ Prognosis   Favorable<br>Questionable   Mental<br>Physical

Additional care advised: Clinic<br>Physician

Signature ..............................
Rosina Volk, R.N.
Esther Alger, R.N.
Evelyn Johnson, R.N.
Martha Smith, R.N.

As my agent repeat Rx P.R.N. ......

Date completed ................................................................

Signature .............................

Date of Recheck ...................    Easy, difficult, comfortable to both ........
Physical or mental effect .................

# Maternal Health Association Patient Information Form

## Schedule for Case Analysis

Record Number
     Color
     Religion
     Source of Referral
     Education

Occupation
     Skilled and semi-skilled labor
     Unskilled labor
     Transportation
     Trade
     Agriculture
     Professional
     Clerical
     Personal Service
     Public Service
     Not given

Weekly Income
     $0–$9
     $10–$14
     $15–$19
     $20–$24
     $25–$29
     $30–$34
     $35–$39
     $40–$44
     $45–$49
     $50 or more
     Savings
     Agency Active
     Dependent on Relatives

Age
     0–19 years
     20–24
     25–29
     30–34
     35–39
     40–44
     45–49
     50 or more

Number in the family
Number of years married

# Maternal Health Association Patient Information Form

## Schedule (cont'd.)

Housing
> Very spacious
> Spacious
> Crowded
> Overcrowded
> Greatly Overcrowded

Patient Employed or not
Number of Pregnancies
Number of Miscarriages and Stillborn
Number of Children Born Alive
Contraceptives Previously Used
Contraceptive method recommended at Clinic
> 1.
> 2.
> 3.
> 4.
> 5.
> 6.
> 7.

Reasons for Admittance
> Tuberculosis
> Recent Pregnancy
> Asthenia
> Poor Inheritance Prognosis
> Spacing
> Recent Operation
> Acute Economic Stress
> Husband's mental or physical disability
> Pelvic Pathology
> Other reasons

Cost to Patient
> $0–$0.99
> $1–$4.99
> $5–$9.99
> $10 or more

# List of Abbreviations of Sources

| | |
|---|---|
| ACOG | American College of Obstetricians and Gynecologists |
| *AHR* | *American Historical Review* |
| *AJOG* | *American Journal of Obstetrics and Gynecology* |
| *AJDWC* | *American Journal of Diseases of Women and Children* |
| *BCR* | *Birth Control Review* |
| BCS | Birth Control Society of Hamilton, Ontario, Canada |
| BF | Brush Foundation Archives |
| BrI | Brush Inquiry Scrapbooks |
| CFB | Charles F. Brush Sr., Papers |
| C.F.B. | Charles Francis Brush Sr. |
| CWRU | Case Western Reserve University |
| *DCB* | *Dictionary of Cleveland Biography* |
| DHB | Dorothy Hamilton Brush Papers |
| D.H.B. | Dorothy Hamilton Brush (Dorothy Dick, Dorothy Walmsley) |
| DMHC | Dittrick Medical History Center |
| *ECH* | *Encyclopedia of Cleveland History* |
| *JAH* | *Journal of American History* |
| *JAMA* | *Journal of the American Medical Association* |
| MHA | Maternal Health Association, Cleveland |
| MS-LC | Margaret Sanger Papers, Library of Congress |
| *MSPCDM* | *Margaret Sanger Papers Microfilm Edition: Collected Documents* |
| MS-SS | Margaret Sanger Papers, Sophia Smith Collection, Smith College |
| MS-WIA | Margaret Sanger, Part 1: Diaries, Speeches and Writings, Microfilm, Women in America: Core Primary Sources for Women's Studies |
| OHS | Ohio Historical Society |
| PPCO | Planned Parenthood of Central Ohio Archives (originally Columbus Maternal Health Clinic) |

| | |
|---|---|
| PPFA | Planned Parenthood Federation of America |
| PPGC | Planned Parenthood of Greater Cleveland (formerly MHA) |
| PPLM | Planned Parenthood League of Massachusetts |
| SCA | Smith College Archives |
| *SGO* | *Surgery, Gynecology, and Obstetrics* |
| WCC | Women's City Club of Cleveland Records |
| WRHS | Western Reserve Historical Society |

# Notes

## Notes to Introduction

1. For woman-to-woman spreading of birth control knowledge, see Angus McLaren and Arlene Tigar McLaren, *The Bedroom and the State*, 28–30; Linda Gordon, *Woman's Body*, 1990, 26, 47; and Dyer, "Curiosities of Contraception," 2818–19. Letter quoted in Ladd-Taylor, *Raising a Baby the Government Way*, 183. For other references to birth control as a rich woman's secret, see Margaret Sanger, *My Fight for Birth Control*, 49; Ray and Gosling, "American Physicians and Birth Control," 400; and Lynd and Lynd, *Middletown*, 123–24.

Letters from Maternal Health Association (MHA) clients taken from the clinic's scrapbook are not placed in quotation marks. For birth rates see Reed, *The Birth Control Movement*, x; R. R. Kuczynski, "Births," *Encyclopaedia of Social Sciences*, vol. 2 (New York: Macmillan, 1937), 569. Also see Grossberg, *Governing the Hearth*, esp. chapter 5.

2. Angus McLaren bases his history of contraception on the premise that "reproductive decisions are of greater significance to women than to men." McLaren, *A History of Contraception*, 6. Linda Gordon and Rosalind Pollack Petchesky pursue a similar argument. See Gordon, *Woman's Body*, and Petchesky, *Abortion and Woman's Choice*. For culture as affecting the regulation and perception of sexuality, see D'Emilio and Freedman, *Intimate Matters*, xviii–xix.

For the purposes of this work, "family limitation" and "birth control" refer only to methods used during or immediately following sexual intercourse to prevent conception, although couples have used and continue to use sterilization, abortion, and even infanticide for family limitation. "Natural" methods include extended nursing, abstinence, withdrawal, and variations on the rhythm method. "Mechanical" methods include using douches, suppositories, sponges or tampons (purchased or homemade), spermicides, condoms, cervical caps, and diaphragms. Linda Gordon points out that there's nothing natural about society's treatment of birth control. See *The*

*Moral Property of Women: A History of Birth Control Politics in America* (Urbana: University of Illinois Press, 2002), 8. Since the term "birth control" was not used before 1914, I use "family limitation" or "contraception" for previous eras. Margaret Sanger claimed to have coined the term birth control, but evidence—including her own autobiography—strongly suggests that in fact she only popularized another's inspiration. See *Margaret Sanger: An Autobiography*, 108; and Chesler, *Woman of Valor*, 97.

3. The birth control clinics studied here are those begun by private individuals rather than those run by manufacturers. For information on the latter, see Rosemarie Petra Holz, "The Birth Control Clinic in America: Life Within, Life Without, 1923–1972" (Ph.D. diss., University of Illinois at Urbana-Champaign, 2002), 96–101.

4. Petchesky, *Abortion and Woman's Choice*, 10; *Margaret Sanger Centennial Conference, November 13 & 14, 1979*, 34–35; Suzanne Lebsock, *The Free Women of Petersburg*, xii.

5. Brush Foundation, Deed of Gift, chapter 3, fig. 13. Petchesky, *Abortion and Woman's Choice*, 5. See also Molly Ladd-Taylor, *Mother-work: Women, Child Welfare, and the State, 1890–1930* (Urbana and Chicago: University of Illinois Press, 1994).

6. Todd, "Women's Bodies as Diseased and Deviant," 83–95; Emily Martin, "The Egg and the Sperm," 485–501.

7. Michael Grossberg explores the blurred rules of the socially acceptable and emphasizes the role of nineteenth-century male legislators and judges in codifying cultural ambiguities about sexuality, women, and the family. In a broader context Morton Keller roots the twentieth-century polity in nineteenth-century tensions around social control and anxieties about social order. See Grossberg, *Governing the Hearth*, and Morton Keller, *Affairs of the State: Public Life in Late Nineteenth Century America* (Cambridge, Mass.: Belknap Press, 1977).

8. Martin, *The Woman in the Body*. Adrienne Rich claims that the politicization of the female body has resulted in woman's experience of it being "cruelly disorganized." She is quoted in Donchin, "The Future of Mothering," 135. See also Corea, *The Mother Machine*.

9. For the general lack of reference to birth control in diaries, see Jane H. Pease and William Pease, *Ladies, Women and Wenches: Choice and Constraint in Antebellum Charleston and Boston* (Chapel Hill: University of North Carolina, 1990), 26. Two published compilations of mothers' letters about birth control are Margaret Sanger, *Motherhood in Bondage*, and Ruth Hall, ed., *Dear Dr. Stopes*. Petchesky, *Abortion and Woman's Choice*, 10.

10. Patricia Cornwell digs beneath the accepted version of an account in the history of crime against women to find "the story within the story." Cornwell, *Portrait of a Killer: Jack the Ripper—Case Closed* (New York: G. P. Putnam's Sons, 2002).

11. Sandra Morgen, *Into Our Own Hands: The Women's Health Movement in the United States, 1969–1990* (New Brunswick, N.J.: Rutgers University Press, 2002), xvi. Michael Grossberg, *A Judgment for Solomon: The D'Hauteville Case and the Legal Experience in Antebellum America* (Cambridge: Cambridge University Press, 1996), ix–x.

Grossberg cites Joan Scott, who analyzes the importance of "experience" and of the discourse about that experience to the study of history. She asserts, "Experience is a subject's history. Language is the site of history's enactment. Historical explanation cannot, therefore, separate the two." Scott, "The Evidence of Experience."

12. Gordon, *The Moral Property of Women*, 3; Scott, "Evidence of Experience."

13. Jessie May Rodrique has called for more attention to African American birth control clinics and notes the obstacles to finding such informations. I offer this work as a stepping stone to the job of attending to the diversity of experiences among clients of a single agency. Rodrique, "The Afro-American Community and the Birth Control Movement, 1918–1942" (Ph.D. diss., University of Massachusetts, 1991), esp. 10–11, 222.

14. *Cleveland Plain Dealer,* November 22, 1922, 15.

15. Felicia A. Kornbluh outlines recent historical work on women and state building in "The New Literature on Gender and the Welfare State: The U.S. Case." She distinguishes between "mother-oriented" reformers and social feminists, noting that the former did not necessarily support suffrage—see p. 179. Kornbluh mentions the understudied significance of "sexuality and the politics of maternity"—see pp. 192–193. Thanks to Mike Grossberg for bringing this article to my attention. Gladys Gaylord, Rosina Volk, R. N., and board member Virginia Wing are the single women mentioned. MHA annual reports, 1928–1943, unprocessed records of Planned Parenthood of Greater Cleveland (hereafter PPGC) in the Western Reserve Historical Society, Cleveland, Ohio (hereafter WRHS), box 2.

16. McCarthy, *Lady Bountiful Revisited,* x–xi.

17. Gloria Feldt, with Carol Trickett Jennings, *Behind Every Choice Is a Story* (Denton: University of North Texas Press, 2003).

18. Nancy Cott speculates that possibly the "greatest extent of associational activity in the whole history of American women took place between the two wars" and sees that period as one of crisis and transition for women's activity. She notes that, in the late 1920s and 1930s, individualistic rather than collective assertion of woman's equality to and difference from men prevailed. See Cott, *The Grounding of Modern Feminism,* 10, 97, 280. Cott quotes a self-proclaimed feminist of the 1930s, Miriam Allen de Ford, as saying that "there was no organized [feminist] movement outside of birth control," implying that birth control supporters acted as feminists. See ibid., 281–82.

19. Anne G. Balay discusses the 1911 novella *Mother* by Kathleen Norris, for example. Balay, "'Hands Full of Living': Birth Control, Nostalgia, and Kathleen Norris," *American Literary History* 8, no. 3 (1996): 471–96.

20. Tone, *Devices and Desires,* 151–200, and Gordon, *Woman's Body,* 249–340.

21. This period falls in the third stage of the birth control movement, as identified by Linda Gordon. Gordon notes that in the first stage, beginning in the mid-nineteenth century, feminists called for "voluntary motherhood." In the second stage, from 1910 to 1920, proponents turned away from feminism to emphasize "birth control."

Between 1920 and 1940, the "professionalization" stage, Gordon says, birth control evolved into family planning, institutionalized in 1942 in Planned Parenthood. See Gordon, *Woman's Body*, xix–xx.

## Notes to Chapter 1

1. Comstock, *Traps for the Young*, 136.

2. Many publications ran afoul of the law for their explicit descriptions of sexual reproduction and their advocacy of family limitation. See "A Chronology of the use and impact of civil disobedience and related strategies on the reproductive rights movement in America," Finding Aid, February 11, 1991, 1, the records of the Planned Parenthood Federation of America, Sophia Smith Archives, Smith College, Northampton, Massachusetts (hereafter PPFA). For example, in 1876 a judge found Edward Bliss Foote guilty of breaking the law by mailing a copy of a pamphlet, *Words in Pearl for the Married*, which detailed contraceptive technique. After this indictment, Foote removed much of the contraceptive information from later editions of *Medical Common Sense*. See Peter Fryer, *The Birth Controllers* (New York: Stein and Day, 1965), 116–17. For Charles Knowlton see Robert E. Riegel, "The American Father of Birth Control," *The New England Quarterly* 6, no. 3 (September 1933): 470–90; Fryer, *Birth Controllers*, 99–106; and Grossberg, *Governing the Hearth*, 157–59. See also Paul S. Boyer, *Purity in Print: Book Censorship in America from the Gilded Age to the Computer Age*, 2d ed. (Madison: University of Wisconsin Press, 2002), chapters 1 and 2.

3. D'Emilio and Freedman, *Intimate Matters*, 59–60. For the business opportunities in birth control see Tone, *Devices and Desires;* Tone, "Contraceptive Consumers," 485–506; and Holz, "The Birth Control Clinic in America," Ph.D. diss., esp. chapter 2. For a contemporaneous source on commercialization and details about the dangers of some common abortifacients, see Palmer and Greenberg, *Facts and Frauds*, 165–75.

4. Tone, *Devices and Desires*, 14–15.

5. Grossberg, *Governing the Hearth*, 161. For the history of abortion practice and regulation, see Reagan, *When Abortion Was a Crime*, Mohr, *Abortion in America*, Brodie, *Contraception and Abortion in 19th Century America* (Ithaca, N.Y.: Cornell University Press, 1994), and Joffe, *Doctors of Conscience*. For anti-abortion law in Ohio see *Acts of a General Nature Passed at the First Session of the Thirty Second General Assembly of the State of Ohio*, vol. 23 (Columbus: David Smith, 1834), 20–21.

6. Ernst and Schwartz, *Censorship*, esp. 18–22. See also Dienes, *Law, Politics and Birth Control*, and Dennett, *Birth Control Laws*.

7. D'Emilio and Freedman, *Intimate Matters*, 59–60, 65; Grossberg, *Governing the Hearth*, 170; McLaren, *A History of Contraception*, 73.

8. Mosher, *The Mosher Survey*, and D'Emilio and Freedman, *Intimate Matters*, 55–56.

9. D'Emilio and Freedman, *Intimate Matters,* 55–84; Biesel, *Imperiled Innocents,* esp. the introduction and chapter 1. Laipson, "From Boudoir to Bookstore," 641. For changes in courtship during this era, see Karen Lystra, *Searching the Heart: Women, Men, and Romantic Love in Nineteenth-Century America* (New York: Oxford University Press, 1989), and Beth L. Bailey, *From Front Porch to Back Seat: Courtship in Twentieth-Century America* (Baltimore, Md.: Johns Hopkins University Press, 1988).

10. Nancy Cott, *Public Vows: A History of Marriage and the Nation* (Cambridge, Mass.: Harvard University Press, 2000), 50–51, 105–7. "Shivers" quote on p. 50. For other analyses of motherhood over time, see Curry, *Modern Mothers in the Heartland;* Rima D. Apple and Janet Golden, eds., *Mothers and Motherhood: Readings in American History* (Columbus: Ohio State University Press, 1997); Theda Skocpol, *Protecting Soldiers and Mothers: The Political Origins of Social Policy in the United States* (Cambridge, Mass.: Belknap Press, 1992); and Linda Gordon, *Pitied But Not Entitled: Single Mothers and the History of Welfare* (New York: Free Press, 1994).

11. The first quote refers to the conditions in the 1850s that led to the creation of the Cleveland Children's Aid Society. See Cleveland Industrial School and Home, "Annual Report, 1880," 13–14, WRHS. For the second quote see Anne Lee Lavin, "They do go home again," master's thesis, 8.

12. David D. Van Tassel and John Grabowski, eds., "Herrick, Maria M. Smith," *Dictionary of Cleveland Biography* (hereafter *DCB*), (Bloomington: Indiana University Press, 1996), 217–18; David D. Van Tassel and John Grabowski, eds., "Mothers and Young Ladies Guide," *Encyclopedia of Cleveland History* (hereafter *ECH*), 2d ed. (Bloomington: Indiana University Press, 1996), 711. One nineteenth-century mothers' handbook went through seven editions in England before being published in the United States. See Pye Henry Chavasse, *Woman as a Wife and Mother* (Philadelphia: William D. Evans and Company, 1871), a combination of two previous works by Chavasse, *Advice to a Wife* and *Advice to a Mother.* Mothers' guides of the early twentieth century include Ellen Key, *The Renaissance of Motherhood* (New York: Putnam's, 1914) and *Mother's Own Book* (New York: The Parents' Publishing Association, 1928).

13. For Comstock's supporters see Biesel, *Imperiled Innocents,* 49–75. Colgate is mentioned on page 53. See also Johnson, "Anthony Comstock: Reform, Vice, and the American Way," Ph.D. diss., 64–69. For the number of items seized, see Reed, *Birth Control Movement,* 38. The record is unclear as to the intentionality of the last-minute inclusion of the provisions against birth control information in the obscenity legislation. Some scholars insist that Comstock himself did not realize that the phrase had been included. See Louise Bates, *Weeder in the Garden of the Lord: Anthony Comstock's Life and Career* (Lanham, Md.: University Press of America, 1995), 153. Biesel, on the other hand, claims that contraception was inseparably linked with obscenity during the late nineteenth century. Biesel, *Imperiled Innocents,* 38–42.

14. Cleveland Industrial School, "Annual Report 1880," 17. For Cleveland purity groups see *The Search Light* (1908–1911), the monthly organ of the Christian League

for the Promotion of Purity, and "Report of the Vice Commission of the Cleveland Baptist Brotherhood" (1911), WRHS. David Pivar mentions the Cleveland Purity Alliance and the Cleveland Moral Education Society, but little evidence of their work has been located. See David J. Pivar, *Purity Crusade: Sexual Morality and Social Control, 1868–1900* (Westport, Conn.: Greenwood Press, 1973), 148 and 174 respectively. The same lack of evidence holds true for the short-lived Cleveland Female Moral Reform Society, which disbanded in 1844. See Van Tassel and Grabowski, eds., "Herrick," *DCB*, and Marian J. Morton, "Temperance Reform in the 'Providential Environment,' Cleveland, 1830–1934," in *Cleveland: A Tradition of Reform*, ed. David D. Van Tassel and John J. Grabowski (Kent, Ohio: Kent State University Press, 1986), 50–66, and Jimmy Wilkinson Meyer, "Children and Youth," *ECH*, 176–78.

15. Comstock Act, chap. 258, 17 Stat. 598 (1873); Brodie, *Contraception and Abortion*, 255–56; Tone, *Devices and Desires*, chapter 1.

16. Quote is from the Tariff Act of 1930. See Ernst and Schwartz, *Censorship*, 163–64, also 105–106; and Brooks, "The Early History of the Anti-contraceptive Laws," 12. On amending the Comstock Act in 1971 see Reed, *Birth Control Movement*, 102, 121, and Brief *amicus curiae* of 281 American Historians, *Webster v. Reproductive Health Services*, et al. (October 1988): 19, note 60. For present status of federal obscenity ban see the *Webster* case and *United States Code*, title 18, ch. 71, sections 1460–1468 (Washington, DC: United States Government Printing Office, 2001). In 2000–01, legislation against indecency in the media, including the Internet, spurred some observers to recall the efforts of Anthony Comstock. See David E. Rosenbaum, "Raw Rap May Stir a Fuss but Hist'ry Shows 'Twas Ever Thus," *New York Times*, September 21, 2000, sec. 1, p. 1, and Christopher Gray, "1892 House Built by a Famous Crusader Against Vice," *New York Times*, May 27, 2001, sec. 11, p. 7. See also LaMay, "America's Censor," 1–59. Bates analyzes Comstock's impact on women in "Protective Custody: A Feminist Interpretation of Anthony Comstock's Life and Laws," Ph.D. diss., and in *Weeder in the Garden*. See also Biesel, *Imperiled Innocents*, and Johnson, "Anthony Comstock," Ph.D. diss.

17. *Hicklin* case quoted in Grossberg, *Governing the Hearth*, 189. The *Hicklin* case also allowed judges to decide that a work was obscene based on isolated passages, passages that might incite lustful thoughts in the "young and inexperienced." The item's purpose or social value became irrelevant. In the late 1870s Judge Samuel Blatchford even prohibited discussion of the item in question in the courtroom. Beisel, *Imperiled Innocents*, 91–92.

18. Beisel, *Imperiled Innocents*, 50–52.

19. Dienes, *Law Politics, and Birth Control*, 103.

20. Ernst and Schwartz, *Censorship*, 30–33; LaMay, "America's Censor"; and Anthony Comstock, *Traps for the Young*, 137. United States postal inspectors still used entrapment in the 1990s. See the *Cleveland Plain Dealer*, March 21, 1992, 1-B, 3-B.

21. *U.S. v. Bott* (1873) and *U.S. v. Whittier* (1878), cited in Tone, *Devices and Desires,* 36–37.

22. *Acts of a General Nature and Local Laws and Joint Resolutions Passed by the Fifty-fifth General Assembly of the State of Ohio,* vol. 59 (Columbus: Richard Nevins, 1862), 64. The 1862 ruling contradicts Andrea Tone's assertion that obscenity laws did not address contraception before 1873. See Tone, *Devices and Desires,* 16. For other states see Dennett, *Birth Control Laws,* 268–70. For abortion law, see *Acts of a General Nature,* vol. 23 (1834), 20–21. This anti-abortion law was apparently among the most stringent of the era. See Brodie, *Contraception and Abortion,* 254.

23. Dennett, *Birth Control Laws,* 268–70.

24. *Acts of a General Nature,* vol. 59 (1862), 64.

25. *The General and Local Laws and Joint Resolutions passed by the Sixty-Second General Assembly of the State of Ohio,* vol. 73 (Columbus: Nevins and Myers, State Printers, 1876), 158–59. For 1872 law see *The State of Ohio General and Local Laws and Joint Resolutions Passed by the Sixtieth General Assembly,* vol. 69 (Columbus: Nevins and Myers, 1872), 174–75. Opponents of the Comstock laws often argued on the basis of the right to free speech. For a contemporaneous example, see Heywood Broun and Margaret Leech, *Anthony Comstock: Roundsman of the Lord* (New York: Albert and Charles Boni, 1927), 265–72.

26. On Ohio law see Dennett, *Birth Control Laws,* 270, and *General and Local Laws,* vol. 73 (1876), 158–59. One of the few legal articles discussing the evolution of obscenity law in Ohio focuses on sexually provocative printed matter and film rather than information about contraception or abortion, suggesting perhaps a dearth of cases in that area. Richard H. Harris, "Obscenity Law in Ohio," *Akron Law Review* 13, no. 3 (winter 1980): 520–39.

27. The Cleveland Medical College was begun as a department of Western Reserve College, and is the ancestor of the School of Medicine of Case Western Reserve University. Mark Gottlieb, *The Lives of University Hospitals of Cleveland* (Cleveland: Wilson Street Press, 1991), 19; and Cramer, *Case Western Reserve,* 76. Charity Hospital Medical College became the Cleveland College of Physicians and Surgeons and, in 1896, affiliated with Ohio Wesleyan University in Delaware, Ohio, before merging into Western Reserve's School of Medicine in 1910. See Brown, ed., *The History of Medicine in Cleveland,* 626–28. The Starling-Ohio Medical College, predecessor of the College of Medicine and Public Health at The Ohio State University, opened in 1848 and trained students in conjunction within St. Francis Hospital in Columbus, Ohio. <http://www.osu.edu>.

28. Brodie, *Contraception and Abortion,* 70–73. For drugstores as marketers of contraception see Brodie, *Contraception and Abortion,* and Tone, *Devices and Desires.*

29. McCann, *Birth Control Politics,* 27–28, 71.

30. Johnson, "Anthony Comstock," Ph.D. diss., 111, and Tone, *Devices and Desires,* 28–29.

31. For 1862 Ohio law see J. R. Sayler, ed., *Statutes of the State of Ohio*, vol. 1, 1861–1865 (Cincinnati, Ohio: Robert Clarke, 1876), 268–69. For the Ohio abortion law, passed on February 27, 1834, see *Acts of a General Nature*, vol. 23 (1834), 20–21. Also see Dennett, *Birth Control Laws*, 10. Dennett's work was a popular rather than a legal analysis. Vermont passed the first state law against indecent literature in 1821, followed by Connecticut (1834) and Massachusetts (1835). See Ernst and Schwartz, *Censorship*, 18. For a chart showing the number of states with laws against birth control devices generally and condoms specifically in 1973, see Murphy, *The Condom Industry*, 9.

32. Dennett, *Birth Control Laws*, 268–70. The Connecticut prohibition was not lifted until 1965, in *Griswold v. The State of Connecticut*, 381 U.S. 479 (1965). From studying drafts of the Connecticut bill, Carol Brooks speculates that adding the prohibition of "use" may have been unintentional. See Brooks, "The Early History," 12.

33. Reagan, *When Abortion Was a Crime*, 117. Tone, *Devices and Desires*, chapter 2, esp. 26–28. For the widespread sale and use of contraceptives, see McLaren, *A History of Contraception*, 178–251, and Brodie, *Contraception and Abortion*. A contemporaneous work listing manufacturers of contraceptives is Palmer and Greenberg, *Facts and Frauds*. For birth rate see Reed, *Birth Control Movement*, x. Also see Grossberg, *Governing the Hearth*, esp. chapter 5.

34. Joseph L. Baer, "Discussion," in *Surgery, Gynecology, and Obstetrics* (hereafter *SGO*) 36, no. 3 (March 1923): 438.

35. *Recent Social Trends in the United States: Report of the President's Research Committee on Social Trends*, vol. 1 (New York: McGraw-Hill Book Company, 1933), 53.

36. Rachel Yarros, "Discussion," in *SGO* 36, no. 3 (March 1923): 437. See also Reed, *Birth Control Movement*, 29–33, 40, 124. Aletta Jacobs, a Dutch physician and early birth control advocate, described a similar situation overseas: "It was an age steeped in hypocrisy! . . . Clergymen would denounce contraception from the pulpit and then pack their wives off to my office. I also remember women who were only too pleased to use the means I prescribed for them yet never lost a chance to condemn me at every tea party and sewing circle. And, while publicly denouncing my work, some doctors would still expect me to instruct them in the practical application of birth control!" See Jacobs, *Memories*, 50.

37. Histories of contraception that detail techniques are John M. Riddle, *Eve's Herbs: A History of Contraception and Abortion in the West* (Cambridge, Mass.: Harvard University Press, 1997); McLaren, *A History of Contraception*; Brodie, *Contraception and Abortion*, esp. 212–24; Tone, *Devices and Desires*; and Himes, *Medical History*. A brief overview can be found in Robertson, *An Illustrated History of Contraception*. For a detailed description of methods known to North American women, complete with diagrams and recipes, see Margaret Sanger, *Family Limitation* (1914), in Jensen, "The Evolution of Margaret Sanger's *Family Limitation* Pamphlet," 556–67; McLaren and McLaren, *The Bedroom and the State*, 28–30; and "Some Suggestions Concerning Contraceptives; Birth Control Information for Lay

Readers," (n.p., n.d.) in the papers of Sarah Marcus, M.D. (hereafter SM), at the Dittrick Medical History Center (hereafter DMHC), Cleveland, Ohio. See also Cooper, *Technique of Contraception.* Harvey Green includes illustrations of pessaries and their use in *The Light of the Home: An Intimate View of the Lives of Women in Victorian America* (New York: Pantheon Books, 1983), 123–25. For abortion as birth control see Reagan, *When Abortion Was a Crime,* chapter 1, and Sanger, *Motherhood in Bondage,* 359–93, esp. 394–410; for infanticide see D'Emilio and Freedman, *Intimate Matters,* 27, 51. For the Comstock syringe see Brodie, "Family Limitation," Ph.D. diss., 162–63, and Tone, *Devices and Desires,* 37–39. Brodie notes that any asymmetry of the uterus was considered a serious health problem in the nineteenth century and describes the wide and prolonged use of pessaries as womb supporters. Brodie, *Contraception and Abortion,* 221–22. For a contemporaneous view of pessaries, with illustrations, see Grace Peckham Murray, "Pessaries, Their Use and Abuse," *The Woman's Medical Journal* 18, no. 12 (December 1908): 249–53. This article does not mention the contraceptive nature of pessaries.

38. Andrea Tone, "Making Room for Rubbers: Gender, Technology, and Birth Control Before the Pill," *History and Technology* 18, no. 1 (2002): 51. For description of the changes after vulcanization see Brodie, *Contraception and Abortion,* 209–10; McLaren, *A History of Contraception,* 157–58; Gordon, *Woman's Body,* 44; Gamson, "Rubber Wars," 265; and Murphy, *The Condom Industry,* 7.

39. For latex and testing see Tone, *Devices and Desires,* 188–200. Tone cites the 1938 study as Randolph Cautley, Gilbert W. Beebe, and Robert L. Dickinson, "Rubber Sheaths as Venereal Disease Prophylactics," *American Journal of the Medical Sciences* (February 1938): 156–58. See Tone, *Devices and Desires,* 196, note 36. For an earlier study by Cecil Voge that found similar results, see Palmer and Greenberg, *Facts and Frauds,* 271–72.

40. On the diaphragm see Robert A. Hatcher et al., eds., *Contraceptive Technology, 1988–89,* 14th rev. ed. (New York: Irvington Publishers, 1989), 303–5, and "The Use of the Pessary," Margaret Sanger Papers Project Newsletter, 27 (spring 2001), 5, note 2. For Mensinga see Tone, *Devices and Desires,* 121. For the diaphragm's use in British and North American clinics see Gordon, *Woman's Body,* 179; Kennedy, *Birth Control in America,* 32; McLaren and McLaren, *The Bedroom and the State,* 107–8. For Cleveland see MHA, Annual Reports, 1928–1943, PPGC, box 2; MHA, "Report of Three Years' Work, March 22, 1928–March 21, 1931," 12, Papers of Margaret Sanger in the Sophia Smith Archives (hereafter MS-SS) at Smith College, Northampton, Massachusetts, Clinics-Ohio; MHA, Report of Fourth Year, March, 1931–March, 1932, Records of the Hamilton Birth Control Society (hereafter BCS), Hamilton Public Library Special Collections, Hamilton, Ontario, Canada, record group 2, series A. The Mensinga pessary was not available in the United States when Sanger began her work; she popularized the Mizpah and Ramses diaphragms instead. See Tone, *Devices and Desires,* 122–23. For Jacobs see Jacobs, *Memories.* Janet Brodie found

American patents for items similar to Mensinga's dating from the 1840s. See Brodie, *Contraception and Abortion*, 216–18. Sources differ as to the date of Mensinga's invention. For the use of the diaphragm in America, see Tone, *Devices and Desires*, 153, and The Boston Women's Health Collective, *The New Our Bodies, Ourselves, Updated and Expanded for the Nineties* (New York: Simon and Schuster, c. 1984, 1992), 265.

The history and implication of the woman-centered focus of birth control technology and rhetoric has yet to be written. For a call for scholarship on other woman-centered technology see Ruth Schwartz Cowan, "From Virginia Dare to Virginia Slims: Women and Technology in America," in *Dynamos and Virgins Revisited: Women and Technological Change in History*, ed. Martha Moore Trescott (Metuchen, N.J.: Scarecrow, 1979), 30–44. For a scientific look at the topic, see Jessika van Kammen, "Representing Users' Bodies: The Gendered Development of Anti-Fertility Vaccines," *Science, Technology, and Human Values* 24, no. 3 (summer 1999): 307–37.

41. Brodie, *Contraception and Abortion*, 73. A 1996 study found a correlation between douching and reduced fertility but would not go so far as to assume causality. Donna Day Baird, Clarice R. Weinberg, Lynda F. Voigt, and Janet R. Daling, "Vaginal Douching and Reduced Fertility," *American Journal of Public Health* 86, no. 6 (June 1996): 844–50. Stix quoted in Gordon, *Woman's Body*, 317. By the 1990s, after years of disparaging so-called primitive contraceptive techniques such as withdrawal or the use of spermicidal jelly alone, birth control activists and manufacturers had finally recognized the widespread use—and relative effectiveness—of these family limitation methods. A patient education flyer printed by Wyeth-Ayerst Laboratories detailed "contraceptive options" and listed them in order of efficacy in preventing conception. Just below the condom, diaphragm, and cervical cap (all rated as between 82 percent and 98 percent effective), the following options appear: periodic abstinence, 80 percent to 99 percent effective; spermicide (alone), 79 percent to 97 percent; withdrawal, 72 percent. See "contraceptive options" flyer, Wyeth-Ayerst Laboratories, n.d. The effectiveness ratings vary greatly from source to source.

42. Unless otherwise indicated (by notes and quotation marks), all letters quoted are from Scrapbook-Letters from Patients, 1928–1938, PPGC, box 6. Spelling is unchanged from the original letters.

43. Ellen Chesler, interview with Sarah Marcus. For effects of Lysol douche, see Tone, *Devices and Desires*, 170, and personal conversation with Janice Falk Harclerode, March 18, 1997, Clinton, South Carolina. Lysol ad from Himes, *Medical History*, 329, quoted in Gordon, *Woman's Body*, 318; Brodie, *Contraception and Abortion*, 68. For other Lysol ads see Tone, *Devices and Desires*, 158, 161.

44. Elizabeth Jameson, "Women as Workers, Women as Civilizers: True Womanhood in the American West," in *The Women's West*, ed. Susan Armitage and Elizabeth Jameson (Norman: University of Oklahoma Press, 1987), 152. Jameson also describes a woman on the frontier who attempted to use the "safe period" method of birth control. See pp. 151–52.

45. Gordon, *Woman's Body*, 45, 63, 317. For a discussion of nineteenth-century theories of ovulation see Brodie, *Contraception and Abortion*, 80–89; for twentieth-century theories see Paula Viterbo, "The Promise of Rhythm: The Determinators of the Women's Time of Ovulation and Its Social Impact in the United States, 1920–1940," (Ph.D. diss., State University of New York at Stony Brook, 2000), esp. 114. The responses to Clelia Mosher's survey reveal a wide variety of popular interpretations of the safe period. See Mosher, *The Mosher Survey*. For a brief summary of research on the female reproductive system before 1950, see Bernard Asbell, *The Pill: A Biography of the Drug That Changed the World* (New York: Random House, 1995), 14–18. See also Borell, "Biologists and the Promotion of Birth Control Research," 51–87.

46. Bates, "Protective Custody," Ph.D. diss., 126; Gordon, *Woman's Body*, 161–63, 259–74; D'Emilio and Freedman, *Intimate Matters*, 243–44; Reed, *The Birth Control Movement*, 143–46; Palmer and Greenberg, *Facts and Frauds*, 260–64; and Starr, *The Social Transformation*, 49–50. For physicians campaigning against or supporting abortion see Joffe, "Portraits of Three 'Physicians of Conscience,'" 48–49, and Grossberg, *Governing the Hearth*, 179–87. See also Mohr, *Abortion in America*, and Joffe, *Doctors of Conscience*.

47. Tone, *Devices and Desires*, 22–24, and Jimmy Elaine Wilkinson Meyer, "Motherhood and Morality," *ACOG Clinical Review* (December 1996): 14–16.

48. Quoted in Reed, *Birth Control Movement*, 42–44.

49. Portions of the information in the next five paragraphs appeared in a slightly different form in Meyer, "Motherhood and Morality." Bagshaw is quoted in "Birth Control Clinic Pioneer," *Spectator,* October 25, 1971, Elizabeth Bagshaw Papers. Special Collections, Hamilton Public Library, Hamilton, Ontario, Canada. In the 1995 study that formed the basis for the "Motherhood and Morality" article in the *ACOG Clinical Review,* I examined the tables of contents and indices of every issue of *AJOG* (in all of its name permutations) from 1914 to 1940 and of issues at five-year intervals from 1870 to 1910. In addition to articles on the prevention of conception, I examined most articles on related topics such as infant mortality or criminal abortion. In the *Transactions of the American Association of Obstetricians and Gynecologists,* I checked the indices at five-year intervals beginning with volume 3 (1890) through volume 53 (1940) and found no articles indexed under any topic having to do with the prevention of conception. Checking the indices and contents of most of the textbooks in gynecology and obstetrics in the American College of Obstetricians and Gynecologists History Library located few references to contraception. Most of those were less than one half of a page long.

50. James R. Garber, "A Plea for Prenatal Care and the End-Results of the Hygiene of Pregnancy," *AJOG* 78, no. 4 (October 1918): 575. For "pernicious practices" see Thomas McArdle, "The Physical Evils Arising from the Prevention of Conception," *American Journal of Diseases of Women and Children* (hereafter *AJDWC*) 21, no. 9 (September 1888): 939. Originally presented before the Washington, DC, Obstetrical and

Gynecological Society in May 1888. Edward J. Ill, "The Rights of the Unborn—The Prevention of Conception," *AJDWC* 40, no. 5 (November 1899): 577–84. For the supposed ill effects of the prevention of conception see pp. 583–84.

51. Tone, *Devices and Desires*, 22–24, and Meyer, "Motherhood and Morality," 14–16.

52. Reed, *Birth Control Movement*, 39, 52; Leavitt, *Brought to Bed*, 59, 63.

53. "Summary of the answers to the questionnaire submitted to the members of the New York Obstetrical Society on the 'regulation of conception' [discussion]," *AJOG* 7, no. 3 (1924): 266–69, 339–43. "Resolutions Adopted at the Annual Convention," *Medical Woman's Journal* 37, no. 7 (July 1930): 196–97. Janet Brodie cites letters to the editor of two different 1888 issues of the *Philadelphia Medical and Surgical Reporter* as proof of physicians advising patients about family limitation. Brodie, *Contraception and Abortion*, 278, note 75. For abortion see Joffe, *Doctors of Conscience*, and Reagan, *When Abortion Was a Crime*, esp. chapters 2 and 4. Gosling and Ray, "American Physicians." For evidence of conflict within the profession see Robinson, *Seventy Birth Control Clinics*, 207, and Committee on Legislation for Birth Control, *Removal of Legal Obstacles Opens New Opportunities: A New Day Dawns for Birth Control* (New York: National Committee on Federal Legislation for Birth Control, 1937), 19. For physicians performing illegal abortions see Joffe, "Portraits of Three"; Joffe, *Doctors of Conscience;* and Reagan, *When Abortion Was a Crime.*

54. For the use of condoms by the military and the effect on the industry, see Gordon, *Woman's Body*, 63–64, and Tone, *Devices and Desires*, 189–91. On the effect of the condom's dual roles and the continuity of the respectability conflict see Gamson, "Rubber Wars," 262–82, especially 268, note 20. Quote is from *Youngs Rubber Corporation v. C. I. Lee and Co.*, 45 F.2d 103 (1930), cited in "Rubber Wars," 269, note 21. See also Trumbach, Bravman, and Gamson, "Commentary," 95–105; and Murphy, *The Condom Industry*, esp. 95, 98. Popular histories of the strong Ohio rubber industry do not discuss contraceptives, but some mention "druggist sundries" in passing. See, for example, Steve Love and David Giffels, *Wheels of Fortune: The Story of Rubber in Akron* (Akron, Ohio: Akron University Press, 1999), and Mansel G. Blackford and K. Austin Kerr, *BFGoodrich: Tradition and Transformation, 1870–1995* (Columbus: Ohio State University Press, 1996). For druggist sundries see Blackford and Kerr, *BF Goodrich*, 94, 98–99, 301, and Tone, *Devices and Desires*, 29. For condom conflagrations in the 1990s and in the first decade of the twenty-first century, see, for example, Doug Lifton, "Condoms no longer something to hide," *Cleveland Plain Dealer*, Nov. 19, 1990, 1A–2A; "Hut Conundrum: Drive Through, or Out?" *New York Times*, July 25, 1992; and Nicholas D. Kristof, "The Secret War on Condoms," *New York Times*, Jan. 10, 2003, <www.nytimes.com>.

55. Sanger, *My Fight for Birth Control*, 49–52, and Sanger, *Margaret Sanger: An Autobiography*, 89–92. For research casting doubt on Sanger's sudden conversion to the cause see Cigi B. Dillberger, "From Woman Rebel to Birth Control Advocate," mas-

ter's thesis, and Jensen, "Evolution." For reluctance of doctors to inform "ladies" about birth control, see Dyer, "Curiosities of Contraception," 2818–19, and Meyer, "Motherhood and Morality."

56. The predilection of many physicians to avoid informing even their privileged patients about preventing pregnancy negates the claim of Sanger and other activists that only the poorest of women lacked access to safe contraception. Sanger, *Motherhood in Bondage,* 359–93.

57. For the woman with no surviving children, see ibid., 386. For the woman who would rather die, see p. 392. For fear of intercourse letter, see p. 388.

58. Ibid., 381, 380.

59. For quote about doctors, see ibid., 392. For mothers' questions, see ibid., 370, 377.

60. By the 1940s birth control advocates such as Dr. Lydia DeVilbiss stated, "Every child has the right to be well-born." Kline, *Building a Better Race,* 64.

61. *Encyclopaedia of the Social Sciences,* vol. 3 (1930), 617–21.

62. An earlier version of the material in the next few paragraphs appeared in a paper, "The Quest for the Perfect Child," presented by the author at Case Western Reserve University History Associates, Cleveland, Ohio, April 1999. Adam Kuper, *The Chosen Primate: Human Nature and Cultural Diversity* (Cambridge, Mass.: Harvard University Press, 1994), 114. Thanks to Nicole Wilkinson Duran for pointing out this source. Martin Pernick, *The Black Stork: Eugenics and the Death of Defective Babies in American and Motion Pictures Since 1915* (New York: Oxford University Press, 1996), 32–39; Gordon, *Woman's Body,* 136, 231; Angus McLaren, *Our Own Master Race: Eugenics in Canada, 1885–1945* (Toronto, Ontario: McClelland and Stewart, 1990), 27, 44–46; and McLaren and McLaren, *Bedroom and the State,* 67.

63. For the term "eugenics" see Daniel Kevles, *In the Name of Eugenics: Genetics and the Uses of Human Heredity* (New York: Knopf, 1985), ix; and Chesler, *Woman of Valor,* 122–23. Linda Gordon includes an extensive discussion of eugenics in *Woman's Body,* especially chapters 6, 7, 9, and 10. Kevles lists some prominent scientists involved in the eugenics movement. See Kevles, *In the Name of Eugenics,* 69. Carl N. Degler explains the development of and scientific basis for the concept of feeblemindedness in *In Search of Human Nature: The Decline and Revival of Darwinism in American Social Thought* (New York: Oxford University Press, 1991), 139–45; see also Kevles, *In the Name of Eugenics,* 70–84. Foucault argues that connecting sex with heredity, with "biological responsibility" for the race, contributed to the emphasis on state management of sex and marriage. See Foucault, *The History of Sexuality,* 118. Barry Alan Mehler reinterprets the eugenics movement and provides biographical data for many American Eugenics Society board members in "A History of the American Eugenics Society, 1921–1940" (Ph.D. diss., University of Illinois at Urbana-Champaign, 1988).

64. World War II Nazi experiments in race purification badly tainted eugenics and forced proponents to modify their positions. However, the ideology did not dissipate completely. See Glenn McGee, *The Perfect Baby: A Pragmatic Approach to Eugenics*

(New York: Rowman and Littlefield, 1997), and Meyer, "Quest for the Perfect Child." Lawrence K. Frank, "Towards a Re-orientation of the Birth Control Movement," unpublished speech presented at the Conference on Eugenics and Birth Control, January 28, 1938, New York City, p. 7 PPGC, box 5, pamphlets. In 1946 Frank, a pioneer in the study of aging, became the first editor of the *Journal of Gerontology* (later the *Gerontologist*). See Lawrence K. Frank, "Gerontology," *Journal of Gerontology* 1 (1946): 1–11.

65. McLaren, *Our Own Master Race,* 9.

66. Du Bois, in a 1932 *Birth Control Review* (hereafter *BCR*) article titled "Black Folk and Birth Control," used eugenic language to argue for contraception. He despaired of what he called careless breeding among blacks, especially among those unfit to produce progeny. Margaret Sanger quoted this article verbatim when defending her proposed "Negro Project" (a birth control service specifically for women of color in Harlem) to the Birth Control Federation in 1938. See Dorothy Roberts, *Killing the Black Body: Race Reproduction, and the Meaning of Liberty* (New York: Pantheon, 1997), 77. Sheila Rowbotham states that DuBois supported birth control, but Marcus Garvey feared that it would lead to the extinction of blacks. Rowbotham, *Women in Movement,* 228. In 1919 Burrill published a one-act play, *They That Sit in Darkness,* in the *BCR.* See "Mary Powell Burrill," in *African American Women: A Biographical Dictionary,* ed. Dorothy Salem (Hamden, Conn.: Garland Publishing, 1993), 81. For Cincinnati see Lindenmeyer, "Saving Mothers and Babies," 125.

67. Martin Pernick, "Eugenics and Public Health," *American Journal of Public Health* (November 1997) 87: 1768.

68. Shields chaired the Ohio Social Hygiene Committee. "Race Betterment: A Symposium" (Dayton: Ohio Race Betterment Association, 1929), 25–30. Brush Foundation Publications, no. IV. For letter see Sanger, *Motherhood in Bondage,* 424.

69. Watson, *The Charity Organization Movement in the United States,* 429–36; Bremner, *American Philanthropy,* 118, 224; Campbell and Miggins, eds., *The Birth of Modern Cleveland,* 158, 161–63; Keller, *Affairs of State,* 7–13, 517–18. For Sanitary Fair see "Northern Ohio Sanitary Fair," *ECH,* 747. See also Van Tassel and Grabowski, eds., *Cleveland: A Tradition,* and Ross, "The New Philanthropy," Ph.D. diss. The city's Roman Catholic community also shared the predilection for efficiency, being among the first diocese in the country to have a director of diocesan charities (1910). See Ross, "The New Philanthropy," 234.

70. Campbell and Miggins, eds., *The Birth of Modern Cleveland,* 43–44, and John J. Grabowski, "Immigration and Migration," *ECH,* 557–63. In 1900 Cleveland had 381,768 residents, 5,988 of whom were African American. By 1930 the black population stood at 71,799. Campbell and Miggins, *The Birth of Modern Cleveland,* 38; Kusmer, *A Ghetto Takes Shape,* 10, 54–56. For immigration statistics see Rose, *Cleveland: The Making of a City,* 873. See also Grabowski, "Immigration and Migration," and Tuennerman-Kaplan, *Helping Others, Helping Ourselves.*

71. In November of 1918, at the height of the flu epidemic in Cleveland, 985 Clevelanders were buried in Calvary Cemetery, 81 of them on November 4. "Calvary Cemetery," *ECH*, 147–48. For reactions to immigration in Cleveland, see Edward M. Miggins, "Becoming American: Americanization and the Reform of the Cleveland Public
Schools," in *The Birth of Modern Cleveland*, ed. Campbell and Miggins, 325–44. See
also Grabowski, "Immigration and Migration"; Lloyd P. Gartner, *History of the Jews in
Cleveland*, 2d ed. (Cleveland: Western Reserve Historical Society, 1978); and Carol
Poh Miller and Robert A. Wheeler, *Cleveland: A Concise History, 1796–1996*, 2d ed.
(Bloomington: Indiana University Press, 1997). For the rest of the country see Wiebe,
*The Search for Order*, 50–54, 62–67, 89, 157, 210. See also John Higham, *Strangers in
the Land*, 2d ed. (New Brunswick, N.J.: Rutgers University Press, 1981).

72. Roger A. Bruns, *The Damnedest Radical: The Life and World of Ben Reitman,
Chicago's Celebrated Social Reformer, Hobo King, and Whorehouse Physician* (Urbana:
University of Illinois Press, 1987), 181. The Socialist Labor Party, one of Cleveland's
oldest political organizations, was organized in 1877, the same year that local members founded a Czech language newspaper for Cleveland's "workingman," believed to
be the first Socialist Labor Party newspaper in the country. "Socialist Labor Party,"
*ECH*, 937.

73. "On the Road with Birth Control," Margaret Sanger Papers Project Newsletter,
21 (spring 1999): 1–2.

74. "Poverty Makes for Big Families-Mrs. Sanger," *Cleveland Citizen*, April 24,
1916, p. 9; "What the Birth Control Leagues are Doing," *BCR* 1, no. 1 (February
1917): 10; "Channing Hall; Announcement," *Margaret Sanger Papers Microfilm Edition: Collected Documents Series* (hereafter *MSPCDM*), ed. Esther Katz, Series III,
C17:0454. These pieces do not identify the radical sponsors in Cleveland. "MHA
History" (Cleveland: MHA, 1957), 2, PPGC, box 3.

75. "Chicago Address to Women," 1916, 2–3, emphasis Sanger's, MS-SS, early
speeches. For Sanger's tour see "A 'Birth Control' Lecture Tour," typescript copy for
the *Malthusian*, September 1916, 1–2. MS-SS, correspondence 1913–17.

76. Williams soon left Cleveland but stayed active in the national birth control
movement, helping to found a clinic in Rochester, New York, in 1932–1934. See
David Rhys Williams, "Dear Mrs. Sanger," *Our Margaret Sanger* (privately published,
1959), vol. 2, 315–16. MS-SS, and Guttmacher, comp., *Planned Parenthood Beginnings: Affiliate Histories* (n.p., 1979), 89.

77. Reed, *Birth Control Movement*, 109–110; Kennedy, *Birth Control in America*, 92;
"What the Birth Control Leagues," 3, 10; Sanger, *Autobiography*, 198, 210, 251–55;
Gordon, *Woman's Body*, 257–58; "Jottings," *The Survey* 36, no. 21 (August 19, 1916):
529; News article, *Cleveland Press*, n.d., *Cleveland Press* Collection, Cleveland State
University, Cleveland, Ohio; and Chesler, *Woman of Valor*, 166–67. The International
Workers of the World later discredited Blossom. See Gordon, *Woman's Body*, 258;
Chesler, *Woman of Valor;* and Elizabeth Gurley Flynn, "Published Documents and

Letters Re Investigation of Frederick Blossom, 1923," MS-SS. Chesler points out that FBI director J. Edgar Hoover kept a file on Sanger's association with "alleged subversives" until her death in 1966. See Chesler, *Woman of Valor,* 162. For further evidence of Sanger's close anarchist connections before World War I, see "Margaret Sanger and the Modern School," Margaret Sanger Papers Project Newsletter, no. 19 (fall 1998): 1–3. For the continuity of the radical legacy see also Dorothy Green and Mary-Elizabeth Murdock, eds., *Margaret Sanger Centennial Conference, November 13 & 14, 1979,* 36.

78. Bruns, *The Damnedest Radical,* 183; *Cleveland Plain Dealer,* January 16, 1917.

79. *BCR* 1, no. 1 (February 1917): 3. The local birth control supporters listed were: Alfred F. Bosch, League President; Dr. Thomas Adams; Rev. Dwight J. Bradley; Alice Butler, M.D.; David Gibson; H. G. Wellman; Mrs. Percy W. Cobb; and Miss A. G. Wasweyler. "What the Birth Control Leagues," 10. Bruns mentions Gibson as a Reitman supporter. See *The Damnedest Radical,* 180. Bosch belonged to Williams's Cleveland congregation. See Williams, "Dear Mrs. Sanger," 315. Alice Rosenberger Butler served in the national birth control movement until her death in 1928. See, for example, Butler to Sanger, May 19, 1925, *MSPCDM,* series III, C02:0294. For maiden name see *Representative Clevelanders: A Biographical Directory of Leading Men and Women in the Present-Day Cleveland Community* ([Cleveland]: The Cleveland Topics Company, 1927), 57. See Butler's papers at DMHC.

80. See note 25 above.

81. "What the Birth Control Leagues," 10; and "The Spreading Movement for Birth Control," *The Survey* (October 21, 1916), 60. The *Survey* article confirms the Cleveland pamphlet but puts the figure at ten thousand copies, with a second edition. I have found little other information on these early activities, no copy of the pamphlet, and no corroboration on the hospital clinics.

82. Michael Haines, "Birthrate and Mortality," in *The Reader's Companion to American History,* ed. Eric Foner and John A. Garraty (Boston: Houghton Mifflin, 1991), 104; Reed, *The Birth Control Movement,* x. There are differentials within these figures, for rural/urban, first-generation/later-generation immigrants, etc. For a view of the fertility transition worldwide see McLaren, *A History of Contraception,* 178–207. It is important to note that despite the consistent drop in fertility (except for a couple of baby booms) in the last two centuries, "less than 15% of married women have remained childless in the twentieth century." Van Horn, *Women, Work and Fertility,* 5. The race differential within Van Horn's figure, however, deserves closer scrutiny. Paula Giddings notes that in 1910, one fourth of all black women were childless. See Paula J. Giddings, *Where and When I Enter: The Impact of Black Women on Race and Sex in America* (New York: Bantam Books, 1985, 1984), 137, also 150.

83. These figures do not contain the variable of race. Howard Whipple Green, *Housing in the Cleveland Community: Past—Present—Future* (Cleveland: Real Property Inventory of Metropolitan Cleveland, 1947), appendix, 34.

84. Van Horn, *Women, Work and Fertility*, 2, 33.

85. McLaren, *A History of Contraception*, 178; Brodie, "Family Limitation," Ph.D. diss., 7. Mosher, *Mosher Survey*.

86. Sanger, *Motherhood in Bondage*, 300, 302.

87. Gordon, *Woman's Body*, 317; Robishaw, "A Study of 4,000 Patients," 426–34. MHA, "Report of Fourth Year," 12, BCS, record group 2, series A.

88. McLaren, *History of Contraception*, 207.

## Notes to Chapter 2

1. Untitled typewritten manuscript n.d., 2–4; "MHA History" (Cleveland: MHA, 1957), 1; untitled handwritten history, PPGC, box 3; untitled typewritten manuscript, n.d., 1–2. All in PPGC, box 3, early history. The papers of Dorothy Hamilton Brush, Sophia Smith Archives, Smith College, Northampton, Mass. (hereafter DHB), box 1, folder 17.

2. Ibid.

3. For more about Rublee, see Chesler, *Woman of Valor*, esp. 154, 167–68, 224, 412–13, and Margaret Sanger, ed., *International Aspects of Birth Control: Sixth International Neo-Malthusian and Birth Control Conference* (New York: American Birth Control League, 1925), 221.

4. "Sessions of the Conference, Friday, November 11," The papers of Margaret Sanger, Part 1: Diaries, Speeches and Writings, on microfilm. *Women in America: Core Primary Sources for Women's Studies*, in association with the Margaret Sanger Papers Project, New York University, ed. Esther Katz (hereafter MS-WIA), reel 3; and "The Town Hall Raid," Margaret Sanger Papers Project Newsletter, no. 27 (spring 2001): 1.

5. "Programme of the First American Birth Control Conference," November 11, 12, 13, 1921. PPFA, box 36, folder 28. For accounts of the arrest see Sanger, *Margaret Sanger: An Autobiography*, 301–06; Chesler, *Woman of Valor*, 203; untitled typewritten manuscript, 6–7. PPGC, box 3, early history; untitled typewritten manuscript, 6, and untitled typewritten manuscript, 1. DHB, box 1, folder 17; and "The Town Hall Raid," 1–3. Hayes is quoted on p. 2. The police arrested Rublee the next week but held her for only a few hours before finding a lack of evidence. See "Town Hall Raid," 3. In some accounts, Brush claims that she did not follow Sanger as far as she wanted to because "my mother was not used to street scenes." See untitled typewritten manuscript, 1, DHB, box 1, folder 17.

6. For the Children's Bureau refusal to impart birth control information despite repeated requests on a national level, see Ladd-Taylor, *Raising a Baby the Government Way*, 180–84. In Cleveland, the Children's Bureau was allied for a short time with the Children's Aid Society. See "Children's Aid Society," *ECH*, 179. For Brush's quote see "That Children May be Given Every Chance for Mental and Physical Health" (Cleveland, Ohio: MHA, 1929), PPGC, box 3.

7. McCann, *Birth Control Politics,* 12–13, 59–61, 78, 203; Gordon, *Woman's Body,* 310; Chesler, *Woman of Valor,* 297–98; Martin, "The Egg and the Sperm," 493.

8. McCann, *Birth Control Politics,* 59–60, 78; Andrea Tone, *Devices and Desires,* 134–38; Tone, "Contraceptive Consumers: Gender and the Political Economy of Birth Control in the 1930s," in *American Sexual Histories,* ed. Elizabeth Reis (Oxford: Blackwell Publishers, 2001), 257; Chesler, *Woman of Valor,* 295.

9. Quote by R. Illula Morrison Hansen, M.D., in "Contraception: The Woman's Point of View," p. 1, delivered February 19, 1931, before the Lakewood Clinical Luncheon Club, PPGC, box 2, speeches. Chesler, *Woman of Valor,* 407, 445; Reed, *The Birth Control Movement,* 124–125, 375; Borell, "Biologists and the Promotion of Birth Control," 67, 72, 85; and van Kammen, "Representing Users' Bodies."

10. Untitled typewritten manuscript, 7, DHB, box 1, folder 6, and "Farewell to Mrs. Dorothy Brush," *Planned Parenthood Monthly Bulletin of the Family Planning Association of India* 4, nos. 8–9 (February–March 1957): 1, scrapbook 1956–57, PPGC, box 8.

11. Jensen, "Evolution." See also Gordon, *Woman's Body,* 207–23, and Chesler, *Woman of Valor,* 161–63, 165–67, also 57–59, 231–32, 455.

12. Muncy, *Creating a Female Dominion;* Blair, *A History of Women's Voluntary Organizations;* Scharf and Jensen, eds., *Decades of Discontent;* Hine and Thompson, *A Shining Thread of Hope.*

13. For the limited opportunities for women physicians, see Mary Roth Walsh, *Doctors Wanted: No Women Need Apply: Sexual Barriers in the Medical Profession, 1835–1975* (New Haven, Conn.: Yale University Press, 1977), and Regina Markell Morantz, Cynthia Stodola Pomerleau, and Carol Hansen Fenichel, eds., *In Her Own Words: Oral Histories of Women Physicians* (New Haven, Conn.: Yale University Press, 1982). For women's leadership in the international birth control movement, see Perdita Huston, *Motherhood by Choice: Pioneers in Women's Health and Family Planning* (New York: The Feminist Press at the City University of New York, 1992), and Jacobs, *Memories.* See also the published proceedings of early international birth control conferences for women's involvement, for example, Margaret Sanger, ed., *International Aspects; Religious and Ethical Aspects of Birth Control. Sixth International Neo-Malthusian and Birth Control Conference,* vol. 4 (New York: American Birth Control League, 1926). Guttmacher, comp., *Planned Parenthood Beginnings.* This compilation of brief historical sketches of 101 Planned Parenthood affiliates does not always mention the gender of the founders. For Gaylord's involvement outside of Cleveland see Annette B. Ramirez de Arellano and Conrad Seipp, *Colonialism, Catholicism, and Contraception: A History of Birth Control in Puerto Rico* (Chapel Hill: University of North Carolina Press, 1983), 39–43; G. Gaylord to Mrs. Francis Bangs, December 7, 1934, and Catherine C. Bangs to G. Gaylord, December 26, 1934, PPFA, ser. II, box 30, folder 77. For Brush see "Farewell to Mrs. Dorothy Brush." Brush and Weir served on the boards or as an officer in several birth control groups, along with

Jerome Fisher. See, for example, the printed guide *The Margaret Sanger Papers Microfilm Edition: Collected Documents Series,* ed. Esther Katz (Bethesda, Md.: University Publications of America, 1997), 36, 42, 55, 60, 61, 63, 65, 68, 73, 76.

14. Guttmacher, comp., *Planned Parenthood Beginnings,* 18, 40, 58, 67, 93, 123, 127.

15. For Marie Stopes see McLaren and McLaren, *The Bedroom and the State,* 23–24, 56–58; June Rose, *Marie Stopes and the Sexual Revolution* (London: Faber and Faber, 1992); and Hall, ed., *Dear Dr. Stopes,* 7–10.

16. For Kaufman see Reed, *The Birth Control Movement,* 218–22, 252, and McLaren and McLaren, *The Bedroom and the State,* 100, note 40, 103–16. For DeVilbiss see Reed, *Birth Control Movement,* 252; Gordon, *Woman's Body,* 309; and Chesler, *Woman of Valor,* 379–380. DeVilbiss was asked to direct Sanger's Clinical Research Bureau in 1921 but backed out. See Chesler, *Woman of Valor,* 274, and McCann, *Birth Control Politics,* 77, note 49. For commercial marketing see Tone, "Contraceptive Consumers," 485–506. Some states, such as North Carolina, did perform sterilizations—in the latter case, under the auspices of a state eugenics board. See Johanna Schoen, "Between Choice and Coercion: Women and the Politics of Sterilization in North Carolina, 1929–1975," *Journal of Women's History* 13, no. 1 (2001): 132–56.

17. This was Sanger's second arrest. McCann, *Birth Control Politics,* 23–24.

18. "May Day Riots," *ECH,* 682–83; Miller and Wheeler, *Cleveland,* 120. Robert K. Murray, *Red Scare: A Study in National Hysteria, 1919–1920* (Minneapolis: University of Minnesota Press, 1955), 75–76. For more on the Brownsville clinic see Reed, *The Birth Control Movement,* 106–8; Kennedy, *Birth Control in America;* and Chesler, *Woman of Valor,* 151–52.

19. For Denver see *The History of Planned Parenthood of the Rocky Mountains, 1916 . . .* (Aurora, Colo.: Planned Parenthood of the Rocky Mountains, n.d.), 8.

20. Records for the Ohio Birth Control League or copies of its newsletter have yet to be located. Sanger, *Margaret Sanger,* 417. Ellen Chesler rightly argues that Sanger's autobiographies are "self-aggrandizing books filled with petty deceits and outright duplicity." See *Woman of Valor,* 16. I will use Dorothy Hamilton Brush (D.H.B.) to identify the MHA founder in these notes, although she remarried twice after her first husband's death. Dorothy married Charles Francis Brush Jr. in 1917, was widowed in 1927, married Alexander C. Dick in 1929, was divorced in 1947, and married Lewis C. Walmsley in 1962. See *Who's Who of American Women,* 2d ed. (Chicago: Marquis Who's Who, 1962), 139, and Smith College Archives (hereafter SCA), Northampton, Massachusetts. Brush says she first saw Sanger at the New York birth control conference in 1921. See Dorothy Brush, "I Just Love Margaret," in *Our Margaret Sanger,* vol. 1, 41, MS-SS, and untitled typewritten manuscript, n.d., p. 1, DHB, box 1, folder 17. Brush's recollections are probably more accurate than Sanger's, since in 1916 Brush was still a student at Smith College and not yet married. SCA.

21. Untitled typewritten manuscript, n.d., n.p., DHB, box 1, folder 17.

22. Davis, "Maternal Health," master's thesis, 8.

23. Davis, "Maternal Health," appendix 1, ix, xv. The quotes appear anonymously in the text.

24. "Catholics, Roman," *ECH*, 158, and Michael J. McTighe and Jimmy E. W. Meyer, "Religion," *ECH*, 855.

25. "Statement of Hon. Martin L. Sweeney, a Representative in Congress from the State of Ohio," *Birth Control Hearings Before the Committee on Ways and Means, House of Representatives, Seventy-second Congress. First Session on H.R. 11082, May 19 and 20, 1932* (Washington, DC: United States Government Printing Office, 1932), 71–73. See "Sweeney, Martin L.," *DCB*, 438. Pope Pius XI issued the first papal encyclical in fifty years in 1930, condemning birth control as a "craven sin . . . , against the laws of God and nature." The encyclical also reaffirmed the church's opposition to divorce and companionate unions. *Cleveland News,* Jan. 8, 1931, MHA Scrapbook 1929–1935, PPGC, box 7. Noonan Jr., *Contraception*, 424, 426–32. See also chapter 5 in this work.

26. First Ohio State Conference on Birth Control Program, 1922, *MSPCDM*, S67:0925–28.

27. First Ohio State conference on birth control program. "Associated Charities," *ECH*, 65.

28. Untitled typewritten manuscript, 4, DHB, box 1, folder 17; untitled typewritten manuscript, I, 7, and untitled typewritten manuscript, III, 3–4, both in PPGC, box 3, early histories. No record exists of the arguments founders employed, except that they told "the story." See ibid.

29. On U.S. women's organizations see Estelle Freedman, "Separatism as Strategy: Female Institution Building and American Feminism, 1870–1930," *Feminist Studies* 5, no. 3 (fall 1979): 524, and Vandenberg-Daves, "The Manly Pursuit of a Partnership between the Sexes," 1346. On women's organizations recruiting men, see Deutsch, "Learning to Talk More Like a Man," 379–404. On men and Cleveland reform see Van Tassel and Grabowski, eds., *Cleveland: A Tradition.* For the Men's Equal Suffrage League in Cleveland, see Abbott, *A History of Woman Suffrage,* 16. For Ohio Birth Control League, see "What the Birth Control Leagues Are Doing," *BCR* 1, no. 1 (February 1917): 10. For women's separatist cultural activities in the antebellum years, see Kathleen D. McCarthy, *Women's Culture: American Philanthropy and Art 1830–1930* (Chicago: University of Chicago Press, 1991), 59–79. For philanthropy in Cleveland see Van Tassel and Grabowski, eds., *Cleveland: A Tradition;* Ross, "The New Philanthropy," Ph.D. diss.; and Tuennerman-Kaplan, *Helping Others, Helping Ourselves.* For U.S. trends see Bremner, *American Philanthropy.*

30. Untitled typewritten manuscript, 4, DHB, box 1, folder 17; untitled typewritten manuscript, 7, and untitled typewritten manuscript, 3–4, PPGC, box 3, early history. For the Perkinses and Brushes see "Brush, Dorothy Adams Hamilton," *DCB*, 70; "Perkins, Edna Brush," *DCB*, 350; "Perkins, Roger Griswold," *DCB*, 351; and Charles Brush Perkins, *Ancestors of Charles Brush Perkins and Maurice Perkins* (Baltimore, Md.:

Gateway Press, 1976), 21. For Weir see Brown, ed., *The History of Medicine in Cleveland,* figure 47.

31. Cigliano, *Showplace of America,* 291–306. See also Susan A. Ostrander, *Women of the Upper Class* (Philadelphia: Temple University Press, 1984). The formation of the American Society for the Control of Cancer provides an example of similar networking in health voluntarism elsewhere: after Dr. Clement Cleveland of New York proposed the idea of the society, his daughter, Elsie Cleveland Mead, recruited lay participants, including the law partner of her husband, Robert. As chair of the ways and means for the society, Elsie Mead also established a long-standing cooperative relationship between the cancer society and the General Federation of Women's Clubs. See Carter, *The Gentle Legions,* 144.

32. Garrow, *Liberty and Sexuality,* 9–10, 29, 35.

33. The research base on the history of women's networking has grown exponentially since two key articles appeared in the 1970s: Mary P. Ryan, "The Power of Women's Networks: A Case Study of Female Moral Reform in Antebellum America," *Feminist Studies* 5, no. 1 (1979): 66–85, and Cook, "Female Support Networks and Political Activism," 43–61. The following citations represent only a few random examples of scholars who have uncovered the importance of women's networks in their fields of inquiry. Herbert Gutman maintains that enslaved women would share contraceptive knowledge and abortion methods with each other and lie to their masters about pregnancy. See Gutman cited in Hine and Thompson, *A Shining Thread of Hope,* 98–99. Aletta Jacobs, a Dutch physician, describes the network of women involved in creating the International Woman Suffrage Alliance (est. in Berlin in 1904 with six members). Jacobs, *Memories,* 58–59. Ellen Chesler attributes much of the birth control movement's success to Sanger's access to the broad and influential networks of supporters such as Juliet Rublee. Chesler, *Woman of Valor,* 167, 202. Nicola Beisel notes the role of networks in the nineteenth century anti-vice campaigns, in *Imperiled Innocents.* Allen Cairns focuses on the role of social networks in the anti-abortion movement in "Fighting for Life: Ideology, Social Networks, and Recruitment of Activists to a Pro-Life Movement Organization" (Ph.D. diss., State University of New York at Buffalo, 1981). Disciplines other than history are rediscovering the importance of networks. See Emily Eakin, "Connect, They Say, Only Connect," *New York Times,* January 29, 2003, <www.nytimes.com>.

34. Untitled typewritten manuscript, 3–4, PPGC, box 3, early histories, and "History," typewritten manuscript, 5–6. The records of the Brush Foundation at the WRHS (hereafter BF), ser. IV, cont. 3, folder 46.

35. This only represents a smattering of the causes supported by these women. See these activities summarized in untitled typewritten manuscript, 7, PPGC, box 3. For suffrage activities see Abbott, *A History of Woman Suffrage,* esp. 15, 20. For Women's City Club connections, see Women's City Club of Cleveland records (hereafter WCC), WRHS. For Perkins see *National Cyclopaedia of American Biography,* vol. 26 (New York:

James T. White, 1937), 448–49; *The Ohio Blue Book: Who's Who in the Buckeye State*, comp. C. S. Van Tassel (Norwalk, Ohio: American Publishers, 1917), 291; Rose, *Cleveland: The Making of a City*, 585, 621, 703; and Wood, "Cleveland Medicine's Incredible Ghosts," 60. For Flory see Durward Howes, ed., *American Women*, vol. 3, 1939–40 (Los Angeles: American Publishers, 1939), 296, and Cleveland Day Nursery and Free Kindergarten records, WRHS. For Flory's husband see "City Club of Cleveland," *ECH*, 185; "City Planning," *ECH*, 188; "Thompson, Hine & Flory," *ECH*, 1000–01; and Rose, *Cleveland: The Making of a City*, 748, 788, 1004, 1036. For Goff see *The Fourth General Catalogue of the Officers and Graduates of Vassar College, Pough-keepsie, New York, 1861–1910* (Poughkeepsie, New York: A. V. Haight Company, 1910), 91; *The First 25 Years 1914–1939* (n.p., The Cleveland Foundation, n.d.), 2, 22; *Social Register Cleveland 1927* (New York: Social Register Association, 1927); and Gladys Gaylord to Mrs. Donald McGraw, October 10, 1929, MS-WIA, reel 5. Mr. Goff died in 1923, see "Goff, Frederick H.," *DCB*, 182; *The First 25 Years*, 5; Tittle, *Rebuilding Cleveland;* "Ameritrust," *ECH*, 38–39; "Banking," *ECH*, 82; "Banks and Savings and Loans," *ECH*, 86; "Cleveland Foundation," *ECH*, 240–41; "Glenville Race Track," *ECH*, 479; "Mayor's War Advisory Committee," *ECH*, 684–85; David C. Hammack, "Philanthropy," *ECH*, 787; and Rose, *Cleveland: The Making of a City*, 277, 379, 596, 659, 668, 671, 722, 727, 728, 749, 768, 805, 816. For Wason see *Fourth General Catalogue*, 140; *Social Register Cleveland 1927*, 71; and Rose, *Cleveland: The Making of a City*, 585, 752. For Lenore Black see "Family Service Assn. of Cleveland," *ECH*, 417; Rose, *Cleveland: The Making of a City*, 737; and Gaylord to McGraw, October 10, 1929, MS-WIA, reel 5. For Morris Black see "Chamber of Com-merce–City Plan Committee," *ECH*, 168; "Hebrew Free Loan Assn.," *ECH*, 514–15; "Oakwood Club," *ECH*, 752; "Sterling-Lindner Co.," *ECH*, 957–58; "Black, Morris," *DCB*, 46–47; *Who's Who in American Jewry*, vol. 3, 1938–39 (New York: National News, 1938), 99; and Rose, *Cleveland: The Making of a City*, 690, 722, 732, 787. For Oliver see Florence T. Waite, *A Warm Friend for the Spirit: A History of the Family Ser-vice Association of Cleveland and Its Forebears, 1830–1952* (Cleveland: Family Service Association, 1960), 165–67.

36. Cutler quote in "MHA History," 4, PPGC, box 3. For philanthropy and reform in Cleveland see Ross, "The New Philanthropy," Ph.D. diss, and Hammack, "Philan-thropy," *ECH* 785–90. For ballyhooing see R. L. Duffus, "Cleveland: Paternalism in Excelcis," *New Republic*, April 4, 1928, quoted in Peter Dobkin Hall, "Cultures of Trusteeship in the United States," in *Inventing the Nonprofit Sector and Other Essays on Philanthropy, Voluntarism, and Nonprofit Organizations* (Baltimore: Johns Hopkins Uni-versity Press, 1992), 169. For cooperation see also Bertha B. Herzog, "The President's Message," and Mrs. Emil Brudno, "Co-operation," both in *Bulletin-Cleveland Section, National Council of Jewish Women* 1, no. 5 (1924): 3, 14, WRHS. For another example of a Cleveland organization—the Benjamin Rose Institute, which remained independent from the Community Fund yet networked among other agencies—see Beth DiNatale

Johnson, "Creative Consensus: Elite Volunteers and Health Care Policy for the Aged," unpublished paper presented at Women and Health Care in Cleveland Conference, Cleveland, Ohio, November 9, 1996, 9. Used with permission of the author.

37. Waite, *Warm Friend*, 101, 102–5. The directory's 149 pages included 25 pages of legal suggestions for social workers. James R. Garfield, secretary of the Cleveland Humane Society, described and called for interagency cooperation in the protection of children in "A Program of Action for a Children's Protective Society," *Proceedings of the National Conference of Charities and Correction, June 12–19, 1912*, ed. Alexander Johnson (Fort Wayne, Ind.: Fort Wayne Printing Company, 1912), 33–40.

38. Thomas F. Campbell, *SASS: Fifty Years of Social Work Education* (Cleveland: Case Western Reserve University Press, 1967), especially chapter 2.

39. "MHA History," PPGC, box 3; "Legality of Contraception," 151–52. For more about the legal situation see chapter 1. I have not located the text of Fisher's speech at the Ohio birth control conference in November 1922.

40. "Legality of Contraception," 151.

41. For surveys see Robinson, *Seventy Birth Control Clinics*, 3–41, and "Summary of Replies Received to Questionnaire," MS-WIA, reel 7. For other clinics see Guttmacher, comp., *Planned Parenthood Beginnings;* Losure, "'Motherhood Protection'," 359–61; and Leung, "'Better Babies'," 54–68. For Chicago see Guttmacher, comp., *Planned Parenthood Beginnings*, 40, and Holz, "The Birth Control Clinic in America," Ph.D. diss.; for Rochester see Ruth H. Backus, "Planned Parenthood League of Rochester and Monroe County . . . From the Cradle" (n.p., 1965), 2, 6. Newark's Maternal Health Center "set aside funds for legal proceedings." See Guttmacher, comp., *Planned Parenthood Beginnings*, 68. For Sanger's BCCRB see McCann, *Birth Control Politics*, 76–77. Of course, other clinics paid close attention to legal matters. See Losure, "'Motherhood Protection'," 360, for example. Robinson suggests that a law firm in Missouri may have also published an interpretation. See Robinson, *Seventy Birth Control Clinics*, 171. For the BCLM, see the papers of the Planned Parenthood League of Massachusetts (hereafter PPLM), Sophia Smith Collection, Smith College, Northampton, Massachusetts, esp. "Massachusetts Dates of Birth Control Movement," n.d., box 30, and "A Brief Summary of the Legal Opinions That Were Published in the *New England Journal of Medicine*, Jan. 23, 1930," box 83. The BCLM sought advice from Cleveland MHA's Jerome Fisher. See Fisher to Greenbaum, Wolff & Ernst, January 26, 1938, and Fisher to Harriet Pilpel, February 7, 1938, in PPLM, box 89. A 1922 report described Fisher's paper at the Columbus conference and stated, "We have opinions from other law firms, but this one has been considered the best." PPFA, ser. I, box 1, folder 100.

42. "History," typewritten manuscript, 8. BF, ser. IV, cont. 3, folder 46. The date of Kennedy's first trip to Cleveland is unclear. The ABCL was founded in 1921. See Reed, *Birth Control Movement*, 110.

43. For Perkins, Black, and Flory see note 35 above. For Women's City Club of

Cleveland see "Women's City Club," *ECH,* 1098; "The Women's City Club of Cleveland, 1916–1933" (The William Feather Company, n.d.), 10–11; and "Women's City Club History," typewritten manuscript, n.d., Cleveland Public Library. Katherine Fisher to "Gals," n.d. PPGC, box 3, early histories. Unfortunately, the WCC collection at the WRHS does not include the text of Hooker's talk. For the Women's City Club elsewhere see Maureen A. Flanagan, "Gender and Urban Political Reform: The City Club and the Women's City Club of Chicago in the Progressive Era," *American History Review* 95, no. 4 (October 1990): 1032–50.

44. "History," typewritten manuscript, 8, BF, ser. IV, cont. 3, folder 46; "Miss Rowe's Report-Pittsburgh, Cleveland, and Detroit," n.d., PPFA, ser. I, box 1, folder 100.

45. Others present at the organizational meeting included Dorothy Brush, Hortense Shepard, Julia Flory, Jane Hamilton, May Oliver, and Caroline Fisher Sawyer. See "History," typewritten manuscript, 9, BF, ser. IV, cont. 3, folder 46. The names on this officer list differ slightly from those listed at the clinic's opening in 1928. See figure 14, chapter 3. One of the original officers, the treasurer, Madeline Mather, moved to New York between 1923 and 1928, hence her absence from the later group. Personal conversation with Constance Mather Bishop, October 1995, Cleveland, Ohio. MHA records give no explanation or background for the choice of officers. For information about Brush, see class of 1917 records, SCA.

46. For information on Brush family dinners see Letters of Charles Francis Brush Sr. (C.F.B.), 1927–1929. The papers of Charles Frances Brush, Special Collections, Kelvin Smith Library, Case Western Reserve University, Cleveland, Ohio (hereafter CFB), box 1, folders 9 through 18; Letters between D.H.B. and C.F.B., CFB, box 31, microfilm reel 2; and M. W. Childs, "A Fund for Breeding Better Human Beings," *St. Louis Post-Dispatch* Sunday magazine, August 19, 1928, 6. For information on the physicians see Waite, *Western Reserve University Centennial History.*

47. The superintendent of Lakeside Hospital was A. B. Dennison, M.D. Constance Webb was director of social service there, and Robert Bishop, M.D., was the hospital's director. Bishop also served on the Cleveland Hospital Council board and was a former city health commissioner. Cuyahoga County Health Department director was E. A. Peterson, M.D., the only one of this group to become involved in the MHA. See untitled typewritten manuscript, 4, PPGC, box 3, early histories; "History," typewritten manuscript, 5–6, BF, ser. IV, cont. 3, folder 46. Bishop helped found the local Anti-Tuberculosis League and directed the National Social Hygiene Association as well as Lakeside (1920–1924) and University hospitals (1932–1947). He was also married to a member of the Mather family, Constance. "Bishop, Robert H., Jr." *DCB,* 45–46.

48. David Rosner, *A Once Charitable Enterprise: Hospitals and Health Care in Brooklyn and New York, 1885–1915* (Princeton, N.J.: Princeton University Press, 1982), 146–163; Sheila Rothman, "Women's Clinics or Doctor's Offices: The Sheppard-Towner Act and the Promotion of Preventive Health Care," in *Social History and Social Policy,* ed. David Rothman and Stanton Wheeler (New York: Academic Press,

1981), 175–201; Charles E. Rosenberg, "Social Class and Medical Care in 19th Century America: The Rise and Fall of the Dispensary," in *Sickness and Health in America: Readings in the History of Medicine and Public Health,* 2d ed., ed. Judith Walzer Leavitt and Ronald L. Numbers (Madison: University of Wisconsin, 1985), 273–86; and McCann, *Birth Control Politics,* 85–92. For Ohio physician resistance to layperson control of health agencies, see Kriste Lindenmeyer, "Saving Mothers and Babies," 105–134.

49. McCann, *Birth Control Politics,* 85–92.

50. Earl E. Smith and Ralph I. Fried, "Pediatrics and the Northern Ohio Pediatric Society," in *The History of Medicine in Cleveland,* ed. Brown, 281–86.

51. Mark Gottlieb, *The Lives of University Hospitals of Cleveland* (Cleveland: Wilson Street Press, 1990), 74–75, 146–47, 180–82. For more on early children's health care in Cleveland see Smith and Fried, "Pediatrics." For other Cleveland dispensaries see Meyer, "Children and Youth," *ECH,* 176–78; James Edmundson, "Hospitals and Health Planning," *ECH,* 542; and "University Hospitals of Cleveland," *ECH,* 1034–36. For an example of a dispensary leading to the creation of a hospital in another city see Judith Walzer Leavitt, *The Healthiest City: Milwaukee and the Politics of Health Care Reform* (Madison: University of Wisconsin Press, 1996, 1982), 67–68. Leavitt also highlights the important role of voluntary activity in improving health care.

52. Bing, *Social Work in Greater Cleveland,* 195.

53. "History," typescript manuscript, 9–11, BF, container 3, folder 46.

54. MHA, "History" (1957), 4; "The History of the Maternal Health Association," typewritten manuscript, 14–16, PPGC, box 3, early histories. See also "History," typewritten manuscript, 10–11, BF, container 3, folder 46. For Cleveland cooperation, see note 36 above.

55. Minutes, Lakeside Hospital Management Committee, 1928–1930, Stanley A. Ferguson Archives, University Hospitals of Cleveland.

56. Ibid.

57. Untitled typewritten manuscript, 15–16, PPGC, box 3, early histories; Guttmacher, comp., *Planned Parenthood Beginnings,* 103–104; David R. Weir, "The History of Planned Parenthood in Cuyahoga County," in Brown, ed., *The History of Medicine in Cleveland,* 274–80. One 1922 source suggests that Woman's General Hospital already had agreed to sponsor a clinic, but that MHA founders were looking for a hospital "of better standing." See "Miss Rowe's Report," 3, PPFA, ser. I, box 1, folder 100. This is unconfirmed in Woman's General Hospital records (hereafter WGH), DMHC. See Minutes, WGH. For reference to the city health department see untitled typewritten manuscript, 15, PPGC, box 3, early histories.

58. Edmundson, "Hospitals and Health Planning," *ECH,* 542–43. In addition to St. Vincent's, the other hospitals in the city's top six (those that served the most patients, as designated by the Cleveland Hospital Survey of 1921) were: Lakeside, Huron Road, Mt. Sinai (Jewish), St. Luke's (Methodist), and City Hospital. Ibid.

59. The first birth control clinic in Cincinnati, Ohio, opened in that city's public hospital but moved to another site after two years of pressure from the Roman Catholic archbishop. A similar situation occurred in Albany, New York, in 1942. Guttmacher, comp., *Planned Parenthood Beginnings*, 75 (Albany), 101 (Cincinnati). Catholics and other conservative religious groups pressured the Maternal Health Association of Missouri, forcing one of its clinics to close for a time. Katharine T. Corbett, *In Her Place: A Guide to St. Louis Women's History* (St. Louis, MO: Historical Society Press, 1999), 254.

60. D.H.B., speech in Syracuse (n.d.), p. 8, DHB, box 1, folder 4.

61. Stewart quote posted in the Women's Rights National Historical Park Visitor's Center, Seneca Falls, New York, August 1999.

62. Speaking of the history of the condom's acceptance by the American public, Joshua Gamson says, "Clearly, accidents of history (the rise of diseases such as venereal disease and AIDS) provide opportunities for the mobilization of certain interpretive frames." Gamson, "Rubber Wars," 280.

63. Miller and Wheeler, *Cleveland*, esp. chapters 8, 9, and 10; Campbell and Miggins, eds., *The Birth of Modern Cleveland*, esp. 119, 123, 133, 136. See also Phillips, *AlabamaNorth*, and Tuennerman-Kaplan, *Helping Others, Helping Ourselves*.

64. For Associated Charities information from 1927, see "Ours More Than One Fifth," *Cleveland Gazette*, July 14, 1928. African Americans represented 1,497 families among the total assisted by Associated Charities in 1927. Miller and Wheeler, *Cleveland*, 136; Waite, *Warm Friend*, 232. See also Waite, *Warm Friend*, 266–67, for a general description of the problems of unemployment and poverty in Cleveland. For the one-out-of-three statistic see Bing, *Social Work in Greater Cleveland*, 11. Bing graphs the increase in relief dollars expended in Cleveland between 1928 and 1938. See Bing, *Social Work in Greater Cleveland*, 25. For the effect of the Depression on the birth control movement generally see Gordon, *Woman's Body*, chapter 11.

65. For more on the feeding of infants see Janet Golden, *A Social History of Wet Nursing In America: From Breast to Bottle* (Columbus: The Ohio State University Press, 2001), and Rima D. Apple, *Mothers and Medicine: A Social History of Infant Feeding, 1890–1950* (Madison: University of Wisconsin Press, 1987).

66. "A Nation's Babies," *Cleveland Plain Dealer* Sunday magazine, February 27, 1916. Marilyn Irvin Holt, *Linoleum, Better Babies, and the Modern Farm Woman, 1890–1930* (Albuquerque: University of New Mexico Press, 1995), chapter 4.

67. Lydia A. DeVilbiss, "Education for Parenthood," *Proceedings of the First National Conference on Race Betterment, January 8, 9, 10, 11, 12, 1914* (n.p.: n.d.), 267. DeVilbiss chaired the Better Babies Bureau for the *Woman's Home Companion* in 1914. For "maternal efficiency," see Holt, *Linoleum*, 110.

68. Nancy Cott, *Public Vows: A History of Marriage and the Nation* (Cambridge, Mass.: Harvard University Press, 2000).

69. Ben Lindsey and Wainwright Evans popularized the term companionate marriage in their book, *The Companionate Marriage*. Margaret Sanger, *Happiness in Marriage*

(New York: Blue Ribbon Books, 1926). For discussion of Sanger's book, see Chesler, *Woman of Valor*, 263–66. For an interpretation of companionate marriage, see D'Emilio and Freedman, *Intimate Matters*, 265–70. Th. H. Van de Velde, *Ideal Marriage; Its Physiology and Technique* (New York: Random House, 1926, 1930).

70. Ladd-Taylor, *Raising a Baby the Government Way*, 133–34.

71. Interview with Ethel Coulter Meyer, Knoxville, Ohio, 1996.

72. For mothers' letters in general see Ladd-Taylor, *Raising a Baby the Government Way*; Sanger, *Motherhood in Bondage*, and Scrapbook-Letters from Patients 1928–1938, PPGC, box 6. For similar letters in Great Britain, see Hall, ed., *Dear Dr. Stopes*.

## *Notes to Chapter 3*

1. "History," typewritten manuscript, 11, BF, ser. IV, cont. 3, folder 46; Untitled typewritten manuscript, n.d., 5, DHB, box 1, folder 17; and "MHA History," 4, PPGC, box 3. C. F. Brush Jr. died from an infection apparently resulting from a blood transfusion from himself directly to his critically ill daughter, Jane (6), who also died. Perkins, *Ancestors*, 23. The technology of blood transfusion was very primitive at this time. See Rosemary Stevens, *In Sickness and Wealth: American Hospitals in the Twentieth Century* (New York: Basic Books, 1989), 176.

2. "Conference on Contraceptive Research and Clinical Practice, Analysis of Questionnaires," MS-WIA, reel 8, pp. 1–2.

3. Guttmacher, comp., *Planned Parenthood Beginnings;* "Report of the Executive Secretary of the Maternal Health Association to the Brush Foundation, October 7, 1930," 1, PPGC, box 1, Brush Foundation—histories; Robinson, *Seventy Birth Control Clinics*, esp. 8–19; and McLaren and McLaren, *The Bedroom and the State*, 66–67. For Minnesota, see Mary Losure, "'Motherhood Protection'," 359–61. For Arkansas see Leung, "'Better Babies'," 53. A list of reasons for choosing clinic names appears in "Conference on Contraceptive Research," pp. 1–2. The MHA did not adopt the name of Planned Parenthood of Greater Cleveland until 1966, after twenty-four years of being a Planned Parenthood affiliate. See Jean B. Evans, "60 Years of Planned Parenthood in Cleveland," draft II (January 16, 1988), 18. Personal collection of the author.

4. Carole R. McCann, *Birth Control Politics*, 63–64.

5. Reed, *Birth Control Movement*, 143–96, esp. 168.

6. Mary Ware Dennett and others created the NBCL in March 1915. The VPL succeeded this group in 1919, with the particular goal of repealing the Comstock Law. In 1921 Sanger created the ABCL with a broader focus than the VPL. The BCCRB, established by Sanger in 1923, and Dickinson's CMH focused on clinical service and research. Sanger resigned as ABCL president in 1928, taking some supporters with her to the BCCRB. By 1937, however, the rift had healed; the BCCRB and the ABCL merged to form the BCFA, which became PPFA in 1942. Sanger, *Margaret Sanger: An*

*Autobiography*, 108, 180, 300, 360, 395, 414; Gordon, *Woman's Body*, 226, 263, 291–92, 320–21, 329; Reed, *Birth Control Movement*, 100, 163, 265. For quote see "Report of Education and Extension Work of the Executive Secretary of the Maternal Health Association Between July 1, 1938 and July 1, 1939," 2, PPGC, box 1, Brush Foundation–histories.

7. "That Children May be Given," MHA, 1929, PPGC, box 3. Until 1964, like other North American clinics, the MHA adhered to the stipulation that clients be married or carry a statement from their clergy of the intention to marry. See Planned Parenthood of Greater Cleveland, "Every Child a Wanted Child: 60 Years of Planned Parenthood in Cleveland" (Cleveland: PPGC, 1988); Guttmacher, comp., *Planned Parenthood Beginnings;* and chapter 4 in this work.

8. Untitled typewritten manuscript, 9, PPGC, box 3, early history; MHA Annual Report 1939–40, PPGC, box 2.

9. For ABCL's membership requirements see Annual Meeting, ABCL, January 13, 1927, PPFA, ser. I, box 1, folder 105. MHA, "Report of Fourth Year," 20, BCS, record group 2, series A. For the precarious financial status of other clinics, see Losure, "'Motherhood Protection'," 368–369, and Guttmacher, comp., *Planned Parenthood Beginnings*.

10. G. Gaylord, "Philosophies of a Maternal Health Association," West Side Annual Meeting, April 24, 1940, 4, PPGC, box 6, West Side Minutes. MHA, "Report of Three Years' Work," 3, MS-SS, Smith College, Clinics-Ohio.

11. MHA, "Report of Three Years' Work," 3, MS-SS, Smith College, Clinics-Ohio. For propaganda quote, see Davis, "Maternal Health," 34. Federal work quote in "Report of the Executive Secretary," October 15 to November 10, 1923, ABCL, 3, PPFA, series I, box 4, folder 125.

12. For Sanger's separation from the ABCL, see Kennedy, *Birth Control in America*, 103, and Chesler, *Woman of Valor*, 238. For ABCL's reaction to Sanger see McCann, *Birth Control Politics*, 187–88. McCann is a good source for changes within the national movement. For the effects of the Dennett/Sanger controversy on the national movement, see Rachel Brugger, "How Did Animosity Between Margaret Sanger and Mary Ware Dennett Shape the Movement to Legalize Birth Control?" December 1999, Women and Social Movements in the United States, 1830–1930, <http://womhist.binghamton.edu/birth/intro/htm>, and correspondence between Sanger and Dennett, for example, Dennett to Sanger, July 29, 1921, *MSPCDM*, S02:017–18. The printed guide to Sanger's papers offers a good chronology and introduction to the vagaries of the movement. *A Guide to the Microfilm Edition of the Margaret Sanger Papers: Collected Documents Series*.

13. Robinson, *Seventy Birth Control Clinics*, 22; "Report of Extension and Education," 3–4. PPGC, box 1, Brush Foundation–histories; untitled typewritten manuscript, 1, PPGC, box 3, early history. For MHA independence see Annual Reports, 1928–1943, PPGC, box 2. This independent streak stayed with the organization. In

1946 the MHA declined to participate in a national PPFA fund drive. See Mrs. Newell Bolton to R. M. Ruhlman, Cleveland Chamber of Commerce, October 23, 1946, PPGC, box 1. In 1948 the MHA disputed with PPFA about fund-raising and refused to sponsor a citywide fund drive or give one-third of its local funds to the group. See Bernard John Oliver Jr., "Maternal Health Association," unpublished paper, May 15, 1948, 16, PPGC, box 3, early history. The Cleveland facility did separate from PPGC around 1950, rejoining in May 1951. See "'Maternal' Group Rejoins Planned Parenthooders," identified as an article from *Catholic Universe Bulletin*, May 23, 1952, PPGC, box 6, Scrapbook 1951–1953. Annual reports for the 1950s do not always note the MHA's affiliations, adding to the confusion. See, for example, MHA, Annual Report, April 1, 1955–March 31, 1956, PPGC, box 2.

14. For national material used by the MHA see Scrapbook-American Birth Control Leaflets, PPGC, box 3; for participation by Clevelanders in the national scene see, for example, "Stenographic Minutes of Organization Meeting, Middle Western States Conference on Birth Control," November 12, 1929, 17, 36, Margaret Sanger, Part 1: Diaries, Speeches and Writings, reel 5, MS-WIA; and mentions of Jerome Fisher, Roslyn Weir, and Dorothy Brush in the printed guide *A Guide to the Microfilm Edition of the Margaret Sanger Papers: Collected Documents Series*, 36, 42, 55, 60, 61, 63, 65, 68, 73, 76.

15. For Dr. Weir's office address see *Representative Clevelanders*, 391.

16. For other clinics see *The History of Planned Parenthood, of the Rocky Mountains 1916 . . .* (Aurora, Colorado: Planned Parenthood of the Rocky Mountains, n.d.), 11; Planned Parenthood, *A Tradition of Choice*, 18; and Guttmacher, comp., *Planned Parenthood Beginnings*, 15, 54, 59.

17. The influence of the choice of institutional space extends the argument presented by Sara Deutsch in "Learning to Talk More Like a Man."

18. "Conference on Contraceptive Research," 2.

19. The Osborn building is located at 1020 Huron Road/1021 Prospect Street, at the corner of Prospect and Huron, one block south of Ninth Street and Euclid Avenue. The MHA office was on the Prospect side. "History," typewritten manuscript, 16, BF, ser. IV, container 3, folder 46; and "Cleveland Union Terminal," *ECH*, 297–98. The building still stood in 2003, a home to condominiums.

20. "History," typewritten manuscript, 19, and "MHA History," 6–7, PPGC, box 3. Public agitation quote is found in "Report of the Executive Secretary," 1923, ABCL, 2. PPFA, series I, box 4, folder 125. Many other contemporary clinics also discouraged publicity. See Schoen, "Fighting for Child Health," 96, and Guttmacher, comp., *Planned Parenthood Beginnings*, 14, 23, 49, 127, 129. For an example of adverse response to publicity in 1941, see Guttmacher, comp., *Planned Parenthood Beginnings*, 56. By the late 1930s the ABCL was suggesting personal visits by publicity persons of fledgling clinics to newspaper editors, though not exactly for the same purposes. The visits were ostensibly designed to gather information about newspaper deadlines, etc., rather than

to preclude negative publicity. See "Manual of Standard Practices," 26–27, PPFA, series I, box 2, folder 96.

21. For advice to Sanger see Chesler, *Woman of Valor,* 151. For Dickinson see Chesler, *Woman of Valor,* 276, and Reed, *Birth Control Movement,* 167–80. See also D'Emilio and Freedman, *Intimate Matters,* 243. For Buffalo see Guttmacher, comp., *Planned Parenthood Beginnings,* 80. The first woman to enter the Buffalo Maternal Health Clinic walked back out when she saw the nurse smoking a cigarette. She thought the clinic was "an evil place." Guttmacher, comp., *Planned Parenthood Beginnings,* 80.

22. Brush had left Cleveland with her son, trying to start over after the deaths of her daughter and husband. See note 1. D.H.B. to C.F.B., February 6, 1928, CFB, box 1, folder 9. Article from *Cleveland Press,* May 28, 1928; a portion is reprinted in "That Every Child," unp. Brooks Shepard to D.H.B., May 31 [1928], 4, CFB, box 1, folder 9.

23. Scrapbooks, MHA, 1928–1938, PPGC, box 7. The *Bystander* began in 1921 as the *Country Club News* and was published until 1934. See "*Bystander,*" *ECH,* 144. "Parent and Babies," identified as *Cleveland Press* editorial, May 7, 1936, PPGC, box 7, Scrapbook 1935.

24. For raid of Birth Control Clinical Research Bureau, see Chesler, *Woman of Valor,* 282–83. The *Plain Dealer,* December 17, 1929, 1; Thomas Campbell, *Freedom's Forum: The City Club of Cleveland 1912–1962* (Cleveland: City Club, 1963), 24, 57, 121. Sanger's 1929 appearance is mentioned on page 57. City Club of Cleveland records at the WRHS include copies of a few scattered invitations and speeches; Sanger's is not one of them.

25. Campbell, *Freedom's Forum,* 63.

26. "The Brush Foundation, 1928–1980" (Cleveland: The Brush Foundation, n.d.), 1–2.

27. D.H.B. to C.F.B. Sr., December 21, 1927, January 4, 1928, and February 6, 1928, all in CFB, box 1, folder 9. Less than ten years after graduating from the University of Michigan with a degree in mining engineering, Brush left chemical consulting and devoted his energies to experimenting with electricity, specifically the practical application of the electric arc light. At his death, he held fifty patents for instruments including the lead storage battery and the open coil dynamo. He garnered medals, prizes, and worldwide fame. See "C. F. Brush, Who Gave Arc Light to World, Dies," *Cleveland Plain Dealer,* June 16, 1929, 1A, 8A; "Brush, Charles Francis," *DCB,* 70; "Brush Electric Company," *ECH,* 136; "Brush Foundation," *ECH,* 136–137; "Brush-Wellman, Inc.," *ECH,* 137; Peter Diaconoff, "Electrical and Electronics Industries," *ECH,* 381–83; and Darwin Stapleton, "Technology and Industrial Research," *ECH,* 985. Debbie Conti, "Let There Be Light," *Western Reserve Magazine* (March 1982): 30–32. See also Eisenmann III, "Charles F. Brush," Ph.D. diss., University Archives, CWRU, and CFB.

The health of the Brush family may have influenced Brush's particular philanthropic choice. Mary Morris Brush, the inventor's wife, died at age forty-eight of "an attack of malarial fever," according to her obituary, or "dilatation of the heart," according to her death certificate. See *New York Times*, June 26, 1902, 9; Perkins, *Ancestors*, 29. None of the three Brush children lived past midlife. Daughter Helene (1884–1935) spent her adult life in a sanitarium. Both she and her sister, Edna (1880–1930), died after their father, but Charles Jr. preceded Charles Sr. in death by two years. Charles Brush Sr. lost both his son and young granddaughter Jane within a week. See note 1. Another grandchild, Edna's teenage son, was struck by an auto and killed only two months before the deaths of Jane and Charles Jr. See "Charles Francis Brush: Scientist and Inventor," MSS copy for *American Biography*, 11, in CFB, box 21, folder 6; Perkins, *Ancestors*, 20–23; and Wood, "Cleveland Medicine's Incredible Ghosts," 127–30.

As an example of Brush's philanthropy, on the very night of granddaughter Jane's death, he promised Mt. Sinai Hospital fifty thousand dollars in her memory. The grieving inventor, almost an octogenarian, must have wrestled with the inadequacies of medical technology that caused the death of his son and granddaughter, and the infirmities that led to the early demise of his wife and incapacitation of one daughter. Establishing a foundation designed to scientifically improve the quality of human beings just might prevent similar deaths in future generations. Brush kept his grief private, hardly mentioning the deaths in his correspondence. See CFB, box 1, folders 9 through 18 (1927–1929).

James Wood claims that Helene Brush was mentally ill. See Wood, "Cleveland Medicine's Incredible Ghosts," 60. See also Peacock, "Everything You Always Wanted to Know," 100. The grandniece of Charles Brush Sr., Roslyn Campbell Weir, hypothesized that Brush's interest in the inherited quality of people resulted from "an unfortunate marriage." See transcript of interview with Roslyn Weir, January 30, 1963, in CFB, box 25, folder 4.

28. For examples of public response to the creation of the Brush Foundation see C.F.B. to D.H.B., July 18, 1928, in CFB, box 1, folder 9; "Hail Brush Gift as Eugenic Dawn," *Cleveland Plain Dealer*, n.d. in CFB, box 17, scrapbook; and "Money for Birth Control," unidentified news article, n.d., in CFB, box 28, folder 3.

29. Bradley is quoted in a clipping from *Cleveland Plain Dealer*, n.d., MHA scrapbook 1929–1935, PPGC, box 7; "Bishop Throws Irony at Brush Foundation Aim," unidentified news article, n.d., in CFB, box 17, folder 2.

30. Mrs. Maxwell [Winifred E. Rogers] to Friend, n.d., PPGC, box 1, Brush Foundation–histories. This note is written on memo paper with *The Cleveland Press* as a header. Mrs. Maxwell was a columnist answering a query. Thanks to the *Cleveland Press* Collection of Cleveland State University for locating Maxwell's real name.

31. Different documents list slightly different names of the MHA's founding board. My source is MHA's first annual report, "That Children May Have." Other versions are found in "History—Planned Parenthood," Brush Foundation, series IV, container

3, folder 46, and "MHA-History" (MHA, n.d.), PPGC, box 3, early history 1921–57. For the given names of female board members see Rose, *Cleveland: The Making of a City; ECH; DCB; Social Register Cleveland 1927; Social Register Summer 1936* (New York: Social Register Association, 1936); *Who's Who in American Jewry*, vol. 3, 1938–39 (New York: National News, 1938); *American Women*, vol. 3, *1939–40*, ed. Durward Howes (Los Angeles: American Publications, 1939); *The Book of Clevelanders: A Biographical Dictionary of Living Men of the City of Cleveland* (Cleveland: The Burrows Bros. Co., 1914); *Representative Clevelanders;* Ruth J. Neely, *Women of Ohio* (n. p.: S. J. Clarke, n.d.); and the *U.S. Census, 1920*, WRHS. "The Brush Foundation, 1928–1980" (Cleveland: The Brush Foundation, n.d.), 25.

32. "That Children May be Given," MHA, 1929, PPGC, box 3. Brush Foundation purpose appears in the Deed of Gift, figure 13 in this work.

33. For Brush quotes see figure 13.

34. "That Children May be Given," MHA, 1929, PPGC, box 3. Quote about Brush Foundation appears in Todd, "The Registration of Life's Handicaps," Brush Foundation Publications, no. 10 (1931), 8, BF, container 3, series V, folder 49.

35. McCann, *Birth Control Politics*, chapter 4, 99–134, esp. 122, 126, 129–130. McCann quotes Popenoe on 108–9. See also Kline, *Building a Better Race*.

36. Ladd-Taylor, *Raising a Baby the Government Way;* Rothman, "Women's Clinics or Doctor's Offices," 175–201; Lindenmeyer, "Saving Mothers and Babies," 105–34; and Holt, *Lineoleum*, 111–19. The first national race betterment conference in the U.S. in 1914 featured a better baby contest. *Proceedings of the First National Conference on Race Betterment*, 620–25.

37. Ladd-Taylor, *Raising a Baby the Government Way*, 134.

38. MHA, "Report of Three Years' Work," 2, MS-SS, Smith College, clinics-Ohio; Gaylord, "The Eugenic Value," 53. For scientific philanthropy, see Warren Weaver, *U.S. Philanthropic Foundations: Their History, Structure, Management and Record* (New York: Harper and Row, 1967), 24–25, and Barry D. Karl and Stanley N. Katz, "The American Private Philanthropic Foundation and the Public Sphere 1890–1930," *Minerva* 19 (1981): 243–45.

39. For demonstration projects, see Robert H. Bremner, *American Philanthropy*, 128; "The Brush Foundation, 1928–1980," 13, 19; Theodore Hall, "Life in Our Hands, The Story of the Brush Foundation" (Cleveland: Brush Foundation, 1946), 3, BF, series III, container 2, folder 44. Minutes of the Brush Foundation Board of Managers, September 25, 1928, November 5, 1928, December 31, 1928, and March 5, 1929, BF, series I, sub-series A, cont. 1, folder 1.

The second Brush project was the Brush Inquiry, a long-term study of the growth of children. See Todd, "The Aim and Program of the Brush Inquiry," 9, 21; Wood, "Cleveland Medicine's Incredible Ghosts," 56–60, 127–31; and Scrapbooks, the records of the Brush Inquiry, School of Dentistry, Case Western Reserve University, Cleveland, Ohio (hereafter BrI).

40. MHA, "Report of Two Years' Work, March 1928–April 1930," 3, PPGC, box 2, annual reports. For D.H.B.'s opening gift, see note 1. A later report gives a different figure of the number of MHA clients served in 1928–29: 225. See MHA, "Report of Two Years' Work," 4, PPGC, box 2, annual reports.

41. "That Children May be Given," MHA, 1929, PPGC, box 3; Julia C. Brown, "Maternal Health Association Faces the Future," 1. Reprint from *The Bulletin,* Academy of Medicine of Cleveland (April 1957), PPGC, box 8, Scrapbook 1956–57. Unfortunately, no other detailed accounting of contributions and disbursements has been located. For financial surplus, see "That Children May be Given."

42. Karl and Katz, "American Private Philanthropic Foundation," 244, 248, 252, 260–61; Bremner, *American Philanthropy,* 128; and Horace Coon, *Money to Burn: What the Great American Philanthropic Foundations Do with Their Money* (London: Longmans, Green and Co., 1938), 54–55, 231–32.

43. MHA Annual Reports, 1928–30, 1931–32, and 1935 through 1940, PPGC, box 2. MHA, "Report of Fourth Year," BCS, record group 2, series A; and MHA, "Report of Three Years'." Brush Foundation–minutes, BF, series I, sub-series A, container 1, folder 1. For separate mission of the Brush Foundation see "Notes Taken at Board Meeting September, 1938," in Brush Foundation–historical, PPGC, box 1. For indications that private contributions came primarily from trustees, see MHA, "Report of Two Years' Work," 12, PPGC, box 2, annual reports. Robert Bremner notes that foundations provided only about half of the U.S. philanthropic dollars given during this time period. He maintains that individual giving remained the "mainstay of philanthropy." See Bremner, *American Philanthropy,* 139–40. For more on the MHA as a Brush Foundation demonstration center, see chapter 6 in this work. For more on MHA fund-raising see chapter 5 in this work.

44. For Victory Chest Drive and Community Chest, see Rose, *Cleveland: The Making of a City,* 760–61; "Federation for Community Planning," *ECH,* 419; and "United Way Services," *ECH,* 1030. Annual report statement appears in MHA, "Report of Three Years' Work," 14, MS-SS, Smith College, Clinics-Ohio; and MHA, "Report of Fourth Year," 20, for example. PPGC, box 2.

45. Untitled typewritten manuscript, 1, PPGC, box 3, early history.

46. MHA trustees with close connections to the Community Fund included Florence and Herman Moss. One source credits Florence's father, Martin A. Marks, with conceiving the idea for Community Fund in Cleveland. See *Representative Clevelanders,* 262. Guttmacher, comp., *Planned Parenthood Beginnings,* 50, 75. "Newsletter for the friends and supporters of the Maternal Health Association," April 1, 1951, 1, PPGC, box 1.

47. T. W. Todd to G. Gaylord, Dec. 1, 1937, PPGC, box 1, Brush Foundation–historical.

48. "History," typewritten manuscript, (n.d.), 11–12, BF, series IV, container 3, folder 46. For change in the name of the Medical Advisory Staff see MHA Annual

Report, 1934, PPGC, box 2. Minutes from the meetings of both boards are missing from the historical record.

49. Mrs. Walter S. Smith, "History and Information Regarding the Maternal Health Association," typewritten manuscript (1959), 2, PPGC, box 3; and Davis, "Maternal Health," 17–18.

50. MHA, Annual Report 1940–41, PPGC, box 2.

51. Brush expressed his thoughts on the new board in his correspondence, especially to D.H.B. and Edna Brush Perkins (E.B.P.), December 21, 1927, through July 18, 1928, CFB, box 1, folders 9–18, and box 31, microfilm reel 2. Apparently, Brush asked Roger Perkins to serve on the first board, but Perkins declined, saying that he could help more from the outside. He later did become a Brush Foundation trustee. See C.F.B. to E.B.P., February 11, 1928, CFB, box 1, folder 10; "The Brush Foundation, 1928–1980" (Cleveland: The Brush Foundation, n.d.), 25. For information on Todd see "Thomas Wingate Todd," Physical Anthropology Centennial Number, *Journal of the National Medical Association* 51, no. 3 (May 1959): 223–25, 233–46; Wood, "Cleveland Medicine's Incredible Ghosts," 127–28; Scrapbooks, BrI; and Todd's papers at the DMHC.

52. MHA, Annual Report, 1931–32.

53. *Social Register Cleveland 1927.* Jews were not included in this society list; at least five families represented on the first MHA board were Jewish. Clergy were not well represented on the *Register,* either. Of the four members of the clergy on the first MHA board, the *Social Register Cleveland 1927* listed only one, the Rev. T. S. McWilliams. The only Brush board member not listed in this edition of the *Social Register* was the Rev. Joel B. Hayden.

   Sources of educational data include *The Book of Clevelanders; Social Register Cleveland 1927;* Rose, *Cleveland: The Making of a City; ECH; DCB; Social Register Summer 1936; Who's Who in American Jewry* (1938); *American Women,* vol. 3, 1939; *Representative Clevelanders;* and Neely, *Women of Ohio.* Education information was not located for all board members, male or female. The data on Euclid Avenue also is incomplete; this figure is probably low. In addition to above sources, see Cigliano, *Showplace of America,* and Ella Grant Wilson, *Famous Old Euclid Avenue of Cleveland,* vol. 2 (n.p., 1937). For Maxwell, see note 30.

54. "500 Persons Barred at Birth Control Hearing," *St. Louis Star,* April 24, 1929, CFB, box 17, folder 7; "Salem Birth Control Clinic Faces Closing," *Boston Herald,* July 14, 1937; "Three Guilty in Birth Control Case," *Boston American,* July 20, 1937; and unidentified clippings, August 3, 1937, in Scrapbook 1936–41, PPGC, box 7. For Iowa see Guttmacher, comp., *Planned Parenthood Beginnings,* 51.

55. The Municipal Code of the City of Cleveland, 1924, sec. 2951.

56. Unidentified news article, December 28, 1932, PPGC, box 7, scrapbook 1929–1935.

57. "Case Western Reserve University," *ECH,* 154. See also Cramer, *Case Western Reserve.*

58. The foundation rented office space at the Thompson, Hine and Flory law firm for the first few months but moved to WRU in the spring of 1929. "The Brush Foundation, 1928–1980" (Cleveland: The Brush Foundation, n.d.), 13, 19; Minutes of the Brush Foundation Board of Managers, September 25, 1928; December 31, 1928; March 5, 1929; April 17, 1929. BF, ser. I, sub-ser. A, con. 1, folder 1. On the Brush Inquiry, later known as the Bolton-Brush Study, see Bailey, "The Long View of Health," 26–31, and Scrapbooks, BrI.

59. Cramer, *Case Western Reserve,* 69; Trustee Index, University Archives, CWRU.

60. "Mather Advisory Council Members 1888–1970," Mather Advisory Council Records, box 5, folder 1, University Archives, CWRU.

61. Cramer, *Case Western Reserve,* 334; *ECH;* Rose, *Cleveland: The Making of a City; Social Register Cleveland 1927; Social Register Summer 1936; American Medical Directory,* 10th ed. (Chicago: American Medical Association, 1927) and 16th ed. (Chicago: American Medical Association, 1940); Waite, *Western Reserve University Centennial History; Who's Who in American Jewry* (1938); *American Women,* vol. 3, 1939; Neely, *Women of Ohio; Bench and Bar of Northern Ohio: History and Biography,* ed. William Neff (Cleveland: The Historical Publishing Co., 1921); and *U.S. Census 1920,* WRHS, and *U.S. Census 1930.*

62. "MHA History" (Cleveland: MHA, 1957), 10, PPGC, box 3.

63. Ibid.

64. "Tomorrow's Children," 3, no author given, PPGC, box 2, talks; Davis, "Maternal Health," 15; Gladys Gaylord, "Public Acceptance as Related to the Birth Control Field (Talk for Hamilton, Ontario)," February 23, 1939, 2, BCS, record group 62, series H; "MHA History" (Cleveland: MHA, 1957), 5–6, PPGC, box 3. Thanks to the CWRU archives for helping with the information about Rosina Volk.

65. "MHA History" (Cleveland: MHA, 1957), 5–6, PPGC, box 3. Robishaw is listed in the AMA directory, with the specialty of pediatrics. See *American Medical Directory,* 12th ed., 1929. For restrictions against women physicians see Walsh, *Doctors Wanted,* esp. 207–235, 248, and Chesler, interview with Sarah Marcus, M.D., 12–14. See also Morantz, Pomerleau, and Fenichel, eds., *In Her Own Words: Oral Histories of Women Physicians* (New Haven, Conn.: Yale University Press, 1982). Ellen Fitzpatrick found a similar situation with women social scientists. See Fitzpatrick, *Endless Crusade: Women Social Scientists and Progressive Reform* (New York: Oxford University Press, 1990).

In 1918 the WRU School of Medicine began to admit women for the first time since 1884, just in time for Robishaw. See Glen Jenkins, "Women Physicians and Woman's General Hospital," in Brown, ed., *The History of Medicine in Cleveland,* 66–68; and Waite, *Western Reserve University Centennial History,* 125–28. For women WRU medical school graduates before 1884 see Linda Lehmann Goldstein, "'Roses Bloomed in Winter,'": Women Medical Graduates of Western Reserve College, 1852–1856," Ph.D. diss., Case Western Reserve University, 1989. Ruth Robishaw

Rauschkolb used her maiden name in medical practice. See her papers in the CWRU archives.

66. Chesler, interview with Sarah Marcus, ii–iii, 12–13, 15–16. Marcus faced anti-Semitism as well as gender discrimination in medical school and later in her practice. See pages 3 and 9. For a description of the stem pessary, see Cooper, *Technique of Contraception*, 67.

67. See untitled typewritten manuscript, 24, PPGC, box 3, early history; and Oliver, "Maternal Health Association," 17, PPGC, box 3, early history. Chesler, interview with Sarah Marcus, 18. Sanger had trouble finding a physician willing to serve in her clinic in New York City for the same reasons. One physician who worked with Sanger was Hannah Stone. For her association with birth control, Stone suffered "professional ostracism and public humiliation" and was denied membership in the New York Medical Society for years. See Planned Parenthood, *A Tradition of Choice*, 15, 17.

68. MHA, Annual Report, April 1, 1945–March 31, 1946; MHA, Annual Report, April 1, 1950–March 31, 1951; MHA, Annual Report, April 1, 1955–March 31, 1956; and MHA, Annual Report, 1960. PPGC, box 2. See also Chesler, interview with Sarah Marcus; "Marcus, Sarah," *DCB*, 304; and Ruth Robishaw Rauschkolb, *DCB*, 369.

69. Chesler, interview with Sarah Marcus, 32.

70. "MHA History" (Cleveland: MHA, 1957), 5–6, PPGC, box 3.

71. By 1938, the clinic's staff physicians included, in addition to Marcus and Robishaw, Charlotte Kusta, Illula Morrison Hansen, Faith Reed, Edith Hammill, Theodore Zuck, Charles Higley, and Burdette Wylie. Davis, "Maternal Health," 15.

72. For more on research clinic and men's consultations see chapter 4 in this work.

## Notes to Chapter 4

1. MHA Annual Reports, 1929–1939, PPGC, box 2; MHA, "Report of Two Years' Work," 6. WRHS vertical file; MHA, "Report of Three Years' Work," 12, MS-SS, Clinics-Ohio; MHA, "Report of Fourth Year," BCS, record group 2, series A.

2. Margaret Sanger, *Motherhood in Bondage*.

3. Robishaw, "A Study of 4000 Patients," 427.

4. MHA, "Report of Two Years' Work," 6, PPGC, box 2, annual reports; MHA, "Report of Three Years'," MS-SS, Clinics-Ohio.

5. I. M. Rubinow, "Poverty," *Encyclopaedia of Social Sciences* (New York: Macmillan, 1937), 285, and Eric Foner and John A. Garraty, eds., *The Reader's Companion to American History* (Boston: Houghton Mifflin, 1991), 859.

6. For charts indicating family size, see MHA, "Report of Three Years'," MS-SS, Clinics-Ohio; and MHA, "Report of Fourth Year," 9, BCS, record group 2, series A. For census figure see Green, *Housing in the Cleveland Community*, appendix, 24, and Rose, *Cleveland: The Making of a City*, 873. For client income levels see MHA's Annual

Reports, 1929 through 1940, PPGC, box 2, and the 1930, 1931, and 1932 reports cited in note 1. Linda Gordon argues that American birth control clinics of the 1930s served mainly the middle class. While offering contraception in clinics did distance the service from the residents of poor neighborhoods, the MHA letters and statistics prove that some of these same residents found their way to birth control clinics in Cleveland, adding another dimension to Gordon's argument. See Gordon, *Woman's Body*, 249–400, esp. 287.

7. The description "socially and economically handicapped" appears in MHA, "Report of Two Years' Work," 4. WRHS, vertical file. For data, see pp. 7–8, and Maternal Health Association patient information form, appendix to this work. In a talk at the Chicago Birth Control Conference of 1923 about social conditions in Cleveland, Eleanor Rowland Wembridge, referee for Cleveland's Juvenile Court, argued that it would be hard if not impossible to teach "the dull' to use birth control effectively. See Wembridge, "The Seventh Child in the Four-roomed House," in A. Meyer, *Birth Control*, 152; "Wembridge, Eleanor Harris Rowland," *DCB*, 475.

8. MHA, "Report of Two Years' Work," 4. See Chesnutt quoted in Kusmer, *A Ghetto Takes Shape*, 129. See also "Chesnutt, Charles Waddell," *DCB*, 90–91. The WRHS holds a collection of Chesnutt's papers. For the lower rate of racist violence in Cleveland see Kusmer, *A Ghetto Takes Shape*, 128, 263.

9. Marian Morton, "Institutionalizing Inequalities: Black Children and Child Welfare in Cleveland, 1859–1998," *Journal of Social History* 34, no. 1 (2000): 145–46. For Woodland Hills see *Cleveland Gazette*, July 28, 1928; for Luna Park see *Cleveland Gazette*, February 1, 1930. Darlene Clark Hine places discrimination at WRU's nursing school as late as 1941. See Hine, *Black Women in White: Racial Conflict and Cooperation in the Nursing Profession 1890–1950* (Bloomington: Indiana University Press, 1989), 147–150. Hine notes the Cleveland bank's discriminatory hiring practices in *Hine Sight: Black Women and the Re-construction of American History* (Bloomington: Indiana University Press, 1989), 102.

10. Henry R. Pringle and Katherine Pringle, "The Color Line in Medicine," *Saturday Evening Post*, January 24, 1948, 69–70, quoted in Gamble, *Making a Place for Ourselves*, 151. For City Hospital policies see, for example, *Cleveland Gazette*, August 11, 1928, and January 18, 1930. For St. Vincent Charity Hospital see *Cleveland Gazette*, August 21, 1926. For the situation of black physicians and patients in Cleveland see Gamble, *Making a Place for Ourselves*, chapter 6, 151–81, esp. 176–77. Forest City Hospital, Cleveland's first black hospital, did not open until 1957. See Gamble, *Making a Place for Ourselves*, 151, 181.

11. For Garvin see Gamble, *Making a Place for Ourselves*, 154–56; *Cleveland Gazette*, February 6, 1926; Kusmer, "Black Cleveland and the Central-Woodland Community 1865–1930," in *Cleveland: A Metropolitan Reader*, ed. W. Dennis Keating, Norman Krumholz, and David C. Perry (Kent, Ohio: Kent State University Press, 1995), 273; and "Garvin, Charles H.," *DCB*, 171. Garvin's papers are at the WRHS.

12.  MHA, "Report of Two Years' Work," 4; WRHS, vertical file. MHA, "Report of Three Years'," 5, MS-SS, Clinics-Ohio. Later annual reports do not report the race of clients. However, researcher Goldie Davis compared the numbers of "colored" and "white" clients in "Maternal Health," 56, 63. Dickinson and Morris, "Birth Control Centers: Report of 202 in the United States for the Year 1939," *Journal of the American Medical Association* 115 (August 24, 1940): 591–93, cited in Rodrigue, "The Afro-American Community," Ph.D. diss., 132.

13.  Mary Losure, "'Motherhood Protection'," 362; Roberts, *Killing the Black Body*, 82–89; Chesler, *Woman of Valor*, 295–97; and Leung, "'Better Babies'," 54, 65. The Little Rock clinic opened in 1931 but did not accept black women until 1937. For North Carolina see Reed, *The Birth Control Movement*, 252–56, and Gordon, *Woman's Body*, 330, 331. Johanna Schoen suggests that a complexity of motivations, beyond simply racism, contributed to the opening of birth control clinics as public health facilities in North Carolina. See Schoen, "Between Choice and Coercion," 135. A magazine article claimed that public relief funds also supported a birth control clinic in at least one Michigan county in 1935. See "Relief & Babies," *Time*, April 8, 1935, 30–31, PPGC, box 2, Clippings-Duplicate.

14.  C. E. Gehlke, "Statistical Report," in MHA, "Report of Fourth Year," 8, BCS, record group 2, series A; Himes, *Medical History*, 369, note 45. See Gehlke's brief biography in *Who's Who in the Midwest* (Chicago, Illinois: Marquis Who's Who, 1952), 299–300.

15.  Gehlke, "Statistical Report," 8. MHA reports for later years do not provide detailed data on living conditions. For other MHA annual reports, 1934–1940, see PPGC, box 2.

16.  Wandersee, "The Economics of Middle-Income Family Life: Working Women During the Great Depression," in *Decades of Discontent*, ed. Lois Scharf and Joan Jensen, 45–58, esp. 45, 49. For Cleveland see Phillips, *AlabamaNorth*, 143–45. Phillips describes the conditions in general for Clevelanders of African descent in the early twentieth century.

17.  Hine notes a general distrust of hospitals among blacks in *Black Women in White*, 21–22; see also Gamble, *Making a Place for Ourselves*. Roberts, *Killing the Black Body*, 78. Roberts refers to a distrust among women of color of birth control clinics run by whites. As to the clinic's location being a problem, one study found that people of lower income households often rely almost exclusively on neighborhood services. Roger S. Ahlbrandt Jr., cited in Simone M. Caron, "Birth Control and the Black Community in the 1960s," 545–69, note 32. Caron describes birth control services for black women in Pittsburgh, Pennsylvania, beginning in the 1950s, and the efforts of black women to maintain those services. No mention of birth control or the MHA was found in selected issues of the *Cleveland Gazette*, a leading black weekly newspaper (every issue of every other year between 1916 and 1932, and every issue in 1935 and between January and June 1940). For black women's desire for contraception and

their creation of clinics elsewhere during this era see Roberts, *Killing the Black Body*, 78, 82–87; Jessie Rodrigue, "The Black Community and the Birth Control Movement," in *"We Specialize in the Wholly Impossible": A Reader in Black Women's History*, ed. Darlene Clark Hine et al. (New York: Carlson Publishing: 1995), 505–20; and Schoen, "Between Choice and Coercion." See also Rodrigue, "The Afro-American Community," Ph.D. diss. From the late 1930s onward, some black women in North Carolina elected sterilization as a sure way to end their childbearing. Schoen, "Between Choice and Coercion," 136–37.

18. "Maternal Health Clinic-1951," MS-LC, reel 7. As many mothers across the years attest, determination alone does not ensure contraceptive success. The woman's age surely worked in her favor, since she was almost forty when she first came to the clinic.

19. Permission to use Dorothy Brush's name was graciously provided by her family. Dorothy Brush's second husband's name was Alexander Dick, and their daughter was Sylvia Dorothy. See *Who's Who of American Women*, 2d ed., 139. Marriage and birth dates come from DHB and Brush's file, SCA. An address list confirms that Brush lived in Riverdale by 1929. See Margaret Sanger, reel 5, MS-WIA. Patient Register March 1928–November 1938, PPGC, trunk 3. This book of handwritten entries lists name and case number, in chronological order of clinic attendance. Brush (listed under Dick) is case #1718. A cursory scan located seven other MHA board members, whose names are protected by a PPGC request for confidentiality. The register is not included in the unprocessed papers of PPGC at the WRHS. The citation is to its location in 1990.

20. Gordon, *Woman's Body*, 300; Lynd and Lynd, *Middletown*, 125.

21. Davis, "Maternal Health," 63. Gladys Gaylord, "Public Acceptance as Related to the Birth Control Field (Talk for Hamilton, Ontario)," February 23, 1939, 2, BCS, record group 2, series H. Quote about MHA nurse in Davis, "Maternal Health," appendix 2, iii.

22. For other clinics see Johanna Schoen, "Fighting for Child Health," 103–04, and Sullivan, "Walking the Line," master's thesis, 20. For MHA furnishings and screens see "History," typewritten manuscript, n.d., 17, BF, series IV, container 3, folder 46. On atmosphere see "MHA History" (Cleveland: MHA, 1957), 5, 7, PPGC, box 3; and Davis, "Maternal Health," 16–20, appendix 2, iv. The Birth Control Society of Hamilton, Ontario, served tea to its clients. See "Planned Parenthood Society of Hamilton," n.d., 5.

23. Davis, "Maternal Health," 11–13, appendix 2, iii–iv. For Sanger's emphasis on creating a special atmosphere at her clinic see Chesler, *Woman of Valor*, 288–89. For ABCL standards see "Minimum Standards for Clinics Affiliated with the American Birth Control League and Affiliated State Organizations," the records of the Planned Parenthood League of Massachusetts (hereafter PPLM) at the Sophia Smith collection, Smith College, Northampton, Massachusetts, box 120.

24. For an account of Sanger's 1929 entrapment and arrest by an undercover police-woman see Chesler, *Woman of Valor,* 282–83. For MHA rules about contraceptive advice, see Davis, "Maternal Health," 29, 37, appendix 2, iii.

25. Davis, "Maternal Health," 18–19. For fees see p. 21, and MHA, "Report of Two Years' Work," 12. WRHS, vertical files.

26. For lack of advertising for patients see "MHA History" (1957), 6, PPGC, box 3, MHA, "Report of Three Years'," 3, and MS-SS, Clinics-Ohio. For physician disapproval of advertising see "Analysis of State Birth Control Leagues," *BCR* (February 1932): 39–42, and Meyer, "Motherhood and Morality," 14–16. For a statement about coercion see "Six Years With Family Regulation Problems," 1, PPGC, box 2. The clinic purpose appears in "That Children May be Given," MHA, 1929, PPGC, box 3. For married women's statements, see MHA, "Report of Three Years'," 3, and other MHA annual reports, 1934–1941, PPGC, box 2.

27. For married women only and moral constraints see Robinson, *Seventy Birth Control Clinics,* 42–44; Gordon, *Woman's Body,* 310, 364–365, 388, 406. For study results see "Summary of Replies received to Questionnaire," Sanger, reel 7, MS-WIA; for actual questionnaires see Sanger, reel 8, MS-WIA.

28. Backus, "Planned Parenthood League," 14. Copy in author's possession.

29. MHA, "Report of Two Years' Work," 3. WRHS, vertical file. For other U.S. clinics serving married women, see Losure, "'Motherhood Protection'," 361; and "Summary of Replies," Sanger, MS-WIA, reel 7. Statement about pregnant client appears in "The History of the Maternal Health Association," typewritten draft, 32, PPGC, box 3, early history. For examples of MHA attitudes on abortion, see Ruth A. Robishaw, "And There is the Child," talk given during the annual meeting of the Ohio State Nurses Association in Cleveland, May 5, 1939. Reprinted from *Ohio Nurses Review* 14, no. 4 (October 1939): 4, and "Talk Prepared for A.A.U.W. Meeting, Zanesville" (author not provided), November 4, 1940. PPGC, box 2, talks. One off-the-record conversation between the author and a scholar (who wishes to remain anonymous) suggests that some MHA physicians did do abortions in their private practices.

30. MHA, "Report of Three Years'," 3–5, MS-SS, Clinics-Ohio. "The Maternal Health Association," June 1964, 3; "Report of the Executive Secretary of the Maternal Health Association to the Brush Foundation–October 29, 1931"; and "Report of the Executive Secretary of the Maternal Health Association to the Brush Foundation-October 7, 1930," PPGC, box 1, Brush Foundation-historical. Norman Himes compares clinic statistics for Baltimore and Cleveland in *Medical History,* 358–70.

31. MHA, "Report of Three Years'," 4, MS-SS, Clinics-Ohio. Gladys Gaylord, "Premarital and Preconceptional Care," 1939, unidentified article reprint, PPGC, box 5.

32. Gehlke, "Historical and Statistical Report," in "Report of Fourth Year," 4, MS-SS, Cinics-Ohio. It was not until 1964 that the MHA, by then called Planned Par-

enthood, began to admit unmarried women and men who had no wedding plans—as long as they were over twenty-one years of age. See "Every Child a Wanted Child," PPGC (1988). A clinic in Santa Fe, New Mexico, admitted unmarried women and widows in the late 1930s but offered complete medical services, not only birth control. It is unclear whether the Sante Fe clinic dispensed contraceptives to the unwed. See Sullivan, "Walking the Line," master's thesis, 19. For fears around birth control and motherhood see Chesler, *Woman of Valor,* 207–209, and McLaren, *A History of Contraception,* 192–94, 220–22. On the New Woman see Freedman, "'The New Woman',"
372–93.

33. T. Wingate Todd, "Preliminary suggestions for the scientific contribution of a birth control clinic," typescript, PPGC, box 1, Brush Foundation–historical. Todd joined the MHA board in 1931.

34. For copy of record forms see appendix. D'Emilio and Freedman, *Intimate Matters,* 224–25, 248, and Ditzion, *Marriage Morals and Sex in America: A History of Ideas* (New York: W. W. Norton, 1969, 1953), 360–63. For an early example of sex surveys see Mosher, *The Mosher Survey.* See also Alfred Kinsey, *Sexual Behavior in the Human Male* (Philadelphia: W. B. Saunders, 1948). For professionals' interest in sexual matters in the 1930s see, for instance, *Encyclopedia Sexualis: A Comprehensive Encyclopedia-Dictionary of the Sexual Sciences,* ed. Victor Robinson (New York: Dingwall-Rock, 1936).

35. For previous pregnancies of MHA clients, see MHA Annual Reports, 1929 through 1940; MHA, "Report of Two Years' Work." WRHS, vertical file, MHA, "Report of Three Years'," MS-SS, Clinics-Ohio; and MHA, "Report of Fourth Year," BCS, record group 2, series A. Gladys Gaylord, "Building for Tomorrow," May 17, 1944, 2, PPGC, box 1, talks–misc. For the discovery of gynecological problems at other clinics see Robinson, *Seventy Birth Control Clinics,* 154–55, 159; Chesler, *Woman of Valor,* 296–97; and Sullivan, "Walking the Line," master's thesis. The article introducing the vaginal smear as a method for detecting cancer was first published in 1943. See G. N. Papanicalaou and H. F. Traut, "Diagnosis of Uterine Cancer by Vaginal Smear" (New York: Commonwealth Fund, 1943), cited in Novak, *Textbook of Gynecology,* 5th ed. (Baltimore, Md.: Williams and Wilkins, 1956), 260–62.

36. James F. Cooper indicates a condom effectiveness rate of 50 percent among ABCL clients of the 1920s but admits that other couples, who did not need the ABCL's services, might have experienced higher rates of success with the condom. See Cooper, *Technique of Contraception,* 52.

37. Tone, *Devices and Desires,* chapter 6, esp. 129–134; Chesler, *Woman of Valor,* 295–299; Gordon, *Woman's Body,* 309–310.

38. For conditions in Cleveland see Phillips, *Alabama North;* Bing, *Social Work in Greater Cleveland,* 11; and Waite, *Warm Friend,* chapters 6 and 7, esp. 185, 266. For situations elsewhere see, for example, Wandersee, *Women's Work and Family Values 1920–1940* (Cambridge, Mass.: Harvard University Press, 1981); Ladd-Taylor, *Raising a Baby the Government Way;* and Scharf, *To Work and to Wed.* For more on the

diaphragm see Gordon, *Woman's Body*, 310, and Tone, *Devices and Desires*, 153–155.

39. For one example of the embarrassment caused by such intimate attention three decades later, see Tone, *Devices and Desires*, 153–154.

40. MHA, "Report of Two Years' Work," 3. WRHS, vertical file; MHA. "Report of Three Years'," 4, MS-SS, Clinics-Ohio. Davis, "Maternal Health," 16–20. Medical records or patient information forms for the MHA have not been located.

41. Matter-of-fact attitude described in Horner, "The Contribution of the Maternal Health Association," master's thesis, 22. Careful teaching quote from "Report to the Brush Foundation from Gladys Gaylord," October 29, 1931, p. 1, PPGC, box 1, Brush Foundation–historical. Quote about wonted practices appears in "Six Years With Family Regulation Problems," 1, PPGC, box 2; lack of hesitancy in Davis, "Maternal Health," 20. Robishaw, "Medical Report 1930–31," in MHA, "Report of Three Years', 13, MS-SS, Clinics-Ohio. Client quoted in "Founding a Family," speech delivered in Jackson, Michigan, January 1936, 7, PPGC, box 2, misc. speeches.

42. Mohr, *Abortion in America*, vii.

43. Ibid., 39–40, and Grossberg, *Governing the Hearth*, 161–62. *Acts of a General Nature*, vol. 23 (Columbus: David Smith, 1834), 20–21. Ohio strengthened its abortion law with the passage of the state's obscenity restrictions in 1862 and again by passing a tighter abortion law in 1867. For 1862 see chapter 1 in this text. For 1867 see Mohr, *Abortion in America*, 206–10.

44. For women's fear see Reagan, *When Abortion Was a Crime*, 184; Joffe, *Doctors of Conscience*; Lee, *The Search for an Abortionist*; and Ellen Messer and Kathryn E. May, *Back Rooms: Voices from the Illegal Abortion Era* (Buffalo, N.Y.: Prometheus Books, 1994). For general histories of abortion in American see Mohr, *Abortion in America*, and Petchesky, *Abortion and Woman's Choice*.

45. Reagan, *When Abortion Was a Crime*, and Joffe, *Doctors of Conscience*.

46. Ladd-Taylor, *Raising a Baby the Government Way*, 9, 42. Unfortunately, the Children's Bureau ignored women's desire and need for birth control. See p. 9. In 1929 one woman asked the bureau if the government offered any birth control information. She said she already had government pamphlets on child care, as well as "others on floors, leather, heating, plants, goats, bird houses. If the government can't help us now, we'll feel pretty badly," she concluded. Ladd-Taylor, *Raising a Baby the Government Way*, 183–84.

47. For more on condescending "materialism," see Koven and Michel, "Womanly Duties," 1076–1108; Koven and Michel, eds., *Mothers of a New World*; and Mead, "Beneficent Maternalism: Argentine Motherhood in Comparative Perspective, 1880–1920," *Journal of Women's History* 12, no. 3 (2000): 120–45. For MHA statistics, see Robishaw, "Medical Report 1931–1932," in MHA, "Report of Fourth Year," 12–13, BCS, record group 2, series A.

48. MHA, "An Analysis of Pregnancies Among 923 Patients of the Maternal Health Clinic Between March 21, 1928 and February 1, 1931," March 1931, 4, 7, 9, 10, PPGC, box 2, misc. speeches.

49. Scrapbook-Letters from Patients, PPGC, box 6.

50. For another local example of condescending rhetoric beginning a century earlier, see Morton, "'Go and Sin No More': Maternity Homes in Cleveland, 1869–1936," *Ohio History* 93 (summer-autumn 1984): 117–46, and Morton, *And Sin No More: Social Policy and Unwed Mothers in Cleveland, 1855–1990* (Columbus: Ohio State University Press, 1993). "Interviewing" (1935), PPGC, box 2, talks. The conflict was in part engendered by the search for professional status and recognition on the part of early-twentieth-century female social scientists, social workers, and volunteers. See Fitzpatrick, *Endless Crusade,* 118; Walkowitz, "The Making of a Feminine Professional Identity: Social Workers in the 1920s," *AHR* 95, no. 4 (October 1990): 1051–75; and Muncy, *Creating a Female Dominion,* 140–41, 160–61.

51. For women's reaction to medical authority see The Boston Women's Health Collective, *The New Our Bodies, Ourselves: Updated and Expanded for the '90s* (New York: Simon and Schuster, 1992): 657–59, and Barbara Ehrenreich and Deidre English, *For Her Own Good: 150 Years' of the Experts' Advice to Women* (Garden City: Anchor Books, 1969). For a contemporary view of physicians' authority in conflict with that of midwives see Mary M. Lay, *The Rhetoric of Midwifery: Gender, Knowledge and Power* (New Brunswick, N.J.: Rutgers University Press, 2000).

52. For attitudes about abortion, see Edna Rusch, "Talk Given at Sixteenth Annual Meeting, Maternal Health Association," May 17, 1944, p. 3, in PPGC, box 5, talks, and selected letters in Scrapbook-Letters from Patients, 1928–1938, PPGC, box 6.

53. Robinson, *Seventy Birth Control Clinics,* 64. Robinson charts the Catholic population in Cleveland, but her figures are misleading. In 1920 center city Cleveland's population was close to nine hundred thousand, and the population of the greater urban area was 1.25 million (Robinson gives Cleveland's population as over 2 million). The numbers Robinson gives for the Catholic diocese are correct, but the diocese actually extended south, west, and east, well beyond the Cleveland city limits. See Campbell and Miggins, eds., *The Birth of Modern Cleveland,* 298–299. Thanks to Christine Krosel at the Archives of the Diocese of Cleveland for providing an approximation of the 1920 Catholic population in the city of Cleveland: 187,000 (based on parish reports, 1920). *On Christian Marriage,* Casti Connubii, *Encyclical Letter of Pope Pius XI* (New York: Paulist Press, 1941). For discussion of the encyclical see Chesler, *Woman of Valor,* 320–21, and Noonan Jr., *Contraception,* 424–32.

54. Horner, "The Contribution of the Maternal Health Association," 9, 29–30.

55. Scharf, *To Work and to Wed,* 142. For a description of the familial tasks of women who worked at home during the Great Depression, see, for example, Ladd-Taylor, *Raising a Baby the Government Way,* 42–46. See also Wandersee, *Women's Work.*

56. Last quote appears in Horner, "The Contribution of the Maternal Health Association," 31; another reference to clothing appears on p. 23. Other quotes are from Scrapbook-Letters from Clients, PPGC, box 6.

57. Talk Prepared for A.A.U.W., 1.

58. Davis, "Maternal Health," 14; Robishaw, "Medical Report 1930–31," MHA, "Report of Three Years' Work," 12, MS-SS, Clinics-Ohio. For men's luncheons see Gladys Gaylord, "Men and a Maternal Health Program," reprinted from *BCR* (June 1938). PPGC, box 2, miscellaneous speeches. Other descriptions of MHA services to men are found in Charles S. Higley, "Men and Maternal Health" [February 11, 1938], and Burdett Wylie, "Men and Maternal Health," February 11, 1938. PPGC, box 2, miscellaneous speeches. Another version of Higley's speech appeared as "Men's Consultation in a Maternal Health Center," *Journal of Contraception,* 2 (October 1937): 187–88.

59. For a call for men's auxiliaries at birth control clinics, see George Bedborough, "A Men's League for Birth Control," *BCR* 17, no. 7 (July 1933): 175–76. Gaylord, "Men and a Maternal Health Program," and Higley, "Men's Consultation."

60. Tone, *Devices and Desires,* 155–56, 183–84; Kennedy, *Birth Control in America,* 132; Gordon, *Woman's Body,* 237.

61. For letter, see chapter 1 in this text.

62. Higley, "Men and Maternal Health" [February 11, 1938], 2, PPGC, box 2, misc. speeches.

63. H. W. Long, *Sane Sex Life and Sane Sex Living* (New York: Eugenics Publishing, 1919), and B. G. Jefferis and J. L. Nichols, *Safe Counsel or Practical Eugenics, To Which Has Been Added* The Story of Life *by Ozora S. Davis and Emma F. A. Drake,* 38th ed. (Naperville, Ill.: J. L. Nichols, 1925), quote on p. 21. As a note, Long goes into great detail on the art of loving and achieving mutually satisfactory intercourse but does not discuss birth control at all except for a brief mentions of the so-called safe period, which he admits is unproved at the time of his writing. See Long, *Sane Sex,* 119–25. For husbands coming alone to the MHA see Robishaw, "Medical Report 1931–1932," MHA, "Report of Fourth Year," 12, BCS, record group 2, series A.

64. "Projects," MHA Annual Report 1935–36 and "Officers and Projects," MHA Annual Report 1937–38. PPGC, box 2. The 1937–38 report offers no statistics to back up the last few claims.

65. Talk Prepared for A.A.U.W., 2. PPGC, box 2, talks.

66. Hall, ed., *Dear Dr. Stopes,* esp. 25–26, 51, 138–39, 141–42, 143–44, 154, and Sanger, *Motherhood in Bondage,* 246–63.

67. John Hess, "Report of Men's Department 1931–32," in MHA, "Report of Fourth Year," 18–19, BCS, record group 2, series A. For confirmation of this reticence by other researchers see James Leslie McCary, *Human Sexuality: Physiological and Psychological Factors of Sexual Behavior* (New York: Van Nostrand Reinhold, 1967), 205.

68. MHA, "Analysis of Pregnancies," 5, 9, PPGC, box 2, miscellaneous speeches. Similar episodes of sabotage by men happened elsewhere. See for example Schoen, "Fighting for Child Health," 102.

69. Anonymous quote in "Preventive Social Work," *BCR* 14, no. 6 (June 1930): 163.

70. Ibid.

71. "Six Years," 4, PPGC, box 2; Horner, "The Contribution of the Maternal Health Association," 26–27.

72. Brodie, "Family Limitation," Ph.D. diss., 119, 169, 333. On page 119 Brodie cites Edward Bliss Foote, *Medical Common Sense* (1864), 380. See also Brodie, *Contraception and Abortion.*

73. Grossberg, *Governing the Hearth*, 164–65. One study documents intense questioning of women who had procured abortions on the witness stand in the 1940s, which may indicate a reversal of the trend to blame abortion providers rather than clients. See Reagan, *When Abortion Was a Crime.*

## Notes to Chapter 5

1. For Brush and Shephard recruiting family members and Brush family relationships see chapter 2 and figure 6. Ostrander, *Women of the Upper Class*, 112, 128–29, 150–51.

2. Spouses are not counted among the fourteen relatives. Hortense Shepard served on the MHA board with her mother, May Oliver; Frances Goff with her daughter-in-law, Caroline Brewer Goff; and Lenore Black with her sister, Helen Schwab Hellman. Sisters-in-law Kate Hanna Ireland Harvey and Virginia Bonnell Harvey also served as trustees; Kate Harvey was the mother-in-law of MHA board member Margaret Allen Ireland. For Shephard and Oliver see "A History of the Maternal Health Association," typewritten manuscript, PPGC, box 3, drafts of early histories. See *Plain Dealer* obituary for Frances Goff, July 13, 1956, in Scrapbook 1956–57, PPGC, box 8, and *Representative Clevelanders*, 143. For the Holdens, Whites, Ford, and Vail, see Ella White Ford, "Ancestors and Descendants of Thomas H. White" (1928); "Bole, Roberta Holden," *DCB*, 51; "Ford, Horatio," *DCB*, 156; "Holden, Liberty Emery," *DCB*, 223; "Vail, Herman Lansing," *DCB*, 459. For the Irelands and Harveys, see "Harvey, Kate Benedict Hanna," *DCB*, 209; "Ireland, Margaret Allen," *DCB*, 241; and *A Brief Biography of Perry Williams Harvey* (Cleveland: n.p., 1936), 44. For Lenore Schwab Black see obituary in *Jewish Review and Observer* 81, no. 2 (June 3, 1955): 6; for Helen Schwab Hellman see obituary in *Jewish Review and Observer* 83, no. 12 (March 22, 1957): 6.

3. MHA, "Report of Two Years' Work, March 1928–April 1930," 13, vertical file, WRHS. For the Eells family and the Cornings see *Representative Clevelanders*, 110–11, and *Social Register Cleveland* (New York: Social Association,1936), 780. For the Whites, see "Trustees 1934–35," MHA, Annual Report May 1935, PPGC, box 2, and Ford, "Ancestors."

4. James Wallen, *Cleveland's Golden Story* (Cleveland: William Taylor & Son, 1920); David Loth, *A Long Way Forward: The Biography of Congresswoman Frances Payne Bolton* (New York: Longmans, Green, 1957), esp. 6–19. See also Edward P. Whelan, "Cleveland's Mightiest Family," *Cleveland* (December 1976): 52–59, 178,

180. Francie Ostrower, *Why the Wealthy Give: The Culture of Elite Philanthropy* (Princeton, N.J.: Princeton University Press, 1995), 34–35. Ostrander, *Women of the Upper Class*, 129. For culture of trusteeship see Hall, *Inventing the Nonprofit Sector*, 135–206.

5. For examples of women's groups depending on men for public leadership see Sara M. Evans, "Women's History and Political Theory," in *Visible Women: New Essays on American Activism*, ed. Nancy A. Hewitt and Suzanne Lebsock (Urbana and Chicago: University of Illinois Press, 1993), 129. In this article (119–39), Evans articulates the value of "thinking anew" about the critical role of voluntary associations in civil society.

6. Male assistant treasurers of the MHA included Thomas Veach (1928–1931) and Raymond Kelsey (1931–1932); Ferdinand Blanchard filled the office of second vice president from 1931–1932. MHA, Annual Reports 1928–1990, PPGC, box 2; MHA, "Report of Three Years' Work," 12, MS-SS, Smith College, Clinics-Ohio; MHA, "Report of Fourth Year," BCS, record group 2, series A.

7. Lawyers: Jerry Fisher, Walter Flory, Ray Kelsey; physicians: Theodore Herrick, Roger Perkins, William Weir; businessmen: Edgar Adams, Arthur Judson, Herman Moss, Brooks Shepard, Thomas Veach; architect: Alexander Robinson; and engineer: John Webster. Weir and Perkins practiced at Lakeside Hospital; Perkins led the city's health department; and Weir and Perkins taught at WRU's School of Medicine. Attorneys Flory and Fisher practiced at Thompson Hine and Flory; Moss was director and vice president of Great Lakes Engineering as well as a director of Union Trust and a member of the Chamber of Commerce; other chamber members on the MHA board included Adams, Black, Flory, and Webster. Information about board members comes from a variety of biographical sources, including *Representative Clevelanders; Ohio Blue Book; Social Register Cleveland 1940* (New York: Social Register Association, 1940); *Social Register Summer 1936; Who's Who in American Jewry* (1938); *American Medical Directory*, 10th ed., 1927; *American Medical Directory*, 16th ed., 1940; and *American Women*, vol. 3, 1939. For Great Lakes Engineering and Union Trust see *Representative Clevelanders*, 262; for Chamber of Commerce see "Social Service Club," *ECH*, 936 (Adams); "Chamber of Commerce–City Plan Committee," *ECH*, 168 (Black); *Bench and Bar of Northern Ohio*, ed. William Neff, 396 (Flory); and *Representative Clevelanders*, 262 (Moss) and 389 (Webster). Nonprofit manager Virginia Wing seems to be the only woman on the first MHA board who held a paying job in the MHA's early years. She worked as executive secretary of the Anti-Tuberculosis League of Cleveland and Cuyahoga County. See obituary, *Plain Dealer*, January 22, 1951, in BrI, Scrapbook 1936. See also the papers of Virginia's sister, Marie Wing, WRHS.

8. MHA Annual Report, May 1934; MHA Annual Reports 1935–36 through 1941–42, PPGC, box 2. No other record has been found regarding the restructuring.

9. MHA, Annual Reports 1928–1990, PPGC, box 2. The first male MHA trustee since 1935, Meacham Hitchcock served as vice president of the PPGC board in 1966 and later as president. MHA, Annual Reports 1928–1966, PPGC, box 2.

10. Unidentified [possibly Mrs. Walter Smith], MHA treasurer, to Rupert Knoepf, February 12, 1960, PPGC, box 2.

11. Historians as well as other scholars and the general public struggle with the term "feminism." Suzanne Lebsock analyzes the "theory of the decline of feminism" and presents a brief overview of the historiography in *Free Women*, 48–53. For definition quoted see Linda Gordon, "What's New in Women's History," in *Feminist Studies, Critical Studies*, ed. Teresa de Lauretis (Bloomington: Indiana University Press, 1986), 29. Gordon distinguishes between feminism and a female, or bodily, consciousness, claiming that feminism "arises out of a desire to escape the female." Gordon, "What's New," 30. I contend that feminism does not necessarily represent the desire to escape but rather to come to terms with the female.

12. Ostrander, *Women of the Upper Class*, 135–36, and Ostrower, *Why the Wealthy Give*, chapter 3, 69–85.

13. "MHA History" (Cleveland: MHA, 1957), 3, PPGC, box 3; clippings in Scrapbook 1929–35, Scrapbook 1935, PPGC, box 7. See also "Blanchard, Ferdinand Q.," *DCB*, 47, and "Family Service Association," *ECH*, 417; "Bird, Philip Smead," *DCB*, 44–45; "Silver, Abba Hillel," *DCB*, 414; and "Temple-Tifereth Israel," *ECH*, 993–94.

14. MHA, Annual Reports 1928–30, 1938–39, PPGC, box 2; "Brush-Wellman, Inc.," *ECH*, 137 for Sawyer; "Unitarian-Universalism," *ECH*, 1026 for Lupton. Brush Beryllium (later Brush-Wellman, Inc.) was associated with the business interests of Charles Brush Sr.

15. Although the clergy served upper-class congregations, they were not necessarily seen as members of that privileged social group. As noted in chapter 3, clergy generally did not make the *Social Register*. McWilliams is the only pastor in this group whose name appears in the *Social Register* for 1927. Lupton made the book in 1938. See *Social Register Cleveland 1927*, 45, and *Social Register Cleveland* (New York: Social Register Association, 1938): 42.

16. For given names of Ethel Blanchard, Mary Lupton, Susan McWilliams, Caroline Sawyer, and Virginia Silver, see *Representative Clevelanders*, 35, 230, 239, 318, 336; *U.S. Census, 1920*, WRHS, vol. 48, sheet 9, 18. For Margaret Bird see obituary in *Plain Dealer*, September 10, 1998. MHA, Annual Reports 1928–31, 1937–38, PPGC, box 2.

17. Noonan Jr., *Contraception*, 424–32. The Lambeth Conference 1930, Resolution 15, quoted in Noonan Jr., *Contraception*, 424. See also Noonan Jr., *Contraception*, 409, 414–15. News articles in MHA Scrapbook 1929–35, PPGC, box 7.

18. "Birth, Divorce Position Told by Three Pastors," unidentified news article, January 19, 1931, MHA Scrapbook 1929–35, PPGC, box 7.

19. "Lupton Asks O.K. on Birth Control," unidentified news article, n.d.; "Urges Law to Permit Birth Control Teaching," unidentified news clipping, n.d. [1929?]; Guy Clement, "Tells of Taunts on Birth Control," *Plain Dealer*, July 7, 1930. All in PPGC, Scrapbook, 1929–35, PPGC, box 7. Ferdinand Q. Blanchard, "Address Before Annual Meeting, 1931," PPGC, box 2, talks.

20. Rivers divide Cleveland into distinct parcels, east and west. By 1930 industrial workers, many of them immigrants or migrants, congregated close to factories in what became known as the Flats, just west of the city center. Primarily blue-collar residents comprised the West Side populace during the 1920s and 1930s except in a few new upscale western suburbs such as Lakewood (incorporated as a city in 1911). Maternal Health Association trustees Edgar and Elizabeth Carlton Adams lived in Lakewood. For information on board members see Gladys Gaylord to Mrs. Donald McGraw, October 10, 1929, reel 5, MS-WIA, and note 7 and note 16, above. For development of Cleveland residential patterns in response to industry see Campbell and Miggins, eds., *The Birth of Modern Cleveland*, 34–38, 46–52. See also Miller and Wheeler, *Cleveland*, 102–3, 118–20, 131, 147, and James Borchert, "Suburbs," in *ECH*, 977. See "Lakewood," *ECH*, 628–29. Thanks to Gladys Haddad for pointing out the migration pattern of the city's elites. See also Cigliano, *Showplace of America*, 323–27.

21. For shared values see Ostrander, *Women of the Upper Class*, 105, and Ostrower, *Why the Wealthy Give*, 19–20. Joanne Lewis, *In Our Day; Cleveland Heights: Its People, Its Places, Its Past* (Cleveland: Heights Community Congress, n.d.), 7.

22. The Cleveland Heights residents on the original MHA board included Edna and Roger Perkins, Dorothy Brush (before she moved to New York), John and Estelle Webster, Julia Crowell, Mabel Wason, Bertha Herzog, Helen Hellman, Cliffe Merriam, and Hortense and Brooks Shepard. The Perkinses, Brush, Crowell, the Shepards, and the Wasons had family connections to Euclid Avenue. For addresses of board members see note 7 and note 16. For mileage estimate see *Official Street Atlas of Cleveland and Cuyahoga County*, 1991–92 (Cleveland: Commercial Survey Company, 1990), section 9.

Edna Brush Perkins and her brother, Charles F. Brush Jr. (Dorothy Brush's first husband), grew up in the Brush mansion at 3725 Euclid Avenue. See Perkins, *Ancestors of Charles Brush Perkins*, 28–29, and Cigliano, *Showplace of America*, appendix A, 349. Julia Cobb Crowell's husband, Benedict, also grew up on Euclid Avenue. See Cigliano, *Showplace of America*, 299. Hortense Oliver Shepard lived at 8318 Euclid before her marriage, and Charles and Mabel Wason resided at 6709 Euclid before moving to Cleveland Heights. See Cigliano, *Showplace of America*, appendix A, 356, 359.

23. The lakeshore residents included Frances Goff and her daughter-in-law, Caroline Brewster Goff, Kate Harvey, Florence and Herman Moss, Roberta Holden Bole, and Delia White Vale. MHA Annual Reports, 1930 through 1940, PPGC, box 2; MHA, "Report of Three Years' Work," 12, MS-SS, Clinics-Ohio; MHA, "Report of Fourth Year," BCS, record group 2, series A. There is a street in Bratenahl called Holden Lane. See *Official Street Atlas*, section 8. For addresses of board members, see biographical sources in note 7 and note 16. "Bratenahl," *ECH*, 124–25; "Cleveland Heights," *ECH*, 245–46.

24. Frances Bolton, Ella White Ford, and William and Roslyn Weir lived in the rural Mayfield/Richmond area. Goff's family home, the residence of William and

Louisa Stark Southworth, was located at 1276 Euclid Avenue. Kate Harvey's husband, Perry, grew up on Millionaire's Row, as did Vail. Bole lived in the Holden mansion at 1729 Euclid from her teen years until her marriage. Bolton's marriage united two Euclid Avenue families—the Binghams and the Boltons. Ella Ford's family of origin, the Thomas H. Whites, lived at 1820 and then 8220 Euclid in the late nineteenth and early twentieth centuries, near many others of the White family. See Cigliano, *Showplace of America,* 232 (Bolton), 298 (Harvey), 353 (Holden/Bole), 357 (Southworth/Goff), and 359 (Wason and White/Vail). See also "Bole, Roberta Holden," *DCB,* 51–52. The Mosses and the Weirs had no direct relationship to Euclid Avenue, although Roslyn Campbell Weir was the grandniece of Charles F. Brush Sr., longtime Euclid Avenue resident. C. F. Brush obituary, Brush records, Lakeview Cemetery, Cleveland, Ohio.

25. Rowbotham, *Women in Movement,* 248.

26. Ostrander, *Women of the Upper Class,* 135, see also 103.

27. Peacock, "Everything You Always Wanted to Know," 98; "MHA History" (Cleveland: MHA, 1957), 6, PPGC, box 3; "The History of the Maternal Health Association," typewritten manuscript, 28–29, PPGC, box 3, early history; "History—Planned Parenthood," typewritten manuscript, 18, BF, container 3, folder 46.

28. Stenographic Minutes of Organization Meeting, Middle Western States Conference on Birth Control, November 12, 1929, 17, 36. Margaret Sanger, Part 1: Diaries, Speeches and Writings, reel 5, MS-WIA.

29. "MHA History" (Cleveland: MHA, 1957), 6, PPGC, box 3, and Davis, "Maternal Health," master's thesis, 13–14.

30. By the late 1920s Slee had financed the founding of the Holland Rantos Company by another Sanger admirer, Herbert Simonds. The company proved that it was feasible to manufacture diaphragms in the United States by marketing them solely to medical professionals. Reed, *Birth Control Movement,* 114–115, and Tone, *Devices and Desires,* 126–128.

31. MHA, "History," 9, and W. D. Ellis, Pauline G. Fanslow, and Nancy A. Schneider, *The Home Club: The Cleveland Skating Club Story* (n.p.: n.d.), 2–3.

32. Eells was then the MHA's president. Halle was in charge of public relations for the clinic, Ireland a board member, and Gaylord the executive secretary. See Ellis et al., *Home Club,* 2. John Grabowski mentions the popularity of ice skating among Cleveland's wealthy families beginning in the 1860s, and the appeal of professional ice hockey in Cleveland in the 1930s. The ice hockey team played in the Elysium. Grabowski, *Sports in Cleveland* (Bloomington: Indiana University Press, 1992), 19, 58–59. "Planned Parenthood Chronology," Draft II (1/16/88): 8–9; Planned Parenthood, "Every Child a Wanted Child"; Ellis et al., *Home Club,* 3; Peacock, "Everything You Always Wanted to Know," 99. For other society fund-raising functions see, for example, a description of cabaret held by the Bay Village Women's Club in 1931, in Clarice F. White, "New Directors are Named by Girls' Bureau," unidentified news

clipping, March 27, 1931, in Scrapbook 1931, BrI. "Elysium," *ECH*, 385–86. As for other philanthropy in the city, Cleveland's Community Fund raised $4 million in its first campaign in 1919 and more than $5.65 million in 1931. "United Way Services," *ECH*, 1030. See also David Hammack, "Philanthropy," *ECH*, 785–90.

33. Ellis et al., *Home Club*, 3; Guttmacher, comp., *Planned Parenthood Beginnings*, 66.

34. Ellis et al., *Home Club*, 3; MHA Scrapbook, Skating Carnival 1935; MHA Scrapbook Skating Carnival 1936–37; MHA Scrapbook 1935; MHA Scrapbook 1936–41, all in PPGC, box 7; MHA Annual Report, 1935. PPGC, box 2.

35. "Retiring Health Aide Looks Back 24 Years," article identified as one from *Cleveland Plain Dealer*, July 1, 1953, PPGC, box 6, Scrapbook 1952–1953.

36. Ellis et al., *Home Club*, 2–5; "Down From the North Come Crack Skaters," *Cleveland Plain Dealer*, March 11, 1934, 4. Quote from *Cleveland Press*, March 10, 1934, MHA Scrapbook 1929–35, PPGC, box 7. MHA Annual Reports, 1934, 1935, 1935–36. PPGC, box 2. MHA leaders Fayette and Geraldine Brown, Mary Dana Brown, Gertrude Miller Bole, William Chisholm II, Howard Eells Jr., and Walter Halle joined the figure skating club as charter members, along with E. H. Brandenburg, Alexander Brown, Henry L. F. Kreger, J. E. Lambie Jr., W. P. Palmer Jr., Rosamond Robert, Bill Ireland, and Jay and Caroline Raymond. At least seven of these families were related to each other. The club incorporated on September 12, 1936, and changed its name the next year to the Cleveland Skating Club. The group eventually built a skating rink in Shaker Heights and sponsored its own ice carnivals there. See Peacock, "Everything You Always Wanted to Know," 99; Ellis et al., *Home Club*, 4–6; and "Cleveland Skating Club," *ECH*, 289.

37. Quote found in "Projects," MHA. Annual Report 1935–36. See also MHA, Annual Report 1937–38. Both in PPGC, box 2.

38. Rose, *Cleveland: The Making of a City*, 936–37.

39. "Planned Parenthood Chronology," Draft II (1/16/88): 9.

40. Ad and news article fragment, n.d., MHA Scrapbook 1929–35, PPGC, box 7.

41. Ibid. and other articles, MHA Scrapbook 1929–35, PPGC, box 7.

42. MHA Scrapbook, Press Notices 1938–50, PPGC, box 3.

43. MHA Scrapbook-Letters from Patients, PPGC, box 6, and MHA, Annual Reports, 1934–1940, PPGC, box 2.

44. "Six Years With Family Regulation Problems," PPGC, box 2, talks. The woman described by Horner was African American. See Horner, "The Contribution of the Maternal Health Association," 21, 25.

45. For men's letters to the MHA, Margaret Sanger, and Marie Stopes, see chapter 4 in this book.

46. The letter writer does not mention that her sister would be taking a risk if she mailed the diaphragm. This letter offers an example of public disregard for or perhaps

ignorance of the Comstock Law, which made it a crime for a layperson to send a diaphragm through the U.S. mail.

47. Talk Given by Mrs. Edna Rusch, R.N., at the Sixteenth Meeting, MHA, May 17, 1944, p. 4, PPGC, box 5, miscellaneous speeches.

48. MHA Annual Reports, 1929–1935, PPGC, box 2; MHA, "Report of Three Years' Work," 12, MS-SS, Clinics-Ohio; MHA, "Report of Fourth Year," BCS, record group 2, series A. For the jump in referrals from individuals see MHA, "Report of Fourth Year," 4. This figure may be slightly skewed by the reluctance of some people to name their particular agency or to identify themselves as physicians when referring clients, especially in the clinic's early days. Robishaw's prediction appears in "Medical Report," MHA, "Report of Three Years' Work," 12.

49. "Maternal Health Center, Newark, N.J.," *BCR* 16, no. 7 (December 1932): 307; Clara Taylor Warne, "Making Birth Control Respectable," *BCR* 14, no. 4 (April 1930): 110. Melcher, "'Women's Matters'," 47–56. As evidence of this trend continuing beyond the 1940s, referral records for the Parents' Information Bureau in Kitchener, Ontario, Canada, indicate that the proportion of woman-to-woman referrals increased over those by social workers and physicians, from one out of five in 1946 to one out of three in 1960. McLaren and McLaren, *The Bedroom and the State*, 111–12.

50. For Sioux City see Guttmacher, comp., *Planned Parenthood Beginnings*, 54. For situations elsewhere, see, for example, Schoen, "Fighting for Child Health," 100–101. For black women see Rodrigue, "The Black Community," Ph.D. diss., 341. A scholar who has studied abortion networks is Lee, *The Search for an Abortionist*. See also Messer and May, *Back Rooms*, esp. 11, 72, 79.

51. Marion Howell directed the WRU School of Nursing; Elizabeth Folckemer was the VNA executive secretary; and Hanna Buchanan directed the Children's Fresh Air Camp. "History," typewritten manuscript, 13, BF, container 3, folder 46, and chapter 3 in this text. This history spells Folckemer name incorrectly as Falkower; she's listed as Folckemer in "Lakeside Unit, World War I," *ECH*, 628, as well as in MHA, "History" (1957), 5. For referrals from medical facilities see Horner, "The Contribution of the Maternal Health Association," 8, 19, 23, 30. For relief referrals despite stated policy, see Horner, "The Contribution of the Maternal Health Association," 23, 26. References to MHA's cooperative relationship with the Cuyahoga County Relief Administration and visiting nurses, respectively, appear on 19–20, 21, 40.

52. For specialization as a trend in medicine see Starr, *The Social Transformation*, 223–25. Muncy, *Creating a Female Dominion*.

53. Horner, "The Contribution of the Maternal Health Association," 50.

54. MHA members and trustees Marie Green Edwards, Gertrude Judson, Edna Perkins, Delia White, Rabbi Silver, the Rev. Blanchard, and Virginia Wing all served Associated Charities. Waite, *Warm Friend*, 101, 135, 174, 184, 250, 410, 413. Reports of Associated Charities can be found at Cleveland Public Library. For WRU social work school see Campbell, *SASS*, esp. 14, 16, 49, 65.

55. For one example of the interconnections between agencies see Waite, *Warm Friend*, 102.

56. *Representative Clevelanders* offers a great source for many of the affiliations listed. For Perkins see *National Cyclopaedia*, vol. 26, 448–49; *Ohio Blue Book*, 291; Rose, *Cleveland: The Making of a City*, 585, 621, 703; "Perkins, Edna Brush," *DCB*, 350; Wood, "Cleveland Medicine's Incredible Ghosts," 60. For Fisher see typewritten obituary, BF, series IV, container 3, folder 46. For Narten see *Plain Dealer*, January 27, 1931, in Scrapbook, 1929–31, BrI. For Flory see *American Women*, vol. 3, 1939, 296, and Cleveland Day Nursery and Free Kindergarten records, WRHS. For Goff see *Fourth General Catalogue*, 91; *Social Register Cleveland 1927*; and Gaylord to McGraw, October 10, 1929, MS-WIA, reel 5. For Wason see *Fourth General Catalogue*, 140; *Social Register Cleveland 1927*, 71; and Rose, *Cleveland: The Making of a City*, 586, 752. For Black see "Family Service Assn. of Cleveland," *ECH*, 417, Rose, *Cleveland: The Making of a City*, 737, and Gaylord to McGraw, October 10, 1929, reel 5, MS-WIA. For Associated Charities connections see Waite, *Warm Friend*, 101, 135, 161, 165–67, 174, 184, 240, 250, note 250.

57. Planned Parenthood, *A Tradition of Choice*, vi. McCormick became acquainted with birth control advocates Mary Ware Dennett and Aletta Jacobs through international women's suffrage activities. She smuggled diaphragms for Sanger and later helped fund research for the birth control pill. See Reynolds, *Women Advocates for Reproductive Rights*, 108–9.

58. For biographical information on trustees see note 7 and note 16.

59. Susan Ostrander describes the role of the Junior League in Cleveland in the 1970s in "Knowing Her Place: How Elite Women Preserve the Power," *Cleveland* (May 1979): 77, 193, and more fully in *Women of the Upper Class*, 111–15. For Junior League involvement at the MHA, see Davis, "Maternal Health," 16–17; "MHA History," 1, PPGC, box 3; and chapter 2 in this work. See also "Junior League of Cleveland, Inc.," *ECH*, 605.

60. Untitled typewritten manuscript, 7, PPGC, box 3, early history, and biographical sources in note 7.

61. Davis, "Maternal Health," 33. The Jewish Social Service Bureau of Chicago initiated a "sexual hygiene" program in 1922, in the absence of family limitation services in the city. See Virginia C. Frank, "A Constructive Service," *BCR* 17, no. 7 (July 1933): 176. For the involvement of Jewish women in the birth control cause on an international level see Naomi Shepherd, *A Price Below Rubies: Jewish Women as Rebels and Radicals* (Cambridge, Mass.: Harvard University Press, 1993), 219–22.

62. Davis, "Maternal Health," 31. Cleveland had maintained a Social Service Clearinghouse since 1909, designed to register each case known to each social agency. See Mrs. Charles [Constance] W. Webb, "Community Relationships Involved in 100 Percent Registration in Social Service Exchange: From the Standpoint of Hospital Social Service," in *Proceedings of the National Conference of Social Work, 1932* (Chicago: Uni-

versity of Chicago Press, 1933), 186.

63. Davis, "Maternal Health," 31.

64. "Utilizing Community Resources in a Maternal Health Program," talk given by Mrs. Edna Rusch at nurses meeting in Akron, April 1940, 3–7, PPGC, box 5, misc. speeches.

65. Watson, *The Charity Organization Movement in the United States*, 526–27.

66. For Cleveland hospitals see Burdett Wylie, "Obstetrics and Gynecology and the Cleveland Hospital Obstetric Society," in Brown, ed., *The History of Medicine in Cleveland*, 287. For general trends see Charles E. Rosenberg, *The Care of Strangers: The Rise of America's Hospital System* (New York: Basic Books, 1987), 32, 35, 49, 304–5, and Barbara Melosh, *"The Physician's Hand": Work, Culture and Conflict in American Nursing* (Philadelphia: Temple University Press, 1982), esp. 114–15, 134–35, 140–41. William F. May describes the physician as parent in *The Physician's Covenant: Images of the Healer in Medical Ethics* (Philadelphia: The Westminster Press, 1983), chapter 1, 37–62. The *Encyclopaedia of Social Sciences* insists that attitudes in social work changed by the 1930s, from the "external" viewing of "the poor, the sick, the criminal, or neglected . . . in contrast to the normal" to a more analytic view of each client. See "Social Work," *Encyclopaedia of Social Sciences* (New York: Macmillan, 1934), vol. 14, 168. See also James Leiby, *A History of Social Welfare and Social Work in the United States* (New York: Columbia University Press, 1978) and Roy Lubove, *The Professional Altruist: The Emergence of Social Work as a Career, 1880–1930* (Cambridge, Mass.: Harvard University Press, 1965).

67. Mary L. McClure to Bishop Schrembs, August 14, 1934. Records of Joseph Schrembs, Archives of the Diocese of Cleveland, Cleveland, Ohio.

68. Scrapbook-Letters from Patients, 1928–1938, PPGC, box 6. Davis, "Maternal Health," appendix 1, xxii; Horner, "The Contribution of the Maternal Health Association," 39. Off-the-record conversations also indicate that local knowledge of the clinic was not widespread in the early years.

69. Davis, "Maternal Health," 31–32. For Catholicism in Cleveland see Henry B. Leonard, "Catholics, Roman," *ECH,* 157–59, and Michael J. McTighe and Jimmy E. Wilkinson Meyer, "Religion," *ECH,* 854–58. For Associated Charities and its relationship to Catholic organizations, see "Historical Number of The Associated Charities, Cleveland, Ohio, 1884–1924," 16, and other Associated Charities reports. Cleveland Public Library. In contrast to Cleveland and other northern cities, birth control quickly became a public health matter with governmental support in the southern United States. Worries about the alleged high birth rate of blacks contributed to the success of this public health focus but was not the only factor. See Schoen, "Fighting for Child Health"; Gordon, *Woman's Body,* 330, 331; and Reed, *Birth Control Movement,* 252–56.

70. Davis, "Maternal Health," 33.

71. "Birth Control Advocates Propose Clinic for Akron," unidentified news article, June 18, 1934, PPCO, OHS, box 1, Oversize Scrapbook 1932–38, 16.

72. Wing to Gladys Gaylord, December 15, 1930, PPGC, box 1, Brush Foundation–historical.

## Notes to Chapter 6

1. The West Side branch was located at 6516 Detroit Avenue. "Projects," MHA Annual Report March 24, 1935–March 31, 1936; "West Side Branch," MHA Annual Report April 1, 1936–March 31, 1937, PPGC, box 2. In 1941 Hazel C. Jackson served as executive of the branch. MHA, West Side Branch Annual Report April 1, 1940 to March 31, 1941, PPGC, box 2. This branch expanded in 1971. See Planned Parenthood Timeline, 1921–1983. Copy in author's possession.

2. MHA administrative offices and the main clinic remained at 2101 Adelbert Road in University Circle from 1939 to 1957, when they moved to a new building a few blocks away at 2027 Cornell Road. From 1983 until 1989 the administrative offices of the MHA, now named Planned Parenthood of Greater Cleveland (PPGC), were located downtown, in the Bulkley building, at 1501 Euclid Avenue, separate from a clinic. See Planned Parenthood Timeline and MHA/PPGC Annual Reports, box 2. In 1989 the PPGC administrative offices moved to 3135 Euclid Avenue. Little documentation exists for the Woodhill Branch; annual reports after 1940 do not list that clinic. MHA Annual Report April 1, 1938–March 31, 1939; MHA Annual Report April 1, 1939–March 31, 1940; MHA Annual Report April 1, 1940–March 31, 1941; MHA Annual Report April 1, 1941–March 31, 1942; and "Projects," MHA Annual Report 1935–36. All PPGC, box 2.

3. MHA annual reports, 1939–40, 1940–41, 1941–42. PPGC, box 2. "MHA History" (Cleveland: MHA, 1957), 11, PPGC, box 3. Kusmer, *A Ghetto Takes Shape,* 41, 210–12, 220–22; Phillips, *AlabamaNorth,* 129–36. For a brief summary of Cleveland's residential patterns according to ethnicity, especially in the Central area, see Charles Garvin, "Cleveland's Forest City Hospital Celebrates First Birthday," *Journal of the National Medical Association* 51, no. 2 (March 1959): 151. Reprint in Charles Garvin papers, container 1, folder 10, WRHS. Planned Parenthood Timeline.

4. McCann, *Birth Control Politics,* 205–07; Gordon, *Woman's Body,* 353–54, 398–99; and Roberts, *Killing the Black Body.*

5. Mrs. Walter S. Smith, "History and Information Regarding the Maternal Health Association," April 15, 1959, 2. PPGC, box 3, early history. The MHA undertook premarital counseling in 1931 at the request of local clergy. The service expanded to a more formal basis in 1937 with the hiring of Hazel C. Jackson. See MHA, "Report of Three Years' Work, March 22, 1928–March 21, 1931," 4, in MS-SS, Clinics-Ohio; David Weir, "Planned Parenthood, 1923–1976," in Brown, ed., *The History of Medicine in Cleveland,* 277. Gladys Gaylord, "Premarital and Preconceptional Care," presented before the American Congress of Obstetrics and Gynecology, Cleveland, Ohio, September 11–15, 1939, PPGC, box 5, talks. The West Side branch began a

premarital clinic in 1942 with special funding. See Edna L. Rusch, "West Side Branch Seventh Annual Meeting, April 14, 1943, Clinic Report," 3, PPGC, box 1.

6. "MHA History" (Cleveland: MHA, 1957), 6, 10, PPGC, box 3; Meyer, "Motherhood and Morality," 14–16; Weir, "Planned Parenthood, 1923–1976," 279; Sarah Marcus, "Talk Given at the Sixteenth Annual Meeting of the Maternal Health Association," May 17, 1944, 2, PPGC, box 5; Davis, "Maternal Health," 25. See also outline for "Talk to Public Health Nurses, Nov. 4, [19]40," No author given, PPGC, box 2, talks. For 1948 see John Barnard Oliver Jr., "History and Information Regarding the Maternal Health Association," May 15, 1948, typescript copy, 6, PPGC, box 3, early history. For the 1960s see Betty Porcello, "The Maternal Health Association," June 1964, 6. Porcello claims, "The [Maternal Health] Association is often a training center for the personnel of Planned Parenthood clinics all over the United States and from several foreign countries." PPGC, box 1, history of Planned Parenthood.

A 1944 Clinic Handbook for Planned Parenthood of Columbus, Ohio, advises, "Physicians and medical students should have access to teaching facilities offered by the center, where they can acquire the necessary information and skill in describing contraceptive methods." The handbook then describes the content of a course for physicians and medical students, to be given by the clinic's medical director or medical staff member, depending on "community resources and amount of time available." See "Third Draft, Clinic Manual," 5, PPCO, box 3, folder 12. The Birth Control Clinic in Hamilton, Ontario, Canada, also instructed physicians in contraception. See Dodd, "The Hamilton Birth Control Clinic of the 1930s," 82.

7. Gordon, *Woman's Body*, 256–74. See also Joyce M. Ray and F. G. Gosling, "American Physicians," 399–411. James Reed gives an account of the role of Robert L. Dickinson in changing the attitudes of the medical profession toward birth control in *The Birth Control Movement*, esp. 167–80. Gordon and Reed ignore the role of local birth control clinics in convincing individual physicians to include birth control in their private practices.

8. For teaching as a function of medical facilities see Rosner, *A Once Charitable Enterprise*, 99–101. Margaret Sanger and Hannah M. Stone, eds., *The Practice of Contraception: An International Symposium and Survey* (Baltimore, Md.: Williams and Wilkins, 1931), 237; Mary Losure, "'Motherhood Protection'," 368; Backus, "Planned Parenthood League," 10. Copy in personal possession of the author. *The History of Planned Parenthood*, 19. The Cromer Welfare Center in London, England, was training doctors in birth control techniques by 1930. See *Practice of Contraception*, 221. Weir, "History of Planned Parenthood in Cuyahoga County," 279.

9. For a brief description of the origins of the teaching hospital and the conflict over patient rights, see Edward C. Atwater, "Touching the Patient: The Teaching of Internal Medicine in America," in *Sickness and Health in America*, 132–34. See also Susan E. Lederer, *Subjected to Science: Human Experimentation in America before the Second World War* (Baltimore, Md.: The Johns Hopkins University Press, 1995), 37,

74, 115–16. Medical authority and autonomy garnered respect and awe for medical research, especially during the early decades of the twentieth century. See James H. Jones, *Bad Blood: The Tuskegee Syphilis Experiment* (New York: The Free Press, 1981), 97. See also Susan M. Reverby, ed., *Tuskegee's Truths: Rethinking the Tuskegee Syphilis Study* (Chapel Hill: University of North Carolina Press, 2000).

10. "Report of the Executive Secretary of the Maternal Health Association to the Brush Foundation–October 7, 1930," 1, PPGC, box 1, Brush Foundation-historical.

11. Backus and Gladys Gaylord became lifelong friends. Backus, "Planned Parenthood League," 3. The MHA's Medical Advisory Board functioned as a clearinghouse for professional queries. In 1938, describing the responsibilities of the medical board, Goldie Davis stated that the board's chairperson investigated the qualifications and records of physicians "from another locality" who requested instruction in contraceptive technique. See Davis, "Maternal Health," 17.

12. MHA Annual Reports, 1929–39, PPGC, box 2. For examples of speeches in Cleveland see "Family and Sex Education–Theme of Cleveland PTA Council Program," the *Cleveland Plain Dealer,* March 19, 1939, in Scrapbook 1936–41, PPGC, box 7; "Gladys Gaylord Speaks at Onaway School PTA," n.d., and "Speaks on Health Clinic," March 21, 1931, both in Scrapbook 1929–1935, PPGC, box 7. See also MHA Annual Report 1937, PPGC, box 2. Higley, "Men and Maternal Health," February 11, 1938. Printed in the *BCR* (June 1938). R. Illula Hansen, R.N., "Contraception: The Woman's Point of View," talk given October 19, 1931, before the Lakewood Clinical Luncheon Club. Gladys Gaylord, "The Eugenic Value of a Maternal Health Center," May 27, 1939. Printed in the *Journal of Heredity* 30 (1939). All PPGC, box 2, miscellaneous speeches. For family regulation quote, see Report of the Executive Secretary of the MHA to the Brush Foundation–Oct. 29, 1931," 2, in PPGC, box 1, Brush Foundation–historical.

13. See chapter 3 in this text. "The Brush Foundation, 1928–1980" (Cleveland: The Brush Foundation, n.d.), 1–2, 25; MHA Annual Reports, 1928–1936, PPGC, box 2.

14. Louise Stevens Bryant, "Clinical Development," *BCR* 16, no. 10 (December 1932): 299. The Baltimore Bureau of Contraceptive Service was noted in this article along with the Cleveland MHA. For another description of the MHA as a demonstration center and a concise statement of its three-fold purpose see Henry M. Busch, "Historical and Statistical Report of the Maternal Health Association," in MHA, "Report of Two Years' Work, March 1928–April 1930," 3, WRHS vertical file. Gladys Gaylord also delineates the clinic's purpose in "Eugenic Value."

15. Reed, *Birth Control Movement,* 147–48; Van de Velde, *Ideal Marriage;* Lindsey and Evans, *The Companionate Marriage.* Davis, *Factors in the Sex Life;* Robert Latou Dickinson, M.D., "Medical Aspects of Human Fertility: A Survey and Report" (New York: National Committee on Maternal Health, 1932), PPGC, box 3, pamphlets; Reed, *Birth Control Movement,* 143–96; Chesler, *Woman of Valor,* 71–72, note 72; Irvine, *Disorders of Desire,* 33–35. Mosher, *The Mosher Survey.* For a general view of

the development and the ends of social research see Leiby, *A History of Social Welfare*, esp. 180–85.

16. For foundation goals see "The Brush Foundation, 1928–1980" (Cleveland: The Brush Foundation, n.d.), 1–2, and figure 13, chapter 3 in this work.

17. Correspondence and reports on the ovulation research project are located in PPGC, box 1, Brush Foundation–historical. See especially T. W. Todd to G. Gaylord, Sept. 23, 1930 and Dec. 3, 1930; T. Zuck to G. Gaylord, Jan. 12, 1931; and "Report of the Executive Secretary of the MHA to the Brush Foundation–Oct. 29, 1931," 1. Zuck, "The Relation of Basal Body Temperature," 1001.

18. MHA/Brush cooperation is outlined in "Report of the Joint Committee of the Cleveland Maternal Health Clinic and the Brush Foundation," November 21, 1929, 1, in PPGC, box 1, Brush Foundation–historical, and Gaylord, "Premarital," 3.

19. Zuck, "The Relation of Basal Body Temperature," 998–1005, quote appears on page 1004. For the manner of determining ovulation patterns, see page 999.

20. T. Zuck to G. Gaylord, January 12, 1931, PPGC, box 1, Brush Foundation-historical; Zuck, "The Relation of Basal Body Temperature," 1004.

21. See also Paula Viterbo, "The Promise of Rhythm," Ph.D. diss

22. For a brief synopsis of the trials of birth control pills on poor Puerto Rican women see Reed, *Birth Control Movement*, 359–61; for A. R. Kaufman's indiscriminate distribution of contraceptive jelly to the "unfortunate classes" of Canada see McLaren and McLaren, *The Bedroom and the State*, 107, and A. R. Kaufman to Mrs. Leslie D. Hawkridge, February 18, 1938, PPLM, box 13.

23. T. W. Todd to Mrs. Brooks Shepard, President, Maternal Health Association, December 3, 1930, PPGC, box 1, Brush Foundation–historical. Yet Zuck states that "There has been no selection on the basis of economic status." Zuck, "The Relation of Basal Body Temperature," 1001.

24. Italics added. Report of the Executive Secretary of the Maternal Health Association to the Brush Foundation–October 29, 1931, 1, in PPGC, box 1, Brush Foundation–historical. "Map Birth Control With Thermometer," *Plain Dealer*, December 11, 1938, PPGC, box 6, Scrapbook-International.

25. For eugenics as an application of empiricism to social problems see Kevles, *In the Name of Eugenics*, and chapter 1 in this text. For Sanger's clinic see Reed, *Birth Control Movement*, 114, and Chesler, *Woman of Valor*, 226. An early book-length study of contraceptive clinics is Robinson, *Seventy Birth Control Clinics*. Other contemporaneous reports include Robishaw, "A Study of 4,000 Patients," 427–34, and Stix, "Birth Control in a Midwestern City," I, 69–91; II, 152–71. For Gamble's efforts in North Carolina, see Schoen, "'A great thing for poor folks'," Ph.D. diss., 61–65. See also Williams and Williams, *Every Child a Wanted Child*. "Third Draft, Clinical Manual" (November 1944), 6, PPCO, box 3, folder 12. For Denver see Palmer and Greenberg, *Facts and Frauds*, 236. This source does not say more about the Denver experiments, leaving one to question whether the doctor was performing them within the clinic.

26. Research statement in Horner, "The Contribution of the Maternal Health Association," 51.

27. For medical research in other areas see Jones, *Bad Blood,* and Lederer, *Subjected to Science.*

28. Personal interview by the author with a social worker and former Cleveland MHA client, who preferred to remain anonymous. Report of the Executive Secretary of the Maternal Health Association to the Brush Foundation–October 29, 1931, 1; Client to G. Gaylord, December 16, 1939, PPLM, box 51; and Gladys Gaylord to Virginia Wing at the Brush Foundation, Jan. 22, 1940, both in PPGC, box 1, Brush Foundation–historical.

29. Loretta McLaughlin, *The Pill, John Rock, and the Church: The Biography of a Revolution* (Boston: Little, Brown and Company, 1982), 40–44, 48–50; May, *Barren in the Promised Land,* 75–78, 156–57.

30. Weir, "Planned Parenthood, 1923–1976," 279–80; MHA Annual Report 1939–40. PPGC, box 2. For fertility services as a trend in other clinics, see Gordon, *Woman's Body,* 307; Guttmacher, comp., *Planned Parenthood Beginnings,* 27, 50, 142; and May, *Barren in the Promised Land,* 156–57.

31. May, *Barren in the Promised Land,* 72–75.

32. MHA, "Report of Two Years' Work," 2. WRHS, vertical file.

33. Smith, *Sick and Tired,* 24. Charles Garvin, "The New Negro Physician," typescript copy of speech given at the Howard University School of Medicine, n.d., 8, Charles Garvin papers, WRHS, container 1, folder 2.

34. "Pajama Ensembles as Popular for Children as for Grown-ups," *Cleveland Gazette,* March 3, 1930. The piece included an illustraton of a white child, a girl, dressed in what looks to be a pricey ensemble, standing next to a baby carriage.

35. Schoen, "'A great thing'," Ph.D. diss., 219. Roberts, *Killing the Black Body,* 9; McCann, *Birth Control Politics,* chapter 4, esp. 108–9; Edward J. Larson, *Sex, Race, and Science: Eugenics in the Deep South* (Baltimore, Md.: The Johns Hopkins University Press, 1995), 157.

36. MHA, "Report of Three Years,'" 9–10. MS-SS, Clinics-Ohio.

37. MHA, "Report of Fourth Year," 7, BCS, record group 2, series A. See also "Program and Figures," MHA, Annual Report, May 1935. PPGC, box 2. For the prejudice of specific MHA staff members against blacks, see, for example, Chesler, interview with Sarah Marcus, 5, WRHS. Alice Malone served as the MHA's first black nurse. See "70 Years of Excellence 1928–1998," Planned Parenthood of Greater Cleveland, June 24, 1999, 11.

38. For Hawkins see Dodd, "Hamilton Birth Control Clinic," 73; for Brush see *Our Margaret Sanger* (privately published, 1959), vol. 1, 41–52, MS-SS; for Cunningham see "The History of Planned Parenthood of the Rocky Mountains" (Denver: Planned Parenthood of the Rocky Mountains, 1991), 3–4. A 1932 meeting in the Buffalo, New York, home of Mrs. J. F. Schoellkopf Jr., with Schoellkopf's long-time friend, Mar-

garet Sanger, sparked the formation of the Maternal Health Clinic there. See Guttmacher, comp., *Planned Parenthood Beginnings*, 79. Board members of clinics in Hamilton, Ontario, Canada, and in Cleveland, Ohio, attended Vassar College during the 1890s: Mabel Breckinridge Wason of the MHA graduated from Vassar one year before Mary Chambers Hawkins and lived in Hamilton before her marriage brought her to Cleveland. See *Fourth General Catalogue*, 140, 154. MHA board member Mary Dunning graduated from Vassar in Hawkins's class (1897). A New Yorker, Dunning moved to Cleveland to marry Charles Thwing, Western Reserve University president from 1890 to 1921. See *Fourth General Catalogue*, 140, 154; "Thwing, Charles Franklin," *DCB*, 447–48; C. H. Cramer, *Case Western Reserve*, 113–20. Mary Thwing served on the MHA board from its founding until her death in 1931. See MHA Annual Reports, 1929–32, PPGC, box 2. At least two other MHA board members were Vassar graduates: Frances Southworth Goff (1886) and Helene North Narten (1910). See *Fourth General Catalogue*, 91, 324.

39. Minutes of the Brush Foundation Board of Managers, December 3, 1930; Minutes 1931–1949, BF, series I, sub-series A, container 1, folder 1. The Brush Foundation paid Gaylord a pension until her death in 1985. See BF, sub-series B, container 1, folder 7, Gaylord–Pension. For other models of providing birth control see Reed, *Birth Control Movement*, 218–22, 252; McLaren and McLaren, *Bedroom and the State*, 103–16; and chapter 2 in this work. Another example of the MHA's larger influence is that at least four other archival collections—the BCS in Hamilton, Ontario; PPCO, Columbus, Ohio; PPLM, Smith College; and PPFA, Smith College—include Cleveland MHA material. For later International Planned Parenthood activities of the Brush Foundation and D.H.B. see Reed, *The Birth Control Movement*, 292–93; "Dorothy Brush—Founder and First Editor of the News," *International Planned Parenthood News*, 175 (September 1968): 8; "The Brush Foundation, 1928–1980" (Cleveland: The Brush Foundation, n.d.), 7–8, 19–21; and DHB, boxes 2 and 4.

40. Weir, "Planned Parenthood, 1923–1976," 276; Minutes of the Brush Foundation Board of Managers, December 3, 1930; Minutes April 26, 1937. This statement is repeated in the 1939 budget. See Minutes, June 23, 1939, BF, series I, sub-series A, container 1, folder 1; G. Gaylord to MHA, November 20, 1947, PPGC, box 3.

41. "Report of the Executive Secretary of the MHA to the Brush Foundation–Oct. 29, 1931," 2, in PPGC, box 1, Brush Foundation–historical. Maternal Health Association, Ohio, Clinic Report, Oct. 1938 (Aug. 21, 1939). MS-SS, clinics-Ohio; MHA of Ohio, Annual Reports 1938–39, 1940–41. PPCO, box 1, Scrapbook 1939–40. For the Springfield, Ohio, clinic (now Planned Parenthood of West Central Ohio) see Guttmacher, comp., *Planned Parenthood Beginnings*, 112. For Gamble see Williams and Williams, *Every Child a Wanted Child*, 101–2, and Kriste Lindenmeyer, "Expanding Birth Control to the Hinterland: Cincinnati's First Contraceptive Clinic as a Case Study, 1929–1931," *Mid-America* 77, no. 2 (spring/summer 1995): 145–73. Oliver Jr., "History and Information," 6, 22.

42. "Report of the Executive Secretary of the MHA to the Brush Foundation–Oct. 29, 1931," 2, in PPGC, box 1, Brush Foundation–historical. For Cleveland's influence in Canada, see Gertrude Burgar to Mary Chambers Hawkins, April 30, 1931, BCS, record group 1, series H. For another reference to MHA training of Hamilton staff, see unidentified speech, n.d., 2–3, BCS, record group 1, series C. See also Dodd, "Hamilton Birth Control Clinic," 71–86. The Cleveland and Hamilton clinics maintained a close relationship: Gaylord gave a speech in Hamilton at some point in the thirties, see "Public Acceptance as Related to the Birth Control Field (Talk for Hamilton, Ontario)," BCS, record group 2, series H.

43. Oliver Jr., "History and Information," 22; Robishaw, "And There is the Child," talk given during the annual meeting of the Ohio State Nurses Association in Cleveland, May 5, 1939. Reprinted from *Ohio Nurses Review* 14, no. 4 (October 1939), and F. Q. Blanchard, "Brief for Tomorrow's Children," January 3, 1937, PPGC, box 5, talks. Blanchard's quote on page 5.

44. "Centers for Contraceptive Advice in the United States, November 1934," 8–9, PPGC, box 3, Scrapbook-ABCL. The report also lists birth control centers at University and Mt. Sinai Hospitals. No other documentation has been located about these facilities, however. Guttmacher, comp., *Planned Parenthood Beginnings*, 101, 109, 112, 115. Cincinnati and Columbus are 300 and 150 miles from Cleveland, respectively; Dayton, Springfield, and Youngstown are 217, 185, and 76 miles away.

45. Chesler, interview with Sarah Marcus, 23.

46. MHA, Ohio, Clinic Report, October 1938 (August 21, 1939), MS-SS, Clinics-Ohio; MHA of Ohio, Annual Reports 1938–39, 1940–41, PPCO, box 1, Scrapbook-1939–40; G. Gaylord to Kathryn Trent, December 12, 1942, PPFA, box 94, folder 888. Frances W. Bolton to W. W. Greulich, June 8, 1945; Greulich to Bolton, June 26, 1945; and Mrs. Everett R. Castle and Mrs. John T. Webster to Mrs. William Weir, June 22, 1949, all in Brush Foundation–historical, PPGC, box 1. This last letter identifies Castle as both vice president of Planned Parenthood of Ohio and vice president of the Cleveland MHA, and Webster as serving on the finance committee of the state organization and on the board of trustees of the Cleveland group.

47. "Brush Foundation Grant to Maternal Health Association," April 15, 1940, 2; For the Brush Foundation support of the MHA of Ohio activities, see "Report of the Executive Secretary of the MHA to the Brush Foundation-Oct. 7, 1930," 1; "Report of Education and Extension Work of the Executive Secretary of the Maternal Association Between July 1, 1938 and July 1, 1939," 1, 5–6, Brush Foundation–historical. PPGC, box 1.

48. MHA Annual Report, 1936–37, PPGC box 2; Gaylord, "Public Acceptance," 3–5, BCS, record group 2, series H; Ramirez de Arellano and Seipp, *Colonialism, Catholicism, and Contraception*, 30–47. See also Reuben Hill, J. Mayone Stycos, and Kurt W. Back, *The Family and Population Control: A Puerto Rican Experiment in Social Change* (Chapel Hill: University of North Carolina Press, 1959).

49. Brush Foundation minutes are silent about Gaylord's Central American trips. See Minutes, 1934–36, BF, series I, sub-series A, container 1, folder 1.

50. Ramirez de Arellano and Seipp, *Colonialism, Catholicism, and Contraception,* 30–47.

51. Reed, *The Birth Control Movement,* 259–60; and Hill, Stycos, and Back, *Family and Population Control.*

52. MHA Annual Reports, 1928–1939, PPGC, box 2; "Report of Three Years,'" MS-SS, Clinics-Ohio.

53. MHA Annual Report, 1936–37, PPGC, box 2; Hill, Stycos, and Back, *Family and Population Control,* 116–17; Ramirez de Arellano and Seipp, *Colonialism, Catholicism, and Contraception,* 45. Part of the impetus for controlling Puerto Rico's population lay in fears that residents would begin to flood the United States to escape overcrowding. See Ramirez de Arellano and Seipp, 33–34. For Puerto Rico and the pill trials see Chesler, *Woman of Valor,* 443–44; Reed, *Birth Control Movement,* 359–61; and Bernard Asbell, *The Pill: A Biography of the Drug That Changed the World* (New York: Random House, 1995), 143–47.

54. Robinson, *Seventy Birth Control Clinics,* 14–17.

55. C. E. Gehlke, "Historical and Statistical Report of the Maternal Health Association March 22, 1928-March 21, 1931," in MHA, "Report of Three Years,'" 3, MS-SS, Clinics-Ohio. MHA, "Report of Two Years' Work," 10, PPGC, box 2, annual reports.

56. Report of the Executive Secretary of the Maternal Health Association to the Brush Foundation–October 7, 1930, 2; "Notes Taken at Board Meeting September, 1938," PPGC, box 1, Brush Foundation–historical; and Gaylord, "Public Acceptance," BCS, record group 2, series H; "Founding a Family," speech delivered in Jackson, Michigan, January 1936, 5, PPGC, box 2, talks.

## Notes to Conclusion

1. Jeff Sharlet, "Parlor Politics and Power: A New View of Washington Women," review of *Parlor Politics: in which the ladies of Washington help build a city and a government,* by Catherine Allgor, *The Chronicle of Higher Education,* December 15, 2000, 16–17A. Allgor reinterprets the activities of U.S. First Ladies in terms of power politics. This quote refers to the politicking that these women pursued at lavish nineteenth-century parties. Kathleen D. McCarthy studies the power and limits of women's voluntary action in relationship to cultural institutions in *Women's Culture.*

2. Ralph Locke, "Reflections on Art Music in America, on Stereotypes of the Woman Patron, and on Cha(lle)nges in the Present and Future," in *Cultivating Music in America: Women Patrons and Activists since 1860,* ed. Ralph P. Locke and Cyrilla Barr (Berkeley: University of California Press, 1997), 312. In the same volume and in a similar vein, Linda Whitesitt states that women's "willingness to act as the moral con-

science of capitalistic culture may also have had the function of letting men 'off the hook' for the damaging side effects of industrialization." See Whitesitt, "Women as 'Keepers of Culture': Music Clubs, Community Concert Series, and Symphony Orchestras," in *Cultivating Music in America,* ed. Locke and Barr, 80.

3. Tone, *Devices and Desires,* 153–54.

4. Muncy, *Creating a Female Dominion.*

5. Robishaw, "And There is the Child," PPGC, box 2, talks.

6. "Founding a Family," speech delivered in Jackson, Michigan, January 1936, 3. PPGC, box 2, miscellaneous speeches.

7. D'Emilio and Freedman, *Intimate Matters,* 244.

8. Katherine Kish Sklar has noted the critical influence of the local organizations on the national Consumers' League effort. Sklar, talk delivered at Case Western Reserve University, 1998.

9. MHA, Annual Reports, 1928–43, PPGC, box 2. Gordon, *Woman's Body,* 270.

10. D'Emilio and Freedman, *Intimate Matters,* 166, 245; Gordon, *Woman's Body,* 255; MHA Annual Reports 1928–38, PPGC, box 2; "The Brush Foundation, 1928–1980" (Cleveland: The Brush Foundation, n.d.), 6.

11. Ferdinand Q. Blanchard, "A Brief for Tomorrow's children," address at American Birth Control League Session, National Conference of Social Work, 1937, 1, PPGC, box 5, talks.

12. Betsy Hartmann, *Reproductive Rights and Wrongs; Margaret Sanger Centennial Conference, November 13 & 14, 1979,* 24–28.

13. Leavitt, *Brought to Bed,* 13.

14. Suzanne Amelia Onorato, "Organizational Legitimacy and the Social Construction of Contraceptives: The Politics of Technological Choice" (Ph.D. diss., Duke University, 1990), 180. Onorato cites the report as "Agency Cooperation—Asset or Liability?" October 24, 1961. MS-SS, box 135, folder 1490F.

15. *Cleveland Plain Dealer,* March 27, 1992.

16. Edna Rusch, "Utilizing Community Resources in a Maternal Health Program," talk given at nurses meeting in Akron [Ohio], April 1940, 7. PPGC, box 5, talks.

### Notes to Epilogue

1. The above material comes from Jimmy Wilkinson Meyer, draft of PPGC's seventy-fifth anniversary history, "Celebrating 75 Years of Helping Women Lead Healthier Lives" (2003).

# A Word about Sources

The bulk of my research relied on Cleveland's rich deposit of previously untapped resources in the history of family limitation. The archival records of the MHA include a patient ledger, annual reports, speeches, articles, scrapbooks of clippings, correspondence from clients, and anniversary histories written at twenty, thirty, fifty, sixty, and seventy-five years. Missing from the records, however, are minutes from meetings of the MHA board of trustees and the medical advisory board. In 2003 the collection, Planned Parenthood of Greater Cleveland, awaited processing at the Western Reserve Historical Society; citations are to the boxes of unprocessed papers.

Cleveland MHA materials surfaced in the records of other clinics. The archives of the Birth Control Society of Hamilton, Ontario, Canada, provided clippings, speeches, and correspondence related to the Cleveland MHA—and a couple of annual reports, for example. I began this work just as the Margaret Sanger Papers Project was starting its enormous task; some of the references herein may be duplicated in those many rolls of film.

Finding the given names for all of the women mentioned in this work proved a monumental and frustrating effort. Before the 1970s most contemporaneous sources, subsequent histories based on those sources, and photo collections listed married women by only their husbands' names. A Planned Parenthood donor caught the misidentification of Dorothy Rogers Williams (see figure 26) in the PPGC 2003 anniversary history, just before this book went to press. Dorothy Rogers married Whiting Williams after the death of his first wife, MHA founder Carolyn Harter Williams, in the late 1930s. (I had mistakenly identified Dorothy as Carolyn.) If there are other similar errors, I take full responsibility.

In these perilous times for reproductive rights and women's health, books as well as data procured on the Internet may not be what they seem. See, for example, an edition of Margaret Sanger's *Pivot of Civilization in Historical Perspective: The Birth Control Classic* (Inkling Press, 2001), in which the editor, Michael W. Perry, inserts his own polemic alongside Sanger's text. The field is rich with resources, but proceed with extreme caution.

# Bibliography

## Primary Sources

### Archival Collections

Bagshaw, Elizabeth. Papers. Special Collections, Hamilton Public Library, Hamilton, Ontario, Canada.

Birth Control Society of Hamilton. Special Collections, Hamilton Public Library, Hamilton, Ontario, Canada.

Brush, Charles F. Collection. Euclid Historical Museum, Euclid, Ohio.

Brush, Charles F. Papers. Special Collections, Kelvin Smith Library, Case Western Reserve University, Cleveland, Ohio.

Brush, Dorothy Hamilton. Papers. Sophia Smith Collection, Smith College, Northampton, Massachusetts.

Brush Foundation Archives. Western Reserve Historical Society, Cleveland, Ohio.

Brush Inquiry Scrapbooks. Brush-Bolton Growth Study Center. Case Western Reserve University School of Dentistry. Cleveland, Ohio.

Butler, Alice Rosenberger. Papers. Dittrick Medical History Center, Case Western Reserve University, Cleveland, Ohio.

Case Western Reserve University Archives. Cleveland, Ohio.

Cleveland Day Nursery and Free Kindergarten Records. Western Reserve Historical Society, Cleveland, Ohio.

*Cleveland Press* Collection, Photographs and Clippings, Special Collections, Cleveland State University, Cleveland, Ohio.

Cleveland Public Library, Photograph Collection. Cleveland, Ohio.

Garvin, Charles, M.D. Papers. Western Reserve Historical Society, Cleveland, Ohio.

Lakeview Cemetery. Archives. Cleveland, Ohio.

Marcus, Sarah, M.D. Papers. Dittrick Medical History Center, Case Western Reserve University, Cleveland, Ohio.

———. Papers. Western Reserve Historical Society, Cleveland, Ohio.

Maternal Health Association Archives. Records of Planned Parenthood of Greater Cleveland. Unprocessed collection. Western Reserve Historical Society, Cleveland, Ohio.

Mather Advisory Council (Flora Stone Mather College). Records. Case Western Reserve University Archives, Cleveland, Ohio.

Ohio Historical Society. Columbus, Ohio.

Phillis Wheatley Association Records. Western Reserve Historical Society, Cleveland, Ohio.

Planned Parenthood of Central Ohio Archives. Ohio Historical Society, Columbus, Ohio.

Planned Parenthood Federation of America Archives. Sophia Smith Collection, Smith College, Northampton, Massachusetts.

Rauschkolb, Ruth Robishaw. Papers. Case Western Reserve University Archives. Cleveland, Ohio.

Sanger, Margaret. Papers. Sophia Smith Collection, Smith College, Northampton, Massachusetts.

———. Papers on Microfilm. Library of Congress.

———. Part 1: Diaries, Speeches and Writings, on Microfilm. Women in America: Core Primary Sources for Women's Studies, in association with the Margaret Sanger Papers Project, New York University.

———. *The Margaret Sanger Papers: Collected Documents Series,* ed. Esther Katz (Bethesda, Md.: University Publications of America, 1997).

———. *The Margaret Sanger Papers: Smith Collected Documents Series,* ed. Esther Katz (Bethesda, Md.: University Publications of America, 1995).

Schrembs, Bishop Joseph. Papers. Archives of the Diocese of Cleveland, Cleveland, Ohio.

Stanley A. Ferguson Archives, University Hospitals of Cleveland. Case Western Reserve University, Cleveland, Ohio.

Todd, T. Wingate. Papers. Dittrick Medical History Center, Case Western Reserve University, Cleveland, Ohio.

Woman's General Hospital Records. Dittrick Medical History Center, Case Western Reserve University, Cleveland, Ohio.

Women's City Club Records. Western Reserve Historical Society, Cleveland, Ohio.

## Articles

"Birth Control Clinic Pioneer." *Spectator,* October 25, 1971, Elizabeth Bagshaw Papers. Special Collections, Hamilton Public Library, Hamilton, Ontario, Canada.

"Clinical Contraception in the United States." *The Journal of Contraception* 4 (September 1939): 168–69.

Duffus, R. L. "Cleveland: Paternalism in Excelsis." *New Republic* 54, no. 696 (April 4, 1928): 212–16.

Frank, Lawrence K. "Gerontology." *Journal of Gerontology* 1 (1946): 1–11.

Garber, James R. "A Plea for Prenatal Care and the End-Results of the Hygiene of Pregnancy." *American Journal of Obstetrics and Gynecology* (hereafter *AJOG*) 78, no. 4 (October 1918): 566–75.

Garfield, James R. "A Program of Action for a Children's Protective Society." *Proceedings of the National Conference of Charities and Correction, June 12–19, 1912,* ed. Alexander Johnson. Fort Wayne, Ind.: Fort Wayne Printing Company, 1912.

Gaylord, Gladys. "The Eugenic Value of a Maternal Health Center." *The Journal of Contraception* 3, no. 3 (March 1938): 51–53.

Higley, Charles S. "Men's Consultation in a Maternal Health Center." *The Journal of Contraception* 2 (October 1937): 187–88.

Himes, Norman. "Eugenic Thought in the American Birth Control Movement 100 Years Ago." Reprint from *Eugenics* 2, no. 5 (May 1929).

Ill, Edward J. "The Rights of the Unborn—The Prevention of Conception." *American Journal of Diseases of Women and Children* (hereafter *AJDWC*) 40, no. 5 (November 1899): 577–84.

"The Lay Press Looks at Birth Control." *The Journal of Contraception* 3, no. 3 (March 1938): 60–61.

"Legality of Contraception: Birth Control Information and Methods as Found in State and Federal Statutes." *Ohio State Medical Journal* (February 1930): 151–52.

McArdle, Thomas. "The Physical Evils Arising from the Prevention of Conception." *AJDWC* 21, no. 9 (September 1888): 934–39.

Murray, Grace Peckham. "Pessaries, Their Use and Abuse." *The Woman's Medical Journal* 18, no. 12 (December 1908): 249–53.

Pringle, Henry F. "What Do Women of America Think About Birth Control?" *Ladies Home Journal* (March 1938): 14–15.

"Resolutions Adopted at the Annual Convention." *Medical Woman's Journal* 37, no. 7 (July 1930): 196–97.

Riegel, Robert E. "The American Father of Birth Control." *The New England Quarterly* 6, no. 3 (September 1933): 470–90.

Robishaw, Ruth A. "A Study of 4,000 Patients Admitted for Contraceptive Advice and Treatment." *AJOG* 31, no. 3 (March 1936): 426–34.

"The Spreading Movement for Birth Control." *The Survey* (October 21, 1916): 60–61.

Stix, Regine K. "Birth Control in a Midwestern City: A Study of the Clinics of the Cincinnati Committee of Maternal Health, I, Contraception and Fertility Before Clinic Attendance." *Milbank Memorial Fund Quarterly* 17, no. 1 (January 1939): 69–91.

———. "Birth Control in a Midwestern City: A Study of the Clinics of the Cincinnati Committee of Maternal Health, II, The Effectiveness of Contraception After Clinic Attendance." *Milbank Memorial Fund Quarterly*, 17, no. 2 (April 1939): 152–71.

Todd, T. Wingate. "The Aim and Program of the Brush Inquiry." *Bulletin of the Academy Medicine of Cleveland* 14, no. 3 (March 1930): 9, 21.

"What the Birth Control Leagues are Doing." *BCR* 1, no. 1 (February 1917): 10.

Zuck, Theodore T. "The Relation of Basal Body Temperature to Fertility and Sterility in Women." *AJOG* 36, no. 6 (December 1938): 998–1005.

## Biographical Sources

*African American Women: A Biographical Dictionary.* Edited by Dorothy Salem. Hamden, Conn.: Garland Publishing, 1993.

*American Medical Directory.* 10th ed. Chicago: American Medical Association, 1927.

———. 12th ed. Chicago: American Medical Association, 1929.

———. 16th ed. Chicago: American Medical Association, 1940.

*American Women.* Edited by Durward Howes, vol. 3. Los Angeles: American Publishers, 1939.

*Bench and Bar of Northern Ohio: History and Biography.* Edited by William Neff. Cleveland: Historical Publishing Co., 1921.

*The Book of Clevelanders: A Biographical Dictionary of Living Men of the City of Cleveland.*
    Cleveland: The Burrows Bros. Co., 1914.
*A Brief Biography of Perry Williams Harvey.* Cleveland: n.p., 1936.
"Charles Francis Brush: Scientist and Inventor." MSS copy for *American Biography,*
    CFB, box 21, folder 6.
Cleveland Public Library Biography Clipping File.
Cleveland Public Library Necrology File.
*Dictionary of Cleveland Biography.* Edited by David D. Van Tassel and John
    Grabowski. Bloomington: Indiana University Press, 1996.
*Encyclopedia of Cleveland History.* 2d ed. Edited by David D. Van Tassel and John
    Grabowski. Bloomington: Indiana University Press, 1996.
Ford, Ella White. "Ancestors and Descendants of Thomas H. White." 1928.
*The Fourth General Catalogue of the Officers and Graduates of Vassar College Poughkeep-*
    *sie,* New York 1861–1910. Poughkeepsie: A. V. Haight, 1910.
Loth, David. *A Long Way Forward: The Biography of Congresswoman Frances Payne*
    *Bolton.* New York: Longmans, Green and Co., 1957.
"Mather Advisory Council Members 1888–1970." Mather Advisory Council
    Records, box 5, folder 1, Case Western Reserve University Archives.
*National Cyclopaedia of American Biography.* New York: James T. White, 1937.
Neely, Ruth J. *Women of Ohio.* S. J. Clarke, n.d.
*The Ohio Blue Book: Who's Who in the Buckeye State.* Compiled by C. S. Van Tassel. Nor-
    walk, Ohio: American Publishers, 1917.
Perkins, Charles Brush. *Ancestors of Charles Brush Perkins and Maurice Perkins.* Balti-
    more, Md.: Gateway Press, 1976.
*Representative Clevelanders: A Biographical Directory of Leading Men and Women in the*
    *Present-Day Cleveland Community.* Cleveland: The Cleveland Topics Company,
    1927.
*Social Register Cleveland 1927.* New York: Social Register Association, 1927.
*Social Register Cleveland 1936.* New York: Social Register Association, 1936.
*Social Register Cleveland 1938.* New York: Social Register Association, 1938.
*Social Register Cleveland 1940.* New York: Social Register Association, 1940.
*Social Register Summer 1936.* New York: Social Register Association, 1936.
Trustee Index, Case Western Reserve University Archives.
U.S. Census 1920. Washington, D.C.: Government Printing Office, 1921.
U.S. Census 1930. Washington, D.C.: Government Printing Office, 1931.
*Who's Who in American Jewry,* vol. 3, 1938–39. New York: National News, 1938.
*Who's Who of American Women.* 2d ed. Chicago: Marquis Who's Who, 1962.
*Who's Who in the Midwest.* Chicago: Marquis Who's Who, 1952.

## Books and Pamphlets

Abbott, Virginia Clark. *The History of Woman Suffrage and the League of Women Voters*
    *in Cuyahoga County 1911–1945.* N.p.: William Feather, 1949.
Bing, Lucia Johnson. *Social Work in Greater Cleveland: How Public and Private Agen-*
    *cies are Serving Human Needs.* Cleveland: Welfare Federation of Cleveland, 1938.
Blacker, C. P. *Birth Control and the State, A Plea and a Forecast.* New York: E. P. Dut-
    ton, 1926.

Bromley, Dorothy Dunbar. *Birth Control: Its Use and Misuse.* New York: Harper & Brothers, 1934.

Broun, Heywood, and Margaret Leech. *Anthony Comstock: Roundsman of the Lord.* New York: Albert and Charles Boni, 1927.

Chavasse, Pye Henry. *Woman as a Wife and Mother.* Philadelphia: William D. Evans and Company, 1871.

Chesler, Ellen. Interview with Sarah Marcus, M.D. Transcript of Oral History. N.p.: Schlesinger-Rockefeller Oral History Project, 1976. WRHS.

Committee on Legislation for Birth Control. *Removal of Legal Obstacles Opens New Opportunities: A New Day Dawns for Birth Control.* New York: National Committee on Federal Legislation for Birth Control, 1937.

Comstock, Anthony. *Traps for the Young.* New York: Funk and Wagnall's, 1883. Reprint, ed. Robert Bremner, Cambridge, Mass.: Belknap Press, 1967.

Coon, Horace. *Money to Burn: What the Great American Philanthropic Foundations Do with Their Money.* London: Longmans, Green and Co., 1938.

Cooper, James F. *Technique of Contraception: The Principles and Practice of Anti-Conceptional Methods.* New York: Day-Nichols, 1928.

Davis, Katherine Bement. *Factors in the Sex Life of Twenty-two Hundred Women.* New York: Harper and Brothers, 1929.

Dennett, Mary Ware. *Birth Control Laws: Shall We Keep Them, Change Them, or Abolish Them?* New York: The Grafton Press, 1926. Reprint, New York: Da Capo Press, 1970.

Dickinson, Robert Latou, and Lura Beam. *A Thousand Marriages: A Medical Study of Sex Adjustment.* Baltimore, Md.: Williams and Wilkins, 1931.

*The First 25 Years 1914–1939.* Cleveland: The Cleveland Foundation, n.d.

Green, Howard Whipple. *Housing in the Cleveland Community: Past—Present—Future.* Cleveland: Real Property Inventory of Metropolitan Cleveland, 1947.

Himes, Norman. *A Medical History of Contraception.* New York: Gamut Press, 1936. Reprint, New York: Gamut Press, 1963.

*The History of Planned Parenthood of the Rocky Mountains, 1916 . . .* Aurora, Colo.: Planned Parenthood of the Rocky Mountains, n.d.

Key, Ellen. *Mother's Own Book.* New York: The Parents' Publishing Association, 1928.
———. *The Renaissance of Motherhood.* New York: Putnam's, 1914.

Lindsey, Ben B., and Wainwright Evans. *The Companionate Marriage.* Garden City, N.Y.: Garden City Publishing, 1927, 1929.

Lynd, Robert S., and Helen Merrell Lynd. *Middletown: A Study in Modern American Culture.* New York: Harcourt, Brace, 1929.

"Medical Aspects of Contraception," London: Martin Hopkinson, 1927.

Meyer, Adolf. *Birth Control: Facts and Responsibilities.* Baltimore, Md.: William and Wilkins, 1925.

Moore, Edward Roberts. *The Case Against Birth Control.* New York: The Century Co., 1931.

Mosher, Clelia Duel. *The Mosher Survey: Sexual Attitudes of 45 Victorian Women.* New York: Arno Press, 1980.

*A New Day Dawns for Birth Control.* New York: National Committee on Federal Legislation for Birth Control, 1937.

Palmer, Rachel Lynn, and Sarah K. Greenberg. *Facts and Frauds in Woman's Hygiene: A Medical Guide Against Misleading Claims and Dangerous Products.* New York: Vanguard Press, 1936.

*Recent Social Trends in the United States: Report of the President's Research Committee on Social Trends,* vol. 1. New York: McGraw-Hill, 1933.

Robinson, Caroline Hadley. *Seventy Birth Control Clinics.* Baltimore, Md.: Williams and Wilkins, 1930. Reprint, New York: Arno Press and the *New York Times,* 1972.

Robishaw, Ruth. "The Significance of Maternal Health." Cleveland: Maternal Health Association, 1937.

Sanger, Margaret. *Happiness in Marriage.* New York: Blue Ribbon Books, 1926.

———, ed. *International Aspects of Birth Control: Sixth International Neo-Malthusian and Birth Control Conference.* New York: American Birth Control League, 1925.

———. *Margaret Sanger: An Autobiography.* New York: Norton, 1938. Reprint, New York: Dover, 1971.

———. *Motherhood in Bondage.* New York: Brentano's, 1928. Reprint, Columbus: The Ohio State University Press, 2000.

———. *My Fight for Birth Control.* New York: Farrar and Rinehart, 1931.

———, ed. *International Aspects; Religious and Ethical Aspects of Birth Control. Sixth International Neo-Malthusian and Birth Control Conference,* vol. 4. New York: American Birth Control League, 1926.

Sanger, Margaret, and Hannah M. Stone, eds. *The Practice of Contraception: An International Symposium and Survey.* Baltimore, Md.: Williams and Wilkins, 1931.

Van de Velde, Th. H. *Ideal Marriage; Its Physiology and Technique.* New York: Random House, 1926, 1930.

Watson, Frank Dekker. *The Charity Organization Movement in the United States: A Study in American Philanthropy.* New York: Macmillan, 1922.

## Legal Documents

*Acts of a General Nature and Local Laws and Joint Resolutions Passed by the Fifty-fifth General Assembly of the State of Ohio.* Columbus: Richard Nevins, vol. 59, 1862.

*Acts of a General Nature Passed at the First Session of the Thirty Second General Assembly of the State of Ohio.* Columbus: David Smith, vol. 23, 1834.

*The General and Local Laws and Joint Resolutions passed by the Sixty-Second General Assembly of the State of Ohio,* Columbus: Nevins and Myers, vol. 73, 1876.

*Griswold vs. The State of Connecticut,* 381 U.S. 479 (1965).

The Municipal Code of the City of Cleveland, 1924, Sec. 2951.

Sayler, J. R., ed. *Statutes of the State of Ohio,* vol. 1, 1861–1865. Cincinnati, Ohio: Robert Clarke, 1876.

*The State of Ohio General and Local Laws and Joint Resolutions Passed by the Sixtieth General Assembly.* Columbus: Nevins and Myers, vol. 69, 1872.

*United States Code.* Title 18, Ch. 71, Section 1460–1468. Washington, D.C.: United States Government Printing Office, 2001.

*Youngs Rubber Corporation v. C. I. Lee and Co.,* 45 F.2d 103 (1930).

## Letters

Bangs, Catherine C. to G. Gaylord, December 26, 1934, Planned Parenthood Federation of America Archives. Sophia Smith Collection, Smith College, Northampton, Massachusetts (hereafter PPFA), series II, box 30, folder 77.

Bolton, Frances W. to W. W. Greulich, June 8, 1945, Maternal Health Association/Planned Parenthood of Greater Cleveland Archives (unprocessed). Western Reserve Historical Society, Cleveland, Ohio (hereafter PPGC), box 1, Brush Foundation–historical.

Bolton, Mrs. Newell to R. M. Ruhlman, Cleveland Chamber of Commerce, October 23, 1946, PPGC, box 1.

Brush, Charles Francis, Sr., Letters, 1927–1929. Charles F. Brush Sr. Papers. Special Collections, Kelvin Smith Library, Case Western Reserve University, Cleveland, Ohio (hereafter CFB), box 1, folders 9 through 18.

——— to Dorothy Hamilton Brush and Edna Brush Perkins, CFB, box 31, microfilm reel 2.

——— to Dorothy H. Brush, July 18, 1928, CFB, box 1, folder 9.

——— to Edna Brush Perkins, December 21, 1927 through July 18, 1928, CFB, box 1, folders 9–18.

Brush, Dorothy Hamilton, to Charles F. Brush Sr., CFB, box 31, microfilm reel 2.

——— to Charles F. Brush Sr., Dec. 21, 1927, Jan. 4, 1928, and Feb. 6, 1928, CFB, box 1, folder 9.

——— to Edna Brush Perkins, December 21, 1927 through July 28, 1928, CFB, box 1, folders 9–18, and CFB, box 31, microfilm reel 2.

Burgar, Gertrude, to Mary Chambers Hawkins, April 30, 1931, Birth Control Society of Hamilton. Records. Special Collections, Hamilton Public Library, Hamilton, Ontario, Canada (hereafter BCS), record group 1, series H.

Butler, Alice, to M. Sanger, May 19, 1925, *Margaret Sanger Papers Collected Documents Series:* Microfilm Edition, ed. Esther Katz. New York University (hereafter *MSPCDM*), series III, C02:0294.

Castle, Mrs. Everett R., and Mrs. John T. Webster to Mrs. William Weir, June 22, 1949, PPGC, box 1, Brush Foundation–historical.

Client to G. Gaylord, December 16, 1939, Planned Parenthood League of Massachusetts. Archives. Sophia Smith Collection, Smith College, Northampton, Massachusetts (hereafter PPLM), box 51.

Fisher, Jerome, to Greenbaum, Wolff & Ernst, January 25, 1938, PPFA I, box 89.

Fisher, Katherine, to "Gals," n.d. PPGC, box 3, early history.

Flynn, Elizabeth Gurley. "Published Documents and Letters Re Investigation of Frederick Blossom, 1923." Margaret Sanger. Papers. Sophia Smith Collection, Smith College, Northamption, Massachusetts (hereafter MS-SS).

Gaylord, Gladys, to Kathryn Trent, December 12, 1942. PPFA, box 94, folder 888.

——— to MHA, November 20, 1947, PPGC, box 3.

——— to Mrs. Donald McGraw, October 10, 1929. Margaret Sanger. Part 1: Diaries, Speeches, and Writings, on Microfilm. Women in America: Core Primary Sources for Women's Studies, in association with the Margaret Sanger Papers Project, New York University (hereafter MS-WIA), reel 5.

——— to Mrs. Francis Bangs, December 7, 1934, PPFA, series II, box 30, folder 77.

——— to Virginia Wing at the Brush Foundation, January 22, 1940, PPGC, box 1, Brush Foundation–historical.

Greulich, W. W. to F. P. Bolton, June 26, 1945, PPGC, box 1, Brush Foundation–historical.

Kaufman, A. R. to Mrs. Leslie D. Hawkridge, February 18, 1938, PPLM, box 13.

McClure, Mary L. to Bishop Schrembs, August 14, 1934. Records of Joseph Schrembs, Archives of the Diocese of Cleveland, Cleveland, Ohio.

Maxwell, Mrs. [W. E. Rogers], to Friend, n.d., PPGC, box 1, Brush Foundation–histories.

Shepard, Brooks, to Dorothy H. Brush, May 31 [1928]. CFB, box 1, folder 9.

Todd, T. Wingate, to G. Gaylord, September 23, 1930, December 3, 1930, December 1, 1937, PPGC, box 1, Brush Foundation–historical.

Unidentified [possibly Mrs. Walter Smith], MHA treasurer, to Rupert Knoepf, February 12, 1960. PPGC, box 2.

Wing, Virginia, to G. Gaylord, December 15, 1930. PPGC, box 1, Brush Foundation–historical.

Zuck, T., to G. Gaylord, Jan. 12, 1931, PPGC, box 1, Brush Foundation–historical.

## Maternal Health Association and Brush Foundation Reports, Scrapbooks, and Histories

1928–1938, MHA Scrapbook–Letters from Patients, PPGC, box 6.

1928–1938 Patient Register, PPGC, Trunk 2.

March 21, 1928–February 1, 1931, "An Analysis of Pregnancies Among 923 Patients of the Maternal Health Clinic," PPGC, box 2, miscellaneous speeches.

September 25, 1928, November 5, 1928, December 31, 1928, March 5, 1929, April 17, 1929, Minutes of the Brush Foundation Board of Managers, BF, series I, subseries A, container 1, folder 1.

March 22, 1928–April 1930, "Report of Two Years' Work," MHA, WRHS, vertical file.

March 22, 1928–March 21, 1931, "Report of Three Years' Work," MHA, MS-SS, clinics-Ohio.

[between 1929 and 1938], Todd, T. Wingate, "Preliminary suggestions for the scientific contribution of a birth control clinic," typescript. PPGC, box 1, Brush Foundation–historical.

1929, "That Children May be Given Every Chance for Mental and Physical Health," PPGC, box 2, annual reports.

1929–1935, MHA Scrapbook. PPGC, box 7.

Nov. 21, 1929, "Report of the Joint Committee of the Cleveland Maternal Health Clinic and the Brush Foundation," PPGC, box 1, Brush Foundation–historical.

October 7, 1930, "Report of the Executive Secretary of the Maternal Health Association to the Brush Foundation," PPGC, box 1, Brush Foundation–historical.

December 3, 1930, Minutes of the Brush Foundation Board of Managers, 1931–1949, BF, series I, sub-series A, container 1, folder 1.

March 1931–March 1932, MHA, "Report of Fourth Year," BCS, record group 2, series A.

October 29, 1931, "Report of the Executive Secretary of the Maternal Health Association to the Brush Foundation," PPGC, box 1, Brush Foundation–historical.

1934–1936 Minutes of the Brush Foundation, BF, series I, sub-series A, container 1, folder 1.

May 1934, Annual Report, PPGC, box 2, annual reports.

1935, MHA Scrapbook, PPGC, box 7.

1935, MHA Scrapbook Skating Carnival, PPGC, box 7.

March 24, 1935–March 31, 1936, Annual Report, PPGC, box 2, annual reports.

May 1935, MHA Annual Report, PPGC, box 2, annual reports.

1936–1937, MHA Scrapbook Skating Carnival, PPGC, box 7.

1936–1941, MHA Scrapbook, PPGC, box 7.

April 1, 1936–March 31, 1937, MHA Annual Report, PPGC, box 2, annual reports.

1937, MHA Annual Report, PPGC, box 2, annual reports.

April 1, 1937–March 31, 1938, MHA Annual Report, PPGC, box 2, annual reports.

April 26, 1937, Minutes of the Brush Foundation Board of Managers, BF, series I, sub-series A, container 1, folder 1

1938–1939 MHA of Ohio, Annual Report, PPCO, box 1, Scrapbook 1939–40.

1938–1950 MHA Scrapbook, Press Notices, PPGC, box 3.

April 1, 1938–March 31, 1939 Annual Report, PPGC, box 2, annual reports.

July 1, 1938–July 1, 1939, "Report of Education and Extension Work of the Executive Secretary of the Maternal Health Association," PPGC, box 1, Brush Foundation–historical.

September 1938, "Notes Taken at Board Meeting," PPGC, box 1, Brush Foundation–historical.

October 1938 (August 21, 1939), Maternal Health Association, Ohio. Clinic Report, MS-SS, clinics-Ohio

April 1, 1939–March 31, 1940, MHA Annual Report, PPGC, box 2, annual reports.

June 23, 1939, Minutes of the Brush Foundation Board of Managers, BF, series I, sub-series A, container 1, folder 1.

1940–1941, MHA of Ohio Annual Report, PPCO, box 1, Scrapbook 1939–40.

April 1, 1940–March 31, 1941, MHA Annual Report, PPGC, box 2, annual reports.

April 1, 1940–March 31, 1941, MHA, West Side Branch Annual Report, PPGC, box 2, annual reports.

April 15, 1940, "Brush Foundation Grant to Maternal Health Association," PPGC, box 1, Brush Foundation–historical.

April 1, 1941–March 31, 1942, MHA Annual Report, PPGC, box 2, annual reports.

April 14, 1943, Edna L. Rusch, "West Side Branch Seventh Annual Meeting, Clinic Report," PPGC, box 1.

April 1, 1945–March 31, 1946, MHA Annual Report, PPGC, box 2, annual reports.

1946, Theodore Hall. "Life in Our Hands, the Story of the Brush Foundation" (Cleveland: The Brush Foundation).

May 15, 1948, Bernard John Oliver Jr. "Maternal Health Association," unpublished manuscript, PPGC, box 3, early history.

April 1, 1950–March 31, 1951, MHA Annual Report, PPGC, box 2, annual reports.

1951–1953, MHA Scrapbook, PPGC, box 6.

April 1, 1951, "Newsletter for the friends and supporters of the Maternal Health Association," PPGC, box 1.

January 24, 1953, "Maternal Health Association," PPCO, box 2, folder 32.

1956–1957, MHA Scrapbook, PPGC, box 8.

April 1, 1955–March 31, 1956 MHA Annual Report, PPGC, box 2, annual reports.

1957, MHA, "History," pamphlet, box 3, early history.

1959, Mrs. Walter S. Smith, "History and Information Regarding the Maternal Health Association," typewritten manuscript, PPGC, box 3.

1960, "The Maternal Health Association, a Planned Parenthood Center, Service in 1960," PPGC, box 2, annual reports.

1960–1961, "The Maternal Health Association, Planned Parenthood Center," Thirty-third Annual Report, PPGC, box 2, annual reports.

June 1964, Betty Porcello, "The Maternal Health Association," PPGC, box 1, History of Planned Parenthood.

1966, PPGC Thirty-eighth Annual Report, PPGC, box 2, annual reports.

1970, PPGC Forty-second Annual Report, PPGC, box 2, annual reports.

1975, PPGC Forty-seventh Annual Report, PPGC, box 2, annual reports.

June 1982, PPGC, A Report of Planned Parenthood of Greater Cleveland, Inc., '81–'82, PPGC, box 2, annual reports.

[1984], Planned Parenthood Timeline, 1921–1983, copy in personal possession of the author.

1985, PPGC Annual Report, PPGC, box 2, annual reports.

January 16, 1988, Jean B. Evans, "60 Years of Planned Parenthood in Cleveland," Draft II, copy in personal possession of the author.

January 16, 1988, "Planned Parenthood Chronology, draft II," personal possession of the author.

1988, "Every Child a Wanted Child: 60 Years of Planned Parenthood in Cleveland," personal possession of the author.

1991, PPGC, "Taking a Stand," Annual Report, personal possession of the author.

June 24, 1999, Planned Parenthood of Greater Cleveland, "70 Years of Excellence 1928–1998," copy in personal possession of the author.

2003, Jimmy E. Wilkinson Meyer, Draft of PPGC 75th anniversary history, personal possession of the author.

2003, "Voices from the past, visions for the future," PPGC annual report 2001–2002, personal possession of the author.

2003, "Celebrating 75 years of Helping Women Lead Healthier Lives," PPGC anniversary History, personal possession of the author.

n.d. Brush Foundation, "The Brush Foundation 1928–1980."

n.d. "History," Untitled typewritten manuscript. BF, series IV, container 3, folder 46.

n.d. "The History of the Maternal Health Association," typewritten manuscript. PPGC, box 3, early histories.

n.d. "History—Planned Parenthood," BF, series IV, container 3, folder 46.

n.d. MHA Scrapbook–American Birth Control Leaflets, PPGC, box 3.

n.d. MHA Scrapbook–International, PPGC, box 6.

n.d. Untitled handwritten history, PPGC, box 3, early history.

n.d. [1957?] Untitled typewritten manuscripts [three different manuscripts], probably drafts for 1957 MHA "History," PPGC, box 3, early history.

n.d. Untitled typewritten manuscript, DHB, box 1, folder 17.

## Newspapers and Newsletters

*Bystander*
*Catholic Universe Bulletin*
*Cleveland Citizen*
*Cleveland Gazette*
*Cleveland News*
*Cleveland Plain Dealer*
*Cleveland Press*
*International Planned Parenthood News*
*Jewish Review and Observer*

Margaret Sanger Papers Project Newsletter
*New York Times*
Planned Parenthood. *Monthly Bulletin of the Family Planning Association of India*
*The Search Light,* Christian League for the Promotion of Purity, WRHS

### Speeches

Blanchard, Ferdinand Q. Address before annual meeting 1931, PPGC, box 2, talks.
———. "A Brief for Tomorrow's Children," American Birth Control League Session, National Conference of Social Work, 1937, PPGC, box 5, talks.
Brush, Dorothy Hamilton. Speech in Syracuse, n.d., DHB, box 1, folder 4.
"Founding a Family" (author unknown), Jackson, Michigan, January 1936. PPGC, box 2, miscellaneous speeches.
Frank, Lawrence K. "Towards a Re-orientation of the Birth Control Movement," unpublished speech presented at the Conference on Eugenics and Birth Control, January 28, 1938, New York City. PPGC, box 5, pamphlets.
Garvin, Charles. "The New Negro Physician," typescript, the Howard University School of Medicine, n.d. Charles Garvin papers, WRHS, container 1, folder 2.
Gaylord, Gladys. "Building for Tomorrow," May 17, 1944. PPGC, box 1, talks-miscellaneous.
———. "The Eugenic Value of a Maternal Health Center," May 27, 1939, printed in the *Journal of Heredity* 30 (1939). PPGC, box 2, miscellaneous speeches.
———. "Men and a Maternal Health Program," reprinted from *BCR* (June 1938). PPGC, box 2, miscellaneous speeches.
———. "Philosophies of a Maternal Health Association," West Side Annual Meeting, April 24, 1940. PPGC, box 6, West Side Branch minutes.
———. "Premarital and Preconceptional Care," the American Congress of Obstetrics and Gynecology, Cleveland, Ohio, September 11–15, 1939. PPGC, box 5, talks.
———. "Public Acceptance as Related to the Birth Control Field," Hamilton, Ontario, February 23, 1939. BCS, record group 62, series H.
Hansen, R. Illula Morrison. "Contraception: The Woman's Point of View," February 19, 1931, the Lakewood Clinical Luncheon Club. PPGC, box 2, speeches.
Higley, Charles S. "Men and Maternal Health" [1938]. PPGC, box 2, miscellaneous speeches.
"Interviewing" (author unknown), 1935. PPGC, box 2, talks.
Marcus, Sarah. "Talk Given at the Sixteenth Annual Meeting of the Maternal Health Association," May 17, 1944. PPGC, box 5.
Robishaw, Ruth A. "And There is the Child," talk given during the annual meeting of the Ohio State Nurses Association in Cleveland, May 5, 1939. Reprinted from *Ohio Nurses Review* 14, no. 4 (October 1939). PPGC, box 2, talks.
Rusch, Edna. "Talk Given at Sixteenth Annual Meeting, Maternal Health Association," May 17, 1944. PPGC, box 5, talks.
———. "Utilizing Community Resources in a Maternal Health Program," given at a meeting of nurses in Akron [Ohio], April 1940. PPGC, box 5, miscellaneous speeches.
Sanger, Margaret. "Chicago Address to Women," 1916. MS-SS, early speeches.
"Six Years With Family Regulation Problems" (author unknown), PPGC, box 2.

"Talk Prepared for A.A.U.W. Meeting, Zanesville" (author unknown), November 4, 1940. PPGC, box 2, talks.

"Talk to Public Health Nurses, Nov. 4, [19]40" (outline, author unknown). PPGC, box 2, talks.

"Tomorrow's Children" (author unknown). PPGC, box 2, talks.

Unidentified speech, untitled, n.d. BCS, record group 1, series C.

Wylie, Burdett. "Men and Maternal Health," February 11, 1938. PPGC, box 2, miscellaneous speeches.

## Secondary Sources

### Articles and Chapters

Baer, Joseph L. "Discussion." In *Surgery, Gynecology, and Obstetrics* 36, no. 3 (March 1923): 438.

Bailey, Judith. "The Long View of Health." *CWRU Magazine,* February 1992, 26–31.

Baird, Donna Day, Clarice R. Weinberg, Lynda F. Voigt, and Janet R. Daling. "Vaginal Douching and Reduced Fertility." *American Journal of Public Health* 86, no. 6 (June 1996): 844–50.

Balay, Anne G. "'Hands Full of Living': Birth Control, Nostalgia, and Kathleen Norris." *American Literary History* 8, no. 3 (1996): 471–96.

Borell, Merriley. "Biologists and the Promotion of Birth Control Research, 1918–1938." *Journal of the History of Biology* 20, no. 1 (spring 1987): 51–87.

Brooks, Carol Flora. "The Early History of the Anti-contraceptive Laws in Massachusetts and Connecticut." *American Quarterly* 18, no. 1 (spring 1966): 3–23.

Caron, Simone M. "Birth Control and the Black Community in the 1960s: Genocide or Power Politics?" *Journal of Social History* 31, no. 3 (spring 1998): 545–69.

Cook, Blanche Wiesen. "Female Support Networks and Political Activism: Lillian Wald, Crystal Eastman, Emma Goldman," *Chrysalis* 1 (1977): 43–61.

Cowan, Ruth Schwartz. "From Virginia Dare to Virginia Slims: Women and Technology in America." In *Dynamos and Virgins Revisited: Women and Technological Change in History,* ed. Martha Moore Trescott, 30–44. Metuchen, N.J.: Scarecrow, 1979.

Deutsch, Sara. "Learning to Talk More Like a Man: Boston Women's Class-Bridging Organizations, 1870–1940." *AHR* 97, no. 2 (April 1992): 379–404.

Dodd, Diane. "The Hamilton Birth Control Clinic of the 1930s." *Ontario History* 75, no. 1 (1983): 71–86.

Donchin, Anne. "The Future of Mothering: Reproductive Technology and Feminist Theory." *Hypatia* 1, no. 2 (fall 1986): 121–37.

Dyer, Kirsti A. "Curiosities of Contraception: A Historical Perspective." *JAMA* 264, no. 1 (December 5, 1990): 2818–19.

Flanagan, Maureen A. "Gender and Urban Political Reform: The City Club and the Women's City Club of Chicago in the Progressive Era." *AHR* 95, no. 4 (October 1990): 1032–50.

Freedman, Estelle. "'The New Woman': Changing Views of Women in the 1920s." *JAH* 61 (1974): 372–93.

———. "Separatism as Strategy: Female Institution Building and American Feminism, 1870–1930." *Feminist Studies* 5, no. 3 (fall 1979): 512–49.

Gamson, Joshua. "Commentary." *Journal of the History of Sexuality* 2, no. 1 (1991): 95–105.

———. "Rubber Wars: Struggles over the Condom in the United States." *Journal of the History of Sexuality* 1, no. 2 (1990): 262–82.

Garvin, Charles. "Cleveland's Forest City Hospital Celebrates First Birthday." *Journal of the National Medical Association* 51, no. 2 (March 1959): 150–53.

Gordon, Linda. "What's New in Women's History." In *Feminist Studies, Critical Studies*, ed. Teresa de Lauretis. Bloomington: Indiana University Press, 1986, 20–30.

Gosling, F. G., and Joyce Ray. "American Physicians and Birth Control, 1936–1947." *Journal of Social History* 18 (spring 1985): 399–411.

Haines, Michael. "Birthrate and Mortality." In *The Reader's Companion to American History*, ed. Eric Foner and John A. Garraty. Boston: Houghton Mifflin, 1991, 103–5.

Hall, Peter Dobkin. "Cultures of Trusteeship in the United States." In *Inventing the Nonprofit Sector and Other Essays on Philanthropy, Voluntarism, and Nonprofit Organizations*, 135–206. Baltimore, Md.: Johns Hopkins University Press, 1992.

Harris, Richard H. "Obscenity Law in Ohio." *Akron Law Review* 13, no. 3 (winter 1980): 520–39.

Horowitz, Helen Lefkowitz. "Victoria Woodhull, Anthony Comstock, and Conflict over Sex in the United States in the 1870s." *Journal of American History* 87, no. 2 (September 2000): 403–34.

Jameson, Elizabeth. "Women as Workers, Women as Civilizers: True Womanhood in the American West." In *The Women's West*, ed. Susan Armitage and Elizabeth Jameson, 145–64. Norman: University of Oklahoma Press, 1987.

Jensen, Joan. "The Evolution of Margaret Sanger's *Family Limitation* Pamphlet, 1914–1921." *Signs: Journal of Women in Culture and Society* 6 (spring 1981): 548–67.

Joffe, Carole. "Portraits of Three 'Physicians of Conscience': Abortion Before Legalization in the United States." *Journal of the History of Sexuality* 2, no. 1 (1991): 46–67.

Johnson, Beth DiNatale. "Creative Consensus: Elite Volunteers and Health Care Policy for the Aged." Unpublished paper presented at Women and Health Care in Cleveland Conference, Cleveland, Ohio, November 9, 1996.

Karl, Barry D., and Stanley N. Katz. "The American Private Philanthropic Foundation and the Public Sphere 1890–1930." *Minerva* 19 (1981): 243–45.

Kornbluh, Felicia A. "The New Literature on Gender and the Welfare State: The U.S. Case." *Feminist Studies* 22, no. 1 (spring 1996): 171–97.

Koven, Seth, and Sonya Michel. "Womanly Duties: Maternalist Politics and the Origins of Welfare States in France, Germany, Great Britain, and the United States 1880–1920." *AHR* 95, no. 4 (October 1990): 1076–108.

Kusmer, Kenneth L. "Black Cleveland and the Central-Woodland Community 1865–1930." In *Cleveland: A Metropolitan Reader*, ed. W. Dennis Keating, Norman Krumholz, and David C. Perry, 265–82. Kent, Ohio: Kent State University Press, 1995.

Laipson, Peter. "From Boudoir to Bookstore: Writing the History of Sexuality, A Review Article." *Comparative Study of Society and History* (October 1992): 636–44.

LaMay, Craig. "America's Censor: Anthony Comstock and Free Speech." *Communications and the Law* 19, no. 3 (September 1997): 1–59.

Leung, Marianne. "'Better Babies': Birth Control in Arkansas during the 1930s." In *Hidden Histories of Women in the New South,* edited by Virginia Bernhard et al., 52–68. Columbia: University of Missouri Press, 1994.

Lindenmeyer, Kriste. "Saving Mothers and Babies: The Sheppard-Towner Act in Ohio, 1921–1929." *Ohio History* 99 (summer–autumn 1990): 105–134.

Locke, Ralph. "Reflections on Art Music in America, on Stereotypes of the Woman Patron, and on Cha(lle)nges in the Present and Future." In *Cultivating Music in America: Women Patrons and Activists since 1860,* ed. Ralph P. Locke and Cyrilla Barr, 295–336. Berkeley: University of California Press, 1997.

Losure, Mary. "'Motherhood Protection' and the Minnesota Birth Control League." *Minnesota History* 54, no. 8 (winter 1995): 359–70.

Martin, Emily. "The Egg and the Sperm: How Science Has Constructed a Romance Based on Stereotypical Male-Female Roles." *Signs: Journal of Women in Culture and Society* 16, no. 3 (1991): 485–501.

Mead, Karen. "Beneficent Maternalism: Argentine Motherhood in Comparative Perspective, 1880–1920." *Journal of Women's History* 12, no. 3 (2000): 120–45.

Melcher, Mary. "'Women's Matters': Birth Control, Prenatal Care and Childbirth in Rural Montana 1910–1940." *Montana; the Magazine of Western History* 41 (spring 1991): 47–56.

Meyer, Jimmy Elaine Wilkinson. "Children and Youth." *ECH.* 2d ed. Edited by David D. Van Tassel and John Grabowski, 176–78. Bloomington: Indiana University Press, 1996.

———. "Intimate Connections: Trusteeship in Historical Perspective." In *Taking Trusteeship Seriously,* edited by Richard C. Turner, 47–58. Indianapolis: Indiana University Center on Philanthropy, 1995.

———. "Motherhood and Morality." *ACOG Clinical Review* (December 1996): 14–16.

———. and Michael McTigne. "Religion." *ECH.* 2d ed. Edited by David D. Van Tassel and John Grabowski, 854–58. Bloomington: Indiana University Press, 1996.

Morton, Marian J. "'Go and Sin No More': Maternity Homes in Cleveland, 1869–1936." *Ohio History* 93 (summer–autumn 1984): 117–46.

———. "Institutionalizing Inequalities: Black Children and Child Welfare in Cleveland, 1859–1998." *Journal of Social History* 34, no. 1 (2000): 141–62.

———. "Temperance Reform in the 'Providential Environment,' Cleveland, 1830–1934." In *Cleveland: A Tradition of Reform,* ed. David D. Van Tassel and John J. Grabowski, 50–66. Kent, Ohio: Kent State University Press, 1986.

Ostrander, Susan. "Knowing Her Place: How Elite Women Preserve the Power," *Cleveland* (May 1979): 76–77, 193–96.

Peacock, Nancy. "Everything You Always Wanted to Know About *Noblesse Oblige* but Were Afraid to Ask." *Cleveland,* May 1988, 96–100.

Pernick, Martin. "Eugenics and Public Health." *American Journal of Public Health* (November 1997): 1767–72.

Rodrigue, Jessie. "The Black Community and the Birth Control Movement." In *"We Specialize in the Wholly Impossible": A Reader in Black Women's History,* ed. Darlene Clark Hine et al., 505–20. New York: Carlson Publishing: 1995.

Rosenberg, Charles E. "Social Class and Medical Care in 19th Century America: The Rise and Fall of the Dispensary." In *Sickness and Health in America: Readings in the History of Medicine and Public Health,* 2d ed., ed. Judith Walzer Leavitt and Ronald L. Numbers, 273–86. Madison: University of Wisconsin, 1985.

Rothman, Sheila. "Women's Clinics or Doctor's Offices: The Sheppard-Towner Act and the Promotion of Preventive Health Care." In *Social History and Social Policy,* ed. David Rothman and Stanton Wheeler, 175–201. New York: Academic Press, 1981.

Ryan, Mary P. "The Power of Women's Networks: A Case Study of Female Moral Reform in Antebellum America." *Feminist Studies* 5, no. 1 (1979): 66–85.

Schoen, Johanna. "Between Choice and Coercion: Women and the Politics of Sterilization in North Carolina, 1929–1975," *Journal of Women's History* 13, no. 1 (2001): 132–56.

———. "Fighting for Child Health: Race, Birth Control, and the State in the Jim Crow South." *Social Politics* 4, no. 1(spring 1997): 90–113.

Scott, Joan. "The Evidence of Experience." *Critical Inquiry* 17 (summer 1991): 773–97.

Sharlet, Jeff. "Parlor Politics and Power: A New View of Washington Women." Review of *Parlor Politics: in which the ladies of Washington help build a city and a government,* by Catherine Allgor. *The Chronicle of Higher Education,* December 15, 2000, 16–17A.

"Thomas Wingate Todd." Physical Anthropology Centennial Number, *Journal of the National Medical Association* 51, no. 3 (May 1959): 223–25, 233–46.

Todd, Alexandra Dundas. "Women's Bodies as Diseased and Deviant: Historical and Contemporary Issues." *Research in Law, Deviance and Social Control* 5 (1983): 83–95.

Tone, Andrea. "Black Market Birth Control: Contraceptive Entrepreneurship and Criminality in the Gilded Age." *JAH* 87, no. 2 (September 2000): 435–59.

———. "Contraceptive Consumers: Gender and the Political Economy of Birth Control in the 1930s." *Journal of Social History* 29, no. 3 (spring 1996): 485–506.

———. "Making Room for Rubbers: Gender, Technology, and Birth Control Before the Pill." *History and Technology* 18, no. 1 (2002): 51.

van Kammen, Jessika. "Representing Users' Bodies: The Gendered Development of Anti-Fertility Vaccines." *Science, Technology, and Human Values* 24, no. 3 (summer 1999): 307–37.

Vandenberg-Daves, Jodi. "The Manly Pursuit of a Partnership between the Sexes: The Debate over YMCA Programs for Women and Girls, 1914–1933." *JAH* 78, no. 4 (March 1992): 1324–46.

Walkowitz, Daniel J. "The Making of a Feminine Professional Identity: Social Workers in the 1920s." *AHR* 95, no. 4 (October 1990): 1051–75.

Whelan, Edward P. "Cleveland's Mightiest Family." *Cleveland,* December 1976, 52–59, 178, 180.

Whitesitt, Linda. "Women as 'Keepers of Culture': Music Clubs, Community Concert Series, and Symphony Orchestras." In *Cultivating Music in America: Women Patrons and Activists since 1860,* ed. Ralph P. Locke and Cyrilla Barr, 65–86. Berkeley: University of California Press, 1997.

Wood, James M. "Cleveland Medicine's Incredible Ghosts." *Cleveland* magazine, July 1983, 56–60, 127–30.

## Books and Pamphlets

Apple, Rima D. *Mothers and Medicine: A Social History of Infant Feeding, 1890–1950.* Madison: University of Wisconsin Press, 1987.

Apple, Rima D., and Janet Golden, eds. *Mothers and Motherhood: Readings in American History.* Columbus: Ohio State University Press, 1997.

Asbell, Bernard. *The Pill: A Biography of the Drug That Changed the World.* New York: Random House, 1995.

Bailey, Beth L. *From Front Porch to Back Seat: Courtship in Twentieth-Century America.* Baltimore, Md.: Johns Hopkins University Press, 1988.

Bailey, Thomas. *For the Public Good.* Hamilton, Ontario: Planned Parenthood Society of Hamilton, 1974.

Bates, Louise. *Weeder in the Garden of the Lord: Anthony Comstock's Life and Career.* Lanham, Md.: University Press of America, 1995.

Beisel, Nicola. *Imperiled Innocents: Anthony Comstock and Family Reproduction in Victorian America.* Princeton: Princeton University Press, 1997.

Blackford, Mansel G., and K. Austin Kerr. *BFGoodrich: Tradition and Transformation, 1870–1995.* Columbus: Ohio State University Press, 1996.

Blair, Karen J. *A History of Women's Voluntary Organizations.* Boston: G. K. Hall, 1987.

The Boston Women's Health Collective. *The New Our Bodies, Ourselves: Updated and Expanded for the '90s.* New York: Simon and Schuster, 1992.

Boyer, Paul S. *Purity in Print: Book Censorship in America from the Gilded Age to the Computer Age,* 2d ed. Madison: University of Wisconsin Press, 2002.

Bremner, Robert H. *American Philanthropy.* 2d ed. Chicago: University of Chicago Press, 1960, 1988.

Brief *amicus curiae* of 281 American Historians. *Webster v. Reproductive Health Services,* et al. (October 1988).

Brodie, Janet Farrell. *Contraception and Abortion in 19th Century America.* Ithaca, N.Y.: Cornell University Press, 1994.

Brown, Kent L., ed. *The History of Medicine in Cleveland and Cuyahoga County.* Cleveland: Academy of Medicine, 1977.

Bruns, Roger A. *The Damnedest Radical: The Life and World of Ben Reitman, Chicago's Celebrated Social Reformer, Hobo King, and Whorehouse Physician.* Urbana: University of Illinois Press, 1987.

Campbell, Thomas F. *SASS: Fifty Years of Social Work Education.* Cleveland: Case Western Reserve University Press, 1967.

Campbell, Thomas, and Edward Miggins, eds. *The Birth of Modern Cleveland, 1865–1930.* Cleveland: Western Reserve Historical Society, 1988.

Carter, Richard. *The Gentle Legions.* New York: Doubleday, 1961.

Chafe, William. *The American Woman: Her Changing Social, Economic, and Political Roles, 1920–1970.* New York: Oxford University Press, c. 1972, 1974.

Chesler, Ellen. *Woman of Valor: Margaret Sanger and the Birth Control Movement in America.* New York: Simon and Schuster, 1992.

Cigliano, Jan. *Showplace of America: Cleveland's Euclid Avenue, 1850–1910.* Kent, Ohio: Kent State University Press, 1991.

Corbett, Katharine T. *In Her Place: A Guide to St. Louis Women's History.* St. Louis, Mo.: Historical Society Press, 1999.

Corea, Gena. *The Mother Machine: Reproductive Technologies from Artificial Insemination to Artificial Wombs.* New York: Harper and Row, 1985.

Cott, Nancy. *The Grounding of Modern Feminism.* New Haven, Conn.: Yale University Press, 1987.

———. *Public Vows: A History of Marriage and the Nation.* Cambridge, Mass.: Harvard University Press, 2000.

Cramer, C. H. *Case Western Reserve: A History of the University, 1826–1976.* Boston: Little, Brown, 1976.

Crocker, Ruth Hutchinson. *Social Work and Social Order: The Settlement Movement in Two Industrial Cities, 1889–1930.* Urbana: University of Illinois Press, 1992.

Curry, Lynne. *Modern Mothers in the Heartland: Gender, Health, and Progress in Illinois, 1900–1930.* Columbus: The Ohio State University Press, 1999.

de Arellano, Annette B. Ramirez, and Conrad Seipp. *Colonialism, Catholicism, and Contraception: A History of Birth Control in Puerto Rico.* Chapel Hill: University of North Carolina Press, 1983.

Degler, Carl. *At Odds: Women and the Family in America from the Revolution to the Present.* New York: Oxford University Press, 1980.

———. *In Search of Human Nature: The Decline and Revival of Darwinism in American Social Thought.* New York: Oxford University Press, 1991.

D'Emilio, John, and Estelle Freedman. *Intimate Matters: A History of Sexuality in America.* New York: Harper and Row, 1988.

Dienes, C. Thomas. *Law, Politics and Birth Control.* Urbana: University of Illinois Press, 1972.

Ditzion, Sidney. *Marriage Morals and Sex in America: A History of Ideas.* New York: W. W. Norton, 1969, 1953.

Ehrenreich, Barbara, and Deidre English. *For Her Own Good: 150 Years' of the Experts' Advice to Women.* Garden City, N.Y.: Anchor Books, 1969.

Ellis, W. D., Pauline G. Fanslow, and Nancy A. Schneider. *The Home Club: The Cleveland Skating Club Story.* n.p.: n.d.

Ernst, Morris L., and Alan U. Schwartz. *Censorship: The Search for the Obscene.* New York: Macmillan, 1964.

Evans, Sara. *Born for Liberty: A History of Women In America.* New York: Free Press, 1989.

Farnham, Eleanor. *Pioneering in Public Health Education.* Cleveland: Press of Western Reserve University, 1964.

Feldt, Gloria, with Carol Trickett Jennings. *Behind Every Choice Is a Story.* Denton: University of North Texas Press, 2003.

Fitzpatrick, Ellen. *Endless Crusade: Women Social Scientists and Progressive Reform.* New York: Oxford University Press, 1990.

Foucault, Michael. *The History of Sexuality, Vol. I: An Introduction.* New York: Vintage, c. 1978, 1980.

Fryer, Peter. *The Birth Controllers.* New York: Stein and Day, 1965.

Gamble, Vanessa Northington. *Making a Place for Ourselves: The Black Hospital Movement, 1920–1945.* New York: Oxford University Press, 1995.

Garrow, David J. *Liberty and Sexuality: The Right to Privacy and the Making of Roe v. Wade.* New York: Macmillan, 1994.

Gartner, Lloyd P. *History of the Jews in Cleveland.* 2d ed. Cleveland: Western Reserve Historical Society, 1978.

Gerlach, Luther, and Virginia Hine. *People, Power and Change: Movements of Social Transformation.* Indianapolis: Bobbs-Merrill, 1970.

Golden, Janet. *A Social History of Wet Nursing In America: From Breast to Bottle.* Columbus: The Ohio State University Press, 2001.

Gordon, Linda. *The Moral Property of Women: A History of Birth Control Politics in America.* Urbana: University of Illinois Press, 2002.

————. *Pitied But Not Entitled: Single Mothers and the History of Welfare.* Rev. ed. New York: Free Press, 1994.

————. *Woman's Body, Woman's Right: A Social History of Birth Control in America.* New York: Penguin, 1990, 1974.

Gottlieb, Mark. *The Lives of University Hospitals of Cleveland.* Cleveland: Wilson Street Press, 1991.

Grabowski, John J. *Sports in Cleveland.* Bloomington: Indiana University Press, 1992.

Green, Dorothy, and Mary-Elizabeth Murdock, eds. *Margaret Sanger Centennial Conference, November 13 & 14, 1979.* Northampton, Mass.: Sophia Smith Collection, Smith College, 1982.

Green, Harvey. *The Light of the Home: An Intimate View of the Lives of Women in Victorian America.* New York: Pantheon Books, 1983.

Grossberg, Michael. *Governing the Hearth: Law and the Family in Nineteenth Century America.* Chapel Hill: University of North Carolina, 1986.

————. *A Judgment for Solomon: The D'Hauteville Case and the Legal Experience in Antebellum America.* Cambridge: Cambridge University Press, 1996.

Guttmacher, Mrs. Alan, comp. *Planned Parenthood Beginnings: Affiliate Histories.* N.p., 1979.

Hall, Ruth, ed. *Dear Dr. Stopes: Sex in the 1920s.* Middlesex, England: Penguin Books, 1978.

Hartmann, Betsy. *Reproductive Rights and Wrongs: The Global Politics of Poulation Control.* New York: Harper and Row, 1987.

Hartmann, Mary, and Lois Banner, eds. *Clio's Consciousness Raised: New Perspectives on the History of Women.* New York: Harper Colophon, 1974.

Hatcher, Robert A. et al., eds. *Contraceptive Technology, 1988–89,* 14th rev. ed. New York: Irvington Publishers, 1989.

Hewitt, Nancy. *Women's Activism and Social Change: Rochester, New York, 1822–1872.* Ithaca, N.Y.: Cornell University Press, 1984.

Hewitt, Nancy A., and Suzanne Lebsock. *Visible Women: New Essays on American Activism.* Urbana and Chicago: University of Illinois Press, 1993.

Higham, John. *Strangers in the Land.* 2d ed. New Brunswick, N.J.: Rutgers University Press, 1981.

Hill, Reuben, J. Mayone Stycos, and Kurt W. Back. *The Family and Population Control: A Puerto Rican Experiment in Social Change.* Chapel Hill: University of North Carolina Press, 1959.

Hine, Darlene Clark. *Black Women in White: Racial Conflict and Cooperation in the Nursing Profession 1890–1950.* Bloomington: Indiana University Press, 1989.

————. *Hine Sight: Black Women and the Re-construction of American History.* Bloomington: Indiana University Press, 1989.

Hine, Darlene Clark, and Kathleen Thompson. *A Shining Thread of Hope: The History of Black Women in America.* New York: Broadway Books, 1998.

Holt, Marilyn Irvin. *Linoleum, Better Babies, and the Modern Farm Woman, 1890–1930.* Albuquerque: University of New Mexico Press, 1995.

Huston, Perdita. *Motherhood by Choice: Pioneers in Women's Health and Family Planning.* New York: The Feminist Press at the City University of New York, 1992.

Ireland, Louise Ireland Grimes. *Ligi: A Life in the Twentieth Century.* N.p., 1999.

Irvine, Janice M. *Disorders of Desire: Sex and Gender in Modern American Sexology.* Philadelphia: Temple University Press, 1990.

Jacobs, Aletta. *Memories: My Life as an International Leader in Health, Suffrage, and Peace.* Ed. Harriet Feinberg. New York: Feminist Press, 1996.

Joffe, Carole. *Doctors of Conscience: The Struggle to Provide Abortion Before and After Roe v. Wade.* Boston: Beacon, 1995.

Jones, James H. *Bad Blood: The Tuskegee Syphilis Experiment.* New York: The Free Press, 1981.

Katz, Michael, Michael J. Doucet, and Mark J. Stern. *The Social Organization of Early Industrial Capitalism.* Cambridge, Mass.: Harvard University Press, 1982.

Keller, Morton. *Affairs of the State: Public Life in Late Nineteenth Century America.* Cambridge, Mass.: Belknap Press, 1977.

Kennedy, David. *Birth Control in America: The Career of Margaret Sanger.* New Haven, Conn.: Yale University Press, 1970.

Kevles, Daniel. *In the Name of Eugenics: Genetics and the Uses of Human Heredity.* New York: Knopf, 1985.

Kline, Wendy. *Building a Better Race: Gender, Sexuality, and Eugenics from the Turn of the Century to the Baby Boom.* Berkeley: University of California Press, 2001.

Koven, Seth, and Sonya Michel, eds. *Mothers of a New World: Maternalist Politics and the Origins of Welfare States.* New York: Routledge, 1993.

Kuper, Adam. *The Chosen Primate: Human Nature and Cultural Diversity.* Cambridge, Mass.: Harvard University Press, 1994.

Kusmer, Kenneth L. *A Ghetto Takes Shape: Black Cleveland 1870–1930.* Urbana: Illinois University Press, 1978.

Ladd-Taylor, Molly. *Mother-work: Women, Child Welfare, and the State, 1890–1930.* Urbana and Chicago: University of Illinois Press, 1994.

———. *Raising a Baby the Government Way: Mother's Letters to the Children's Bureau, 1915–1932.* New Brunswick, N.J.: Rutgers University Press, 1986.

Larson, Edward J. *Sex, Race, and Science: Eugenics in the Deep South.* Baltimore, Md.: The Johns Hopkins University Press, 1995.

Lay, Mary M. *The Rhetoric of Midwifery: Gender, Knowledge and Power.* New Brunswick, N.J.: Rutgers University Press, 2000.

Leavitt, Judith Walzer. *Brought to Bed: Childbearing in America, 1750 to 1950.* New York: Oxford University Press, 1986.

———. *The Healthiest City: Milwaukee and the Politics of Health Care Reform.* Madison: University of Wisconsin Press, 1996, 1982.

———, ed. *Women and Health in America: Historical Readings.* Madison: University of Wisconsin Press, 1984.

Leavitt, Judith Walzer, and Ronald L. Numbers, eds. *Sickness and Health in America: Readings in the History of Medicine and Public Health.* Madison: University of Wisconsin Press, 1985.

Lebsock, Suzanne. *Free Women of Petersburg: Status and Culture in a Southern Town, 1784–1860.* New York: Norton, 1984.

Lederer, Susan E. *Subjected to Science: Human Experimentation in America before the Second World War.* Baltimore, Md.: Johns Hopkins University Press, 1995.

Lee, Nancy Howell. *The Search for an Abortionist.* Chicago: University of Chicago Press, 1969.

Leiby, James. *A History of Social Welfare and Social Work in the United States.* New York: Columbia University Press, 1978.

Lerner, Gerda. *The Majority Finds Its Past: Placing Women in History.* New York: Oxford University Press, 1979.

Lewis, Joanne. *In Our Day; Cleveland Heights: Its People, Its Places, Its Past.* Cleveland: Heights Community Congress, n.d.

Love, Steve, and David Giffels. *Wheels of Fortune: The Story of Rubber in Akron.* Akron, Ohio: Akron University Press, 1999.

Lubove, Roy. *The Professional Altruist: The Emergence of Social Work as a Career, 1880–1930.* Cambridge, Mass.: Harvard University Press, 1965.

Lystra, Karen. *Searching the Heart: Women, Men, and Romantic Love in Nineteenth-Century America.* New York: Oxford University Press, 1989.

McCann, Carole R. *Birth Control Politics in the United States, 1916–1945.* Ithaca, N.Y.: Cornell University Press, 1994.

McCary, James Leslie. *Human Sexuality: Physiological and Psychological Factors of Sexual Behavior.* New York: Van Nostrand Reinhold, 1967.

Marcus, George E., with Peter Dobkin Hall. *Lives in Trust: The Fortunes of Dynastic Families in Late Twentieth Century America.* Boulder, Colo.: Westview Press, 1992.

Martin, Emily. *The Woman in the Body: A Cultural Analysis of Reproduction.* Boston: Beacon, 1987.

May, William F. *The Physician's Covenant: Images of the Healer in Medical Ethics.* Philadelphia: The Westminster Press, 1983.

McCarthy, Kathleen. *Women's Culture: American Philanthropy and Art, 1830–1930.* Chicago: University of Chicago Press, 1991.

———, ed. *Lady Bountiful Revisited: Women, Philanthropy, and Power.* New Brunswick, N.J.: Rutgers University Press, 1990.

McGee, Glenn. *The Perfect Baby: A Pragmatic Approach to Eugenics.* New York: Rowman and Littlefield, 1997.

McLaren, Angus. *A History of Contraception: From Antiquity to the Present Day.* London: Basil Blackwell, 1990.

———. *Our Own Master Race: Eugenics in Canada, 1885–1945.* Toronto, Ontario: McClelland and Stewart, 1990.

McLaren, Angus, and Arlene Tigar McLaren. *The Bedroom and the State: Changing Practices and Politics of Contraception and Abortion in Canada, 1880–1980.* Toronto: McClelland and Stewart, 1986.

McLaughlin, Loretta. *The Pill, John Rock, and the Church: The Biography of a Revolution.* Boston: Little, Brown and Company, 1982.

Melosh, Barbara. *"The Physician's Hand": Work, Culture and Conflict in American Nursing.* Philadelphia: Temple University Press, 1982.

Messer, Ellen, and Kathryn E. May. *Back Rooms: Voices from the Illegal Abortion Era.* Buffalo, N.Y.: Prometheus Books, 1994.

Miller, Carol Poh, and Robert A. Wheeler. *Cleveland: A Concise History, 1796–1996.* 2d ed. Bloomington: Indiana University Press, 1997.

Mohr, James. *Abortion in America: The Origins and Evolution of National Policy, 1800–1900.* New York: Oxford University Press, 1978.

Moore, Martha, ed. *Dynamos and Virgins Revisited: Women and Technological Change in History.* Metuchen, N.J.: Scarecrow, 1979.

Morantz, Regina Markell, Cynthia Stodola Pomerleau, and Carol Hansen Fenichel, eds. *In Her Own Words: Oral Histories of Women Physicians.* New Haven, Conn.: Yale University Press, 1982.

Morgen, Sandra. *Into Our Own Hands: The Women's Health Movement in the United States, 1969–1990.* New Brunswick, N.J.: Rutgers University Press, 2002.

Morton, Marian. *And Sin No More: Social Policy and Unwed Mothers in Cleveland, 1855–1990.* Columbus: Ohio State University Press, 1993.

Muncy, Robyn L. *Creating a Female Dominion in American Reform, 1890–1930.* New York: Oxford University Press, 1991.

Murphy, James S. *The Condom Industry in the United States.* Jefferson, N.C.: McFarland, 1990.

Murray, Robert K. *Red Scare: A Study in National Hysteria, 1919–1920.* Minneapolis: University of Minnesota Press, 1955.

Noonan, John T., Jr. *Contraception: A History of Its Treatment by the Catholic Theologians and Canonists.* Cambridge, Mass.: Belknap Press, 1965.

Novak, Emil. *Textbook of Gynecology.* 5th ed. Baltimore, Md.: Williams and Wilkins, 1956.

Ostrander, Susan A. *Women of the Upper Class.* Philadelphia: Temple University Press, 1984.

Ostrower, Francie. *Why the Wealthy Give: The Culture of Elite Philanthropy.* Princeton, N.J.: Princeton University Press, 1995.

Pease, Jane H., and William Pease. *Ladies, Women and Wenches: Choice and Constraint in Antebellum Charleston and Boston.* Chapel Hill: University of North Carolina Press, 1990.

Pernick, Martin. *The Black Stork: Eugenics and the Death of Defective Babies in American and Motion Pictures Since 1915.* New York: Oxford University Press, 1996.

Petchesky, Rosalind Pollack. *Abortion and Woman's Choice: The State, Sexuality and Woman's Freedom.* Boston: Northeastern University Press, 1984.

Phillips, Kimberley. *AlabamaNorth: African-American Migrants, Community, and Working-Class Activism in Cleveland, 1915–45.* Urbana: University of Chicago Press, 1999.

Pivar, David J. *Purity Crusade: Sexual Morality and Social Control, 1868–1900.* Westport, Conn.: Greenwood Press, 1973.

Planned Parenthood Federation of America. *A Tradition of Choice: Planned Parenthood at 75.* New York: Planned Parenthood Federation of America, 1991.

Reagan, Leslie J. *When Abortion Was a Crime: Women, Medicine, and Law in the United States, 1867–1973.* Berkeley: University of California Press, 1997.

Reed, James. *The Birth Control Movement in American Society: From Private Vice to Public Virtue.* Princeton, N.J.: Princeton University Press, 1978, 1984.

Reis, Elizabeth, ed. *American Sexual Histories.* Oxford: Blackwell Publishers, 2001.

Reverby, Susan M., ed. *Tuskegee's Truths: Rethinking the Tuskegee Syphilis Study.* Chapel Hill: University of North Carolina Press, 2000.

Reynolds, Moira Davison. *Women Advocates of Reproductive Rights: Eleven Who Led the Struggle in the United States and Great Britain.* Jefferson, N.C.: McFarland, 1994.

Riddle, John M. *Eve's Herbs: A History of Contraception and Abortion in the West.* Cambridge, Mass.: Harvard University Press, 1997.

Roberts, Dorothy. *Killing the Black Body: Race Reproduction, and the Meaning of Liberty.* New York: Pantheon, 1997.

Robertson, William H. *An Illustrated History of Contraception.* Park Ridge, New Jersey: Parthenon, 1990.

Rose, June. *Marie Stopes and the Sexual Revolution.* London: Faber and Faber, 1992.

Rose, William Ganson. *Cleveland: The Making of A City.* Cleveland: World, 1950. Reprint, Kent, Ohio: Kent State University, 1990.

Rosenberg, Charles E. *The Care of Strangers: The Rise of America's Hospital System.* New York: Basic Books, 1987.

Rosner, David. *A Once Charitable Enterprise: Hospitals and Health Care in Brooklyn and New York, 1885–1915.* Princeton, N.J.: Princeton University Press, 1982.

Rothman, Sheila. *Woman's Proper Place: A History of Changing Ideals and Practices, 1870 to the Present.* New York: Basic Books, 1978.

Rowbotham, Sheila. *Women in Movement: Feminism and Social Action.* New York: Routledge, 1992.

Satter, Beryl. *Each Mind a Kingdom: American Women, Sexual Purity, and the New Thought Movement.* Berkeley: University of California Press, 1999.

Scharf, Lois. *To Work and To Wed: Female Employment, Feminism and the Great Depression.* Westport, Conn.: Greenwood Press, 1980.

Scharf, Lois, and Joan Jensen, eds. *Decades of Discontent: The Women's Movement, 1920–1940.* Boston: Northeastern University Press, 1987.

Scott, Anne Firor. *Making the Invisible Woman Visible.* Urbana: University of Illinois Press, 1984.

———. *Natural Allies: Women's Associations in American History.* Urbana: University of Illinois Press, 1991.

Shepherd, Naomi. *A Price Below Rubies: Jewish Women as Rebels and Radicals.* Cambridge, Mass.: Harvard University Press, 1993.

Skocpol, Theda. *Protecting Soldiers and Mothers: The Political Origins of Social Policy in the United States.* Cambridge, Mass.: Belknap Press, 1992.

Smith, Susan L. *Sick and Tired of Being Sick and Tired: Black Women's Health Activism in America 1890–1950.* Philadelphia: University of Pennsylvania Press, 1995.

Starr, Paul. *The Social Transformation of American Medicine: The Rise of a Sovereign Profession and the Making of a Vast Industry.* New York: Basic Books, 1982.

Stevens, Rosemary. *In Sickness and Wealth: American Hospitals in the Twentieth Century.* New York: Basic Books, 1989.

Tittle, Diana. *Rebuilding Cleveland: The Cleveland Foundation and Its Evolving Urban Strategy.* Columbus: The Ohio State University Press, 1992.

Tone, Andrea. *Devices and Desires: A History of Contraceptives in America.* New York: Hill and Wang, 2001.

Tuennerman-Kaplan, Laura. *Helping Others, Helping Ourselves: Power, Giving, and Community Identity in Cleveland, Ohio, 1880–1930.* Kent, Ohio: Kent State University Press, 2001.

Van Horn, Susan Householder. *Women, Work and Fertility, 1900–1986.* New York: New York University Press, 1988.

Van Tassel, David D., and John J. Grabowski, eds. *Cleveland: A Tradition of Reform.* Kent, Ohio: Kent State University Press, 1986.

Waite, Florence T. *A Warm Friend for the Spirit: A History of the Family Service Association of Cleveland and Its Forebears, 1830–1952.* Cleveland: Family Service Association, 1960.

Waite, Frederick Clayton. *Western Reserve University Centennial History of the School of Medicine.* Cleveland: Western Reserve University Press, 1946.

Walsh, Mary Roth. *Doctors Wanted No Women Need Apply: Sexual Barriers in the Medical Profession, 1835–1975.* New Haven, Conn.: Yale University Press, 1977.

Wandersee, Winifred D. *Women's Work and Family Values 1920–1940.* Cambridge, Mass.: Harvard University Press, 1981.

Ware, Susan. *Beyond Suffrage: Women in the New Deal.* Cambridge, Mass.: Harvard University Press, 1981.

Wattleton, Faye. *Life on the Line.* New York City: Ballantine Books, 1996.

Weaver, Warren. *U.S. Philanthropic Foundations: Their History, Structure, Management and Record.* New York: Harper and Row, 1967.

Weinberg, Roy D. *Laws Governing Family Planning.* Dobbs Ferry, N.Y.: Oceana Publications, 1968.

Wells, Robert. *Revolutions in Americans' Lives: A Demographic Perspective.* Westport, Conn.: Greenwood Press, 1982.

White, Deborah Gray. *Too Heavy a Load: Black Women in Defense of Themselves 1894–1994.* New York: Norton, 1999.

Wiebe, Robert. *The Search for Order, 1877–1920.* New York: Hill and Wang, 1967.

Williams, Doone, and Greer Williams. *Every Child a Wanted Child: Clarence James Gamble, M.D., and His Work in the Birth Control Movement.* Cambridge, Mass.: Harvard University Press, 1978.

## Dissertations and Theses

Aseltine, Gwendolyn Pementer. "The Planned Parenthood Association of Nashville." Ph.D. diss., George Peabody College for Teachers, 1977.

Bates, Anna Louise. "Protective Custody: A Feminist Interpretation of Anthony Comstock's Life and Laws." Ph.D. diss., State University of New York at Binghamton, 1990.

Brodie, Janet Farrell. "Family Limitation in American Culture, 1830–1900." Ph.D. diss., University of Chicago, 1982.

Cairns, Allen. "Fighting for Life: Ideology, Social Networks, and Recruitment of Activists to a Pro-Life Movement Organization." Ph.D. diss., State University of New York at Buffalo, 1981.

Davis, Goldie M. "The Maternal Health Association of Cleveland, Ohio. The Organization, Development and Policies of This Agency and Its Relation to Other Health and Social Agencies in Cleveland." Master's thesis, School of Applied Social Sciences, Western Reserve University, 1938.

Dillberger, Cigi B. "From Woman Rebel to Birth Control Advocate: Margaret Sanger's Transformation, 1914–1915." Master's thesis, Florida Atlantic University, 1987.

Dodd, Diane. "The Canadian Birth Control Movement 1929–1939." Master's thesis, University of Toronto, 1982. Ontario Institute for Studies in Education, Toronto, Ontario.

Eisenmann, Harry J., III. "Charles F. Brush: Pioneer Innovator in Electrical Technology." Ph.D. diss., Case Institute of Technology, 1967.

Goldstein, Linda Lehmann. "Roses Bloomed in Winter: Women Medical Graduates of Western Reserve College, 1852–56." Ph.D. diss., Case Western Reserve University, 1989.

Holz, Rosemarie Petra. "The Birth Control Clinic in America: Life Within, Life Without, 1923–1972." Ph.D. diss., University of Illinois at Urbana-Champaign, 2002.

Horner, Katherine. "The Contribution of the Maternal Health Association of Cleveland, Ohio, to Marital Adjustment." Master's thesis, Western Reserve University, School of Social Sciences, 1939.

Johnson, Richard Christian. "Anthony Comstock: Reform, Vice and the American Way." Ph.D. diss., University of Wisconsin, 1973.

Kaiser, Clara Anne. "Organized Social Work in Cleveland, Its History and Setting." Ph.D. diss., Ohio State University, 1936.

Lavin, Anne Lee. "They do go home again: A follow-up study. . . ." Master's thesis, School of Applied Social Sciences, Western Reserve University, 1946. CWRU Archives.

Mehler, Barry Alan. "A History of the American Eugenics Society, 1921–1940." Ph.D. diss., University of Illinois at Urbana-Champaign, 1988.

Meyer, Jimmy E. Wilkinson. "Birth Control Policy, Practice, and Prohibition in the 1930s: The Maternal Health Association of Cleveland, Ohio." Ph.D. diss., Case Western Reserve University, 1993.

Onorato, Suzanne Amelia. "Organizational Legitimacy and the Social Construction of Contraceptives: The Politics of Technological Choice." Ph.D. diss., Duke University, 1990.

Rodrigue, Jessie May. "The Afro-American Community and the Birth Control Movement, 1918–1942." Ph.D. diss., University of Massachusetts, 1991.

Ross, Brian. "The New Philanthropy: The Reorganization of Charity in Turn of the Century Cleveland." Ph.D diss., Case Western Reserve University, 1989.

Schoen, Johanna. "'A great thing for poor folks': Birth Control, Sterlization, and Abortion in Public Health and Welfare in the Twentieth Century." Ph.D. diss., University of North Carolina at Chapel Hill, 1996.

Sullivan, Michael Anne. "Walking the Line: Birth Control and Women's Health at the Santa Fe Maternal Health Center 1937–1970." Master's thesis, University of New Mexico, 1995.

Turner, William B. "Of Class and Contraceptives: Birth Control in Nashville, Tennessee, 1932–1944." Master's thesis, Vanderbilt University, 1992.

Viterbo, Paula. "The Promise of Rhythm: The Determinators of the Women's Time of Ovulation and Its Social Impact in the United States, 1920–1940." Ph.D. diss., State University of New York at Stony Brook, 2000.

**Websites**

Margaret Sanger Papers Project, New York University, ed. Esther Katz, <http://www.nyu.edu/projects/sanger>.

Women and Social Movements in the United States, 1830–1930, ed. Katherine Sklar, State University of New York-Binghamton, <http://womhist.binghamton.edu/>.

# Index

AAUW. *See* American Association of University Women

abortifacients, 2, 9, 42

abortion, 13–14, 15, 16, 68, 95; attitudes toward, 3, 104; avoiding, 99; as birth control, 10, 18, 99–100; birth control clinics opposed to, 94; debates about, 170; fear of, 99–100; legal prosecution and, 99, 113, 227n. 73; MHA physicians and, 222n. 29; and morality, 100; networks and, 134, 233n. 50; Ohio ban upon, 57 fig. 11, 99, 224n. 43; at PPGC, 174; regulation of, 4–7, 99; U.S. government and, 99, 170; women's experience of, 99–100

abortionists, 13; locating, 134; in Montana, 134; in New York City, 6

abstinence, 3, 10, 18, 25–26; disadvantages of, 112; effectiveness of, 192n. 41

Academy of Medicine, American. *See* American Academy of Medicine

Academy of Medicine of Cleveland, 60, 82, 139 fig. 23, 142

Adams, Edgar E., 228n. 7, 229–30n. 20; as MHA board member, 70 fig. 14

Adams, Elizabeth Carlton, 229–30n. 20; as MHA board member, 70 fig. 14

Adams, Jane. *See* Hamilton, Jane Adams

Adams, Thomas, 198n. 79

advertisement: of birth control, 2, 77, 113; clinic clients as providing, 134; of ice skating shows, 128–30. *See also* Maternal Health Association, advertising of

*Advice to a Mother* (Chavasse), 187n.12

*Advice to a Wife* (Chavasse), 187n.12

African Americans, xv, 21, 22, 50 fig. 10, 208n. 64, 235n. 69; better babies and, 153; birth control and, 90, 169, 185n.13, 196n. 66, 220–21n. 17; birth rate of, 25, 235n. 69; call for separate hospital, 87; childlessness and, 198n. 82; in Cleveland, 22, 86–88, 146, 219n. 9; distrust of white medical institutions, 89, 220n. 17; eugenics and, 146, 196n. 66; as hospital staff, 87; MHA and, 156; as MHA clients, 88, 90, 232n. 44; as MHA staff, 156, 172; as managing branch clinic, 146; as physicians, 87; proportion of population, 88, 188n. 70; race uplift and, 154. *See also* children, African American; *Cleveland Gazette;* eugenics, African Americans and; families, African American; newspapers, African American; nurses, African American; physicians, African American; women, African American

*AJOG. See American Journal of Obstetrics and Gynecology*

Akron (Ohio), 133, 143, 157

Albany (New York), 47, 74, 207n. 59

Allen, Margaret. *See* Ireland, Margaret Allen

Allen de Ford, Miriam, 185n.18

Allgor, Catherine, 164

Almy, Madeleine. *See* Mather, Madeleine Almy

AMA. *See* American Medical Association

American Academy of Medicine, 35

American Association of University Women (AAUW), MHA outreach to, 148–49

American Birth Control Conference (1921), 30, 38, 57 fig. 11

American Birth Control League (ABCL), 38, 60, 149, 158, 211–12n. 21; condom use and, 223n. 36; fund-raising and, 59; letters to, 109, 112, 141; membership fees of, 58; merger into BCFA, 57 fig. 11, 59; MHA lack of affiliation with, 58, 64; as model for MHA, 92; officers of,

# WOMEN AND HEALTH: CULTURAL AND SOCIAL PERSPECTIVES SERIES

Rima D. Apple and Janet Golden, Editors

The series examines the social and cultural construction of health practices and policies, focusing on women as subjects and objects of medical theory, health services, and policy formulation.

*Mothers and Motherhood: Readings in American History*
  Edited by RIMA D. APPLE and JANET GOLDEN

*Modern Mothers in the Heartland: Gender, Health, and Progress in Illinois, 1900–1930*
  LYNNE CURRY

*Making Midwives Legal: Childbirth, Medicine, and the Law, second edition*
  RAYMOND G. DEVRIES

*A Social History of Wet Nursing: From Breast to Bottle*
  JANET GOLDEN

*Travels with the Wolf: A Story of Chronic Illness*
  MELISSA ANNE GOLDSTEIN

*The Selling of Contraception: The Dalkon Shield Case, Sexuality, and Women's Autonomy*
  NICOLE J. GRANT

*Women in Labor: Mothers, Medicine, and Occupational Health in the United States, 1890–1980*
  ALLISON L. HEPLER

*Crack Mothers: Pregnancy, Drugs, and the Media*
  DREW HUMPHRIES

*Sexual Borderlands: Constructing an American Sexual Past*
  Edited by KATHLEEN KENNEDY and SHARON ULLMAN

*Beyond the Reproductive Body: The Politics of Women's Health and Work in Early Victorian England*
  MARJORIE LEVINE-CLARK

*Any Friend of the Movement: Networking for Birth Control, 1920–1940*
  JIMMY ELAINE WILKINSON MEYER

*And Sin No More: Social Policy and Unwed Mothers in Cleveland, 1855–1990*
MARIAN J. MORTON

*Handling the Sick: The Women of St. Luke's and the Nature of Nursing, 1892–1937*
TOM OLSON and EILEEN WALSH

*Reproductive Health, Reproductive Rights: Reformers and the Politics of Maternal Welfare, 1917–1940*
ROBYN L. ROSEN

*Women and Prenatal Testing: Facing the Challenges of Genetic Technology*
Edited by KAREN H. ROTHENBERG and ELIZABETH J. THOMSON

*Women's Health: Complexities and Differences*
Edited by SHERYL BURT RUZEK, VIRGINIA L. OLESEN, and ADELE E. CLARKE

*Bodies of Technology: Women's Involvement with Reproductive Medicine*
Edited by ANN R. SAETNAN, NELLY OUDSHOORN, and MARTY KIREJCZYK

*Motherhood in Bondage*
MARGARET SANGER. Foreword by MARGARET MARSH

*Listen to Me Good: The Life Story of an Alabama Midwife*
MARGARET CHARLES SMITH and LINDA JANET HOLMES

*Don't Kill Your Baby: Public Health and the Decline of Breastfeeding in the Nineteenth and Twentieth Centuries*
JACQUELINE H. WOLF

www.ingramcontent.com/pod-product-compliance
Lightning Source LLC
Chambersburg PA
CBHW020337270326
41926CB00007B/212